613.716 BEDGO
Bedgood, Douglas.
Nalu "the wave" : the art
and science of aquatic fitness

WRIGHT LIBRARY

DISCARD

Nalu

"the wave"

The Art and Science of Aquatic Fitness, Bodywork & Therapy

Douglas Bedgood

Barbara Courtney

Alexander Georgeakopoulos

A.E.I. Press

Key West

A.E.I.Press
division of AquaTherapeutics, Inc.
PO Box 4764, Key West, FL 33041 USA
(800)237-0469
info@aquatherapeutics.com
http://www.aquatherapeutics.com

Copyright © 2004 by Douglas H. Bedgood

Bedgood, Douglas H./ 1942-
Nalu – The Art and Science of Aquatic Fitness, Bodywork & Therapy/
Douglas Bedgood, Barbara Courtney, Alexander Georgeakoupolos/
illustrated by the author; includes index and bibliographical references,
hardcover, color photographs, 400 pages, 8 ½" x 11".

I.	Health—physical fitness—aquatic exercise—therapeutic use
II.	Therapeutics—physical therapy—mechanotherapy
III.	Human physiology—muscles—bones—movement
I.	Title

613.716—d21
GV838.53
ISBN 0-9729963-0-3   Library of Congress 2003095785

All rights reserved. No part of this publication may be reproduced, stored in a
retrieval system, or transmitted in any form or by any means, electronic, mechanical,
photocopying, recording, or otherwise, without the prior written permission of the
copyright owner except in the case of brief quotations embodied in critical articles
and reviews.

Printed in the United States of America.

10   9   8   7   6   5   4   3   2   1

Consult your health practitioner before starting any program of exercise/nutrition
that may relate to a current or recurrent condition.

Nalu is dedicated to Taylor and Mackenzie

Acknowledgements

John Burnham – *Nalu* copy editor
Dina Coyle – cover, charts & imaging
Bill Keough – underwater photographs
Barbara Courtney – text and photographs
Annie Forester – preface, biographical editor
Arjana Brunschwiler – WaterDance photographs
Alexander Georgeakopoulos – text and photographs
Richter-Colella Studios – Wave M'ocean photographs; **Moody Castillo** – Hawaiian paddling photographs
Transtar Productions – Videotape of the 2nd World Championships of Polynesian Canoe, Tahiti
'Iwalani Koide Tasaka: Kapi'olani Community College – English to Hawaiian translations
Aquatic Bodywork Association – photographs; **Patti Loverock** – Shape Magazine
DeAngeles, Bedgood, Gipe, Cooper, and Mahlinger families – inspiration
Milt Huffman-Lee – chemicals & charts; **Wil Hutchinson** – research
Toko Irie, Caroline Dean Edwards, Katja Esser – models
Sharon Wohlmuth – photograph of **Theo Vickery**
Gabriella Detrich – The Fit Body TV show
SkyDive Key West – free-fall photo
Harold Dull – photographs
Mark W. McEachren –
fitness philosophy
Keys Media
imaging

*

Preface

Life is incidental. Stars come and go. Water is but a passing matrix in the reality of invincible silence. The storms that have been will return again. Like passing shadows in a sea of mystery, mortal minds exist without bounds. We are limitless. The empowering sound of the Pacific, the smell of Aegean surf against Santorini cliffs, the salty taste of Kiholo Bay, the unforgettable touch of hurricane driven raindrops, the hypnotic sight of Caribbean blue, these are the woven waves of blended sensory impressions.

On the rising crest of the wave there is infinite freedom of imagination that transcends the rippling chords of post-Renaissance polyphony unfolding in time. Hidden in depths beneath the wave are gems of discovery not to be missed. Between the crest and the depth, the sea of learning listens for your awakening questions.

Comfort is warmth, absence of pain, and protection from trauma, confidence from strength, and the optimism of endurance. As we embark on this shamanic voyage of exploration, Nature reveals a charted course. There are no stop signs on the high seas. Reverse gear does not exist. Only the winds of influence can guide the aging process. There are no miracles to save the forgetfulness of perfect DNA replication over time. The rhythm for nature's turnover and rejuvenation is a sacrifice each organism must accept.

The wave is *Nalu* from the core of the universe. It is comfort for you to be on the crest of the wave, reaching farther and farther to learn from our discoveries, to wait for the calmness of the moment after its passing. As *Nalu* ebbs and flows, it will leave behind a more comprehensive understanding of ourselves and the significance of this beautiful blue spheroid upon which we reside. The quality of our health, mental and physical fitness through aquatic bodywork, therapy and aquatic exercise, is the purpose of this textual and illustrative cohesion.

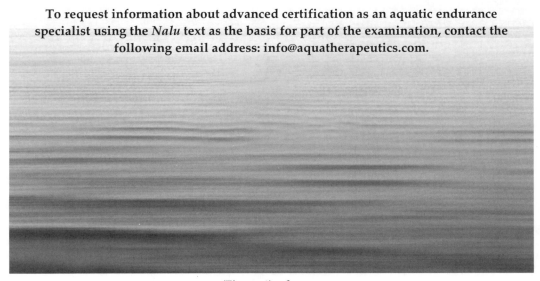

To request information about advanced certification as an aquatic endurance specialist using the *Nalu* text as the basis for part of the examination, contact the following email address: info@aquatherapeutics.com.

(Figure 1) calm seascape

Nalu: The Art and Science of Aquatic Fitness, Bodywork & Therapy

Preparation

A conventional exercise book is not found in this tsunami of seismic origin. The reading will challenge your intellect, awaken your sense of adventure, and lead you at times to the depths of your imagination. **Nalu** surrounds cascading biographical stories of the authors in an exploration of philosophical fitness through water, tissues, bodywork, healing, exercise, and the subconscious mind.

Courtney, in *Healing Waters*, gracefully brings to you the emergence of a new era in aquatic therapy from a psychological and shamanic perspective. Alexander Georgeakopoulos focuses his well-known intellective talents on the popular methods of *Aquatic Bodywork,* and I fill the remainder of **Nalu** with text and illustrations to assist your understanding the farthest reaches of water fitness with ambient art and science.

All the basic sciences bring you *Bone Density and Aquatic Exercise,* where the proximal femur is used as the basic example in a comprehensive cause and effect analysis. *Articular Surroundings* analyzes the rotator cuff and pain syndromes involving joints. The iliopsoas is the example in *Mobility,* as the chapter discovers the nature of the series elastic element and how to keep moving in old age. A solid knowledge of biology and organic chemistry is helpful in *Contractile Physiology in the Pool* as well as in *Nutrition for Aquatic Endurance.* While physics permeates *The Kinetics of Water* and *Aquatic Exercise and the Laws of Physics,* you will find Dr. Igor Burdenko *Floating into Therapy.* Astrophysics, geology, anthropology, Harbin and hydrotherapy are in *Kealawai - The Path of Water.*Two chapters enter the realm of psychology: *Healing Waters* and *Reducing Stress with Water Fitness. Paddling* takes you to the islands. *Water Boxing with Cassius Clay* is an action-packed photo session. An excellent selection of products can be viewed in *Aquatic Exercise Products, Books, and Resources.* The research behind *Nalu* is extensive with over three hundred cited references for further investigation in the *References* section preceding the index.

The supposition is that you are interested and perhaps qualified in a healthcare, physical fitness, instructional, clinical or related occupation and have a formal or self-educated background that includes the relevant sciences needed to absorb *Nalu.* If there is a deficiency, refer to the requisite science texts ancillary to your reading.

There is a need for specialists and diverse certifications in bodywork and in physical fitness. We need in-depth answers to the what, why, and how of every variety of exercise methodology. There is a particular need to know and publicize the immense and greatly varied healing potentials of water. Trained and educated professionals earn the trust and respect of the public. It is the purpose of this book to provide that higher level of training.

The shaded text within *Nalu* contains biographical experiences as they relate to the chapter subjects.

Forward

by Mark W. McEachren

The Greeks were compelled by an equal passion to comprehend the complexities of practical knowledge as well as derive the simple pleasures experienced from viewing, feeling, and replicating the sensual form of the human body. They saw the Mind/Body connection as a physical inspiration, yet simultaneously, a spiritual channel to the eternal dimension of creation and meaning. Their distinct disciplines of philosophy, science, spirituality, physicality, and artistic expression were viewed as integrated elements that made up one divine, unified, whole, a perpetual "conscious" energy... forever flowing in one universal body of knowledge.

Our individual bodies and minds are not simply afterthoughts of this dynamic flow. Each and every one of us comprise and influence this grand consciousness. Our personal actions, thoughts and emotions create the very essence of all that we see, 'All' that is. This understanding opens a profound sense of responsibility: a conscious orientation that our personal values and standards have an essential relationship with the fluid stream of universal thought. We are accountable to the creative life force that lives within us, for it is the cradling buoyancy of life itself.

Once we place a specific orientation on the value of personal/universal existence we may correctly prioritize our thought process, then seek the free and natural flow of a current made up of life giving actions. Life is a harmonic chain of meandering physical and metaphysical events that are seamlessly connected to all thought and action. In order to sustain, perpetuate, and protect the delicate process of universal progress we must engulf our physical being in the amniotic protection of conscious awareness. For, thought is the very essence with (and of) physical creation.

Creation is expression, a discernible or material representation of self while "self" is a representation of the whole. This identifiable organization of metaphysical transcendence is the reflective power of life. We are mirrors of creation gifted with the abilities to honor and contribute to the image of the present moment... forever. Our work, our production, is not merely a marketable trade, or a social interaction, but more so, a color, a stroke, a gesture, and an impression upon the emulsive constitution of an interconnected, interactive, universal progression. Our Awareness, Choice, and Action are the creative and artistic tools of life.

This rough sketch of eternal recapitulation makes a very simple but powerful statement. The pure quality of the universe has produced each one of us, and within the image, or impression, of all that we produce there exists the quality of who and what we are. We are a part of a perfect whole, however we must live up to the pure examples we have the opportunity to represent. The choice to develop the breadth and depth of our intellect, in order to hone life's professional and artistic abilities, is the essential conscious step one must take in order to set the progressive stages of personal development and individual purpose in motion.

The universe is an omnipotent, omnipresent educational institution, forever teaching the students of the mind. The body is a conceptual channel. Within the concept of complete existence are the classrooms where the sacred texts of life are read. The process of Teacher/Student begins from this highest order. The lesson plan is then maternally, patiently, disseminated so it may build upon itself thought by thought, person by person, generation by generation until one day this concept will, once again, recognize and understand itself. It is a beautiful, wondrous event to realize that man recapitulates the universe. To realize that as you read this text you are presently contributing to the outward flow of conscious expression.

If we are to learn from universal laws, and wish to infuse their questing purpose in our lives, we must maintain the integrity of instruction set forth from the very beginning. Instructional concepts must be unveiled in a timely well-structured fashion to ensure they will be perceived, as closely as possible, to their original forms. With newly altered perceptions we must then practice nascent concepts, over and over, within the experiential incubator of trial and error until deft technique and form may repeatably deliver the meaning, and result, of an original concept. You are student of any concept until you have the ability to deliver its purpose.

As fitness professionals we are faced with the same historic conflicts as impressionist artists and the heroes of mythological endeavor. We struggle to defend our ideological identities and artistic expressions while working within the constructs of institutional dogma and financial

necessity. Quality, value and standard are often diminished, even lost, in the translation and transfer of the Teacher/Student channel. As with everything in life there is a homeostasis that must be sought, a consistency maintained by the equal power of two opposing forces. As a teacher it is vital to uphold the integrity of the information you bring forth. As a student it is essential to absorb with an open mind and to constantly contribute the ever-evolving provisional truth. Enjoy the conscious sojourn as you submerge your awareness and thought into the text of this book. In truth, you are neither teacher nor student, but eternally both.

Mark W. McEachren

Mark McEachren has been a fitness trainer and managed, owned, and operated facilities in the fitness industry for the past 25 years. As a philosopher, poet, and exercise instructor, the fitness doctrine for Mark is a philosophy that is as undefinable as the place and space he is evolving towards.

contact: Mceachrenmark@aol.com

Table of Contents

Author Biographies

Douglas Bedgood

B.S. in Health Science from Western Illinois University, Licensed Massage Therapist in Florida, Personal Trainer in Aquatic Exercise, Certified in Neuromuscular Therapy by the Atlanta School of Massage and graduate of the Atlanta School of Massage, Certified by the National Certification Board for Therapeutic Massage and Bodywork, President of AquaTherapeutics, Inc., founder of Aquatic Endurance International and inventor of patented therapy products.

For me, the journey to water fitness began in Melrose Park, Illinois in the late fall of 1942. My family settled in the quaint elm-shaded village of Hinsdale. In my boyhood days there were open fields, wooded lots, meandering creeks and there was room to dream. My parents provided a fertile landscape for my curiosity, imagination and creativity. Early on,

they instilled in me a sense of self-reliance, adventure and a deep reverence for nature. First, curiosity about muscles began when I could do more chin-ups from an apple tree next to our house than my brothers. Then the first real summer job from age 12-18 was to groom twenty-three muscular polo ponies.

So many things sparked my interest that it was difficult to focus on just one calling. In high school I entertained prospects of becoming an artist, a farmer, or perhaps a geologist or a builder. At Western Illinois University, I turned to Physical Education, Biology and Chemistry as major goals. Sports dominated most of my spare time: cross-country running, wrestling, track and power lifting. However, life-altering circumstances put college plans temporarily on hold. It was the 60's. There was a war and a social revolution on the horizon. Unsure of a direction in life, I drifted away one spring in a VW headed for the Yukon Territory.

As the aurora borealis danced across the sky, something about Alaska awakened the wildness in me. I signed on as a fire fighter with the Bureau of Land Management in Fairbanks. Within three years I became responsible for organizing a firefighting force of over 2200 personnel for the entire district. While wintering in Hawaii, I attended Esalen of Big Sur massage classes. With renewed purpose, I returned to W.I.U. in 1970 and completed a degree in Health Science in 1972. At Western, competitive powerlifting became an obsession.

In 1980, I moved from the top of a mountain ridge overlooking Idyllwild, California to the Kona Coast of Hawaii at Keouhou Bay. There I joined a new outrigger canoe club, offered therapeutic massage, made racing paddles and was a competitor in many regattas and long distance races. Kona Paddles, my paddle-making business at Keouhou Bay, began to grow but unexpected circumstances brought me back to the mainland.

The journey continued to bounce all over much of the United States. In the summer of 1982, in a barn near Alden, Illinois, I was shaping wood for a paddle when I had an unusual vision. I thought of when my family tore down our original house in Hinsdale and dug a basement with shovels, then poured the concrete. I remembered the pull of the shovel as a young boy wading in the concrete and how hard it was to cove the concrete with the shovel. I envisioned two long, rectangular troughs on both sides of me as I sat on a platform above and between the troughs. I saw myself with a shovel, paddling the concrete on one side for a while, then on the other side. I then reached down in the real world and picked up some pieces of scrap wood, looked at them for a moment, noticing their size and surface, then nailed on handles in their centers, drilling one surface full of holes, and ran over to the pond, wading in the mud to get to a deeper area. I put the rough octagonal pieces of plywood in the water to see what it would feel like, how close it would be to the feel of vigorous canoe paddling. Creation was at hand.

The design of the device quickly evolved. How unique it was using a radically modified canoe paddle to exercise the legs. I realized that it could be important for disabled people to be able to exercise, people who couldn't do much with weights in a gym.

Returning to the mountains of Idyllwild I set up shop and hand carved Aquatoner® paddles out of hardwoods. It took days of shaping and finishing to make each one. I gave them away to rehabilitation hospitals in southern California to obtain the testimonials that were needed.

When I researched Indian reservations as possible venues to establish manufacturing and possibly to involve a tribe in the venture, the Bureau of Indian Affairs recommended Cherokee, North Carolina. With less than a hundred dollars in my pocket and a bus ticket, I set off across the country to meet with the Cherokee Chief and his tribe's planning department. We arrived at an agreement to make the

Aquatoners at their sheltered workshop. Several tribal business people were willing to participate in the project, Kona Fitness. The Aquatoning exercise program was what I started on the reservation with funding from the Cherokee Health Delivery System and the assistance of Tribal member Jim Cooper. It won a North Carolina Governor's Award in 1986 as Best Fitness Program for Mature Adults. Clients, some young, had all forms of arthritis and other disabling conditions.

As the business grew, it was time to move to Asheville, North Carolina and consolidate the manufacturing into a profitable enterprise. I had added four new designs to the product line. They were variations of bars with Aquatoners and a special product for amputees. I developed more massage techniques from an outstanding therapist, Erin Schone, a graduate of The Florida School of Massage in Gainsville. The Aquatoner steadily continued to spread across the United States. AquaTherapeutics, Inc. came into being in 1989.

In 1997, I moved to Atlanta, Georgia and obtained certification in neuromuscular therapy, a degree in deep tissue structural integration from the Atlanta School of Massage, and passed the National Board exam. Key West was in my sights and proved fertile for more inventions as I developed a private massage practice and provided aquatic exercise instruction to clients and personal trainers. The idea to write *Nalu* began in April 2002 after realizing the need for a higher level of education in the aquatic exercise industry.

Metaphorically speaking, one might say I did not take the journey. The journey took me. As I sat down to write about my life, I suddenly found myself "on the wind," a Native American expression meaning to be open to all possibilities. Clearly the journey has taken me to a place where I can at last see my life's work as a sacred task. I am most grateful to the path and to all those along the way who enlightened and enriched my experience.

Douglas

**The Author, 1948
(Figure 2B)**

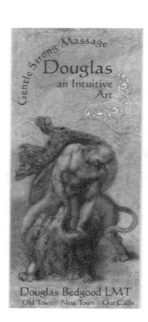

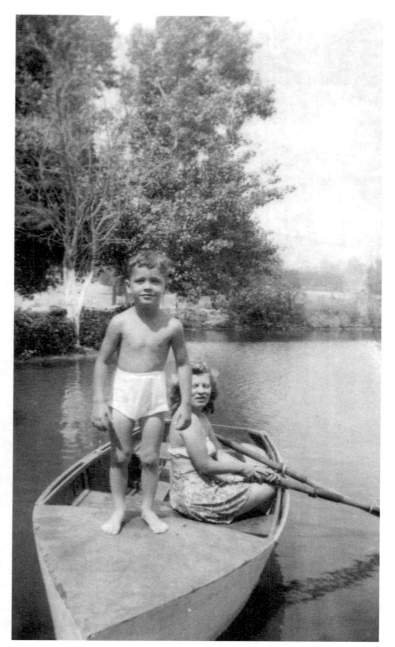

Nalu: The Art and Science of Aquatic Fitness, Bodywork & Therapy

Alexander Georgeakopoulos

It's been about dancing since before I can remember. My mother tells me I used to dance to music on the radio, and that one time in the middle of the night, she was awakened by sounds coming from the living room and there I was, at age two, jumping up and down on the sofa in the dark.

Going out square dancing at age eleven with my divorced mother in southern California was exciting, surrounded by all those big perfumed women in their fluffy dresses as the calls were sung out. "Take your partner by the hand, lead her to the promised land!" Then in the fifth grade we learned ballroom dance and I loved it even more. The waltz and fox trot were great, but ah, to spin around the auditorium doing the polka, my hands firmly on young Mary Tischer's waist… .

At age fifteen my llth grade history teacher, Mr. Stearns, turned me on to culture. I was aflame to learn all I could about the arts. I made a list like the Virgo I was/am and going down it

saw I had written *ballet*. I called a ballet school and began studying on my own initiative, knowing immediately I would be a dancer. Once a week became twice a week became every day. At first it was the challenge, but that turned into the thrill of mastery and finally love for the art. Thanks to Trina Greg and Maria Fielding, my first teachers, and to Patricia Wilde who, as a scout for the Harkness Ballet School in New York City, offered me a full scholarship.

So, after only a year and a half of study, I found myself on scholarship in New York City of the late 60's. Male dancers were a rare species then, and I got scholarships at one ballet school after another, getting kicked out or moving on in search of better teaching. There was plenty of stage experience to be had dancing with small modern groups and regional companies in nearby cities for the next four years. I could jump high and partner well and wanted to be the best dancer in the city. What a place to grow up in! Like all New Yorkers, I have a few cockroach stories to tell,

and like all New Yorkers I thought it was the only place to be, the center of the world. So many amazing dancers and companies performed there. "I'm in New York!" was my astonished mantram for years. I hadn't a clue who I was, but I loved getting high dancing, doing Transcendental Meditation and following an Indian master, Meher Baba.

Married at age 21, my Canadian dancer wife and I moved into an apartment in a decrepit brownstone in the dangerous lower East Side. As we unloaded boxes a street altercation escalated into shouts and bottle throwing in our midst. The building had no front door, but to compensate we installed four different locks on the apartment door and grates over every window. Once, having lost our keys, our next door neighbor helped us get in. It was unsettling how he could wield a screwdriver, rapidly unscrewing each of the locks and opening the door in under three minutes. Those were the days! After a year I auditioned for and was accepted by the National Ballet of Canada in Toronto. They had an excellent school and I was exposed for the first time to solid technical training. I danced lead roles there for a year and a half, then we moved down to Syracuse, New York to a company in which we could both perform. That company went bankrupt after a year, and it was off to Norway for three years with the Norwegian National Ballet. Such a beautiful country! I spent a lot of time skiing and backpacking in the highlands. But falling into a depression and an eating disorder, I lost the will to dance and went to work in a restaurant. My wife and I separated and I moved to Sweden to dance with the Cullberg Ballet, the best troupe I was ever a part of. We were young and idealistic as we performed political and dramatic contemporary ballets. I discovered a new dance identity, interpreting these works in a freer, less classical style.

Back in Canada I had been both thrilled and depressed to read about Primal Therapy. I saw neurosis everywhere, but especially in myself. The world had become a dark and crazy place; my spiritual roots were shaken. While dancing in Sweden I overcame my fears and entered this therapy. It truly saved my life. I learned to feel and remember many things. I was beginning to know myself better and now wanting to get acquainted with the family I had left as a teenager.

After moving back to San Diego I was still performing, but started teaching ballet, too, at the California Ballet Company, San Diego State College, and the Civic Youth Ballet. It was good to think more about others and less about my own technique and career. It was also in this period that I became seriously involved with improvisational dance. I went religiously to the Friday night dance jams, exploring a whole evening of barefoot trance dancing like a meditation, not speaking, not thinking, not repeating the same movement twice.

Then something new entered my life. I received a massage that put me into a feeling space familiar to me from therapy. I wanted to share this. I had been massaging my wife and other dancers prior to this, so it seemed natural to get some training.

In 1980, at age 30, I began the study of holistic massage at the International School of Professional Bodywork in San Diego, completing the 1000 Hour Massage Therapist Training in 1983. My world changed as I experientially understood my body's structure and its embedded feelings from the inside out in a way that had never occurred in dance. I went on to become qualified as a Trager Practitioner in 1986, subsequently studying with Milton Trager himself. I had kept my day job as a ballet teacher, working for companies in San Diego, Germany and Israel until 1989, while massaging a lot of dancers. Aren't the thirties grand? Still with plenty of energy and beginning to mature…

While teaching for the Kibbutz Dance Company in Israel I decided to hang it up and try out living in an intentional community. I moved to Harbin Hot Springs in northern California—an amazing place, a power center where all one's dreams and nightmares come true. There, in my 40's, I had the wild and crazy adolescence I had missed while dancing in the 1960's. I received my first session of aquatic bodywork from Harold Dull, the originator of Watsu. Neither of us realized it was the start of something so momentous for me. I studied Watsu with Harold in 1990. Back then they were teaching in one week what is covered in three weeks now. Even with my dance background I was pretty confused. I tried for a while to get it straight then gave up and started inventing my own moves.

In 1993 I studied WaterDance from one of its founders, Arjana Brunschwiler. I starting teaching anatomy and my own Integrative Massage and Healing Dance techniques, as well as co-teaching WaterDance with Arjana, all at the School of Shiatsu and Massage at Harbin. I worked on the Harbin Healing Staff, doing massages and Watsus and playing in the warm pool for hours. I will always be grateful for the seminal experiences, the healing and the creativity that came to me at Harbin.

I left Harbin in 1997 to spread Watsu, WaterDance and Healing Dance to Brazil, staying there for four years. Ursula Garthoff, who had studied with me at Harbin, invited me down to live with her family in São Paulo and teach the work. I was a long way from the quiet rural community I had spent the previous seven years in. São Paulo is one of the biggest and baddest cities in the world. At first I was terrified to venture out onto the streets, but after three years I had learned Portuguese and could feel comfortable wherever I might be and even teach the trainings without a translator. Like every other *americano* who has ever gone through the Brazilian experience, I was powerfully affected by the people, the culture and the land. *Obrigado, Brasil.*

Since 2001 I have been back in San Diego, my hometown, still a dues paying, certified instructor for the Worldwide Aquatic Bodywork Association, which sponsors trainings in the water modalities that are the topic of my article. I have been collaborating here with local organizer and teacher Theri Thomas.

Soon I will have taught my 100th week-long intensive with WABA.

Life in San Diego is staying balanced and healthy with outdoor exercise in the good weather. I get out of town a few times a year to teach in Europe, Israel and other places in the States. In my fifties now, I am in a quietly productive phase of my life, giving sessions, teaching a lot, writing and helping the Healing Dance to spread.

Whether as dance teacher, bodyworker, or innovator of aquatic bodywork, my desire has always been to give the good movement, that which nurtures, opens the doors to freedom, and inspires dance. It's been a love affair with the living, breathing body, with full and glorious movement, and with benevolent and caring Spirit, guiding us all homeward.

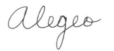

Barbara Courtney

Growing up in Melrose, Massachusetts, my family had a heated pool and I remember the wonderful nurturing feeling of swimming in the steamy warm water at dawn. I now live in Boxford, Massachusetts, and still feel nurtured floating on my back in warm water looking up at the sky and feeling ONE with everything. I am still struck by how powerful this simple experience is and I believe we all seek this kind of connection to ourselves and our environment.

I completed my B.A. in psychology at Boston University, in 1978, and a graduate certificate program in Art Therapy from BU, in 1979. After receiving a MSW in 1984, from Smith College School for Social Work, I went on to become a licensed independent clinical social worker. I worked as a Clinical Coordinator for innovative therapeutic programs for children and families, using a multidisciplinary approach. I found I loved combining the various treatment perspectives to

get a fuller sense of a person and their healing picture. In 1995, I decided to open private practice as a therapist so I could have the freedom to work in a more expanded context. I felt exploring non-traditional ways of healing would allow clients to go deeper into their innate wisdom and come away with more profound results. I began to integrate neuro-linguistic techniques, psychoneuroimmunology, somatic work, and shamanic perspectives and practices into my healing program. The focus for all my work soon became a mind-body integrative orientation, even in my work with movement.

My practice with clients was also influenced by my mentor and teacher, Chonyi Richard Allen, a Cherokee Medicine Man. He truly turned me and my clinical training upside down and shook out many limiting perceptions. His teachings filled me up with faith in the unseen world of guides, spirits and my own ability as a human being to find my way home if given the opportunity. He taught

me how to stay present and open to all the possibilities.

From my personal experiences three important principles emerged and became the conceptual foundation for how I teach movement:

Energy follows attention
During the development of my therapeutic work, my prayers were that I would somehow go deeper into my spiritual growth. As usual, my prayers were answered, but in a most unexpected and unwelcome way. I was diagnosed with leukemia. Without having a clue that I wasn't in perfect health until a few days prior, I was thrust into an experiential lesson in how energy follows attention. I knew immediately this experience had something to do with wanting to go deeper into who I really was. I remember having the sense that something could be created here and that "the something" would depend on where I focused. I realized this experience was going to be about how I decided to engage or not engage with the waking dream I was having about leukemia. After much deep

inner work and many lessons learned, the dream I was having about leukemia started to shift into the prayed-for personal and spiritual growth. I was on my way.

We are mutable beings
The notion that we are capable of recreating ourselves became the next focus of this challenging but enlightening journey. Through exploring movement and its relationship to healing, I discovered at the body level that there was a way to interrupt dysfunctional organismic patterns and holding patterns so that the body was allowed to do what it wanted to do. This fascinated me. Turning to practices such as qigong, wu-chi-in motion and Continuum Movement, I noticed tremendous personal physical improvement. However, I did not yet realize how amplified the effects could be when these self-healing practices were translated into water-based work. That is, not until my husband and I took a vacation to the South Carolina seaside in the summer of 1997. I spent days floating in warm ocean water in an altered state of bliss and

connection to my environment and myself. I put my being in a healing space at every level. It was clear that if I wanted to stay well, I would need to do much of this! Good thing I loved it! This was really the birth of what I now call Wave M'ocean.

We must take full responsibility for our healing
To me, it felt as if I could now take full responsibility for my healing once I realized that I had brought myself to my own healing space. I believe that's what made the difference for me. Through this process, I understood at a deep level that healing is never something done to you or for you. It is a very personal, sacred and empowering experience you create for yourself. This lesson is inherent in the philosophy of Wave M'ocean.

Since 1999, I have offered Wave M'ocean classes and workshops in aquatic settings and movement centers. Preparatory classes on land hold the intention of embracing our aquatic self in motion. The specific focus of each offering appears to be endless and ever changing. Doing

individual work within a Wave M'ocean context has shown great promise for helping a client fully let go into the natural sequencing of movements and into emotional-physical release.

I am committed to exploring the uncharted realm of human transformation which lies somewhere between the depths of our souls and the sacred intelligence of water. This is the calling of Wave M'ocean. To provide an in-depth theoretical and practical exploration of Wave M'ocean, I am putting together a book, *Aquatic Resonant Healing.* This book will explore resonance as an overlighting principle in movement, sound, consciousness and transformation. Through collaboration with originators of related work, the book promises to bring new insights and applications to the holistic practice of aquatic therapy.

It has been exciting for me to work in an aquatic environment helping people discover that fluid movement can be experienced in their bodies, emotions and consciousness. I believe there is an untapped potential in holistic aquatic healing in the areas of somatic awareness, expressive movement, expanded consciousness and sound healing. To access this new wave of aquatic healing, it is evident a specially designed aquatic setting is needed.

With this in mind, I have plans underway for *Atlantis Rising,* an aquatic center for explorations in mutability and human awakening. This indoor facility will be home to pioneers of holistic traditions for research, training and integrated transformational work. Together, we will create an environment where movement in water can be the essential healing medium for all those seeking to further explore their physiology, psychology and resonant nature.

I am grateful for the wisdom shared by teachers of many traditions. The work of movement pioneers Emilie Conrad and Susan Harper, and the shamanic teachings of Rebecca Menard and Chonyi Richard Allen

are among the inspirations for Wave M'ocean. Each has helped me explore the depths of healing and fostered my awareness of my contribution as a healer: to help people enter the wildness and spaciousness of their watery home.

Barbara

Introduction

*U*nrestricted mobility, freedom to move, liberty to explore, ability to create or express and think freely: I have always been drawn to locations that enhanced those birthrights of being.

In the autumn of 1978, lifelong affinities for wood and water guided me to the remoteness of southeastern Arizona. You may wonder how an affinity for water attracted me to the desert. With carpentry tools in a pick-up truck I headed from alpine Idyllwild, California to an ancient Native American spiritual site found along the Gila River. "Healing Waters" is the English translation for this venerable desert oasis of mineral hot springs.

It was a sacred site for tribes of the Apache Nation and indigenous cultures that preceded them. The first inhabitants were the Paleo-Indians, the mastodon hunters of Bearing Land Bridge Siberian migration that dated from 9,000BC back to 40,000 years ago (Cordell, 1989). They were ancestors of the Desert Archaic Indians (9,000BC to 1500 AD) who were agrarian pueblo builders. The Yavapai, who didn't migrate from anywhere, were the truest natives of the area descended from the Archaic Indians. Then came immigrants down the valleys of the Gila River in the 16th century, the Apache Nation of tribes.

Healing at hot springs has a long history (see Chapter 9, *Kealawai* for more information on shamans and hot springs). At Healing Waters, narrow streams interrupted by waterfalls flow down Sonoran slopes, pouring from one steaming natural pool to another like a string of pearls. This healing place was under the wings of the golden eagle for thousands of years. Hot water came from deep within the earth, heated by the spirits of native ancestors. Then came the white invasion sparked by the search for mineral riches. Indians were removed by force abruptly in 1886.

Ben Gardner first developed the homestead that claimed these unusual hot springs. It was known as "The Springs" at the turn of the century. Like at other hot springs stolen from native tribes, a tourist hotel was built, the Indian Hot Springs Resort Hotel. The first group of 325 well-dressed guests arrived in 1903 to have their parties and barbeques. An enormous concrete swimming pool was constructed in 1905 at the base of the springs to contain the steaming mineral water so the tourists could swim. Public use of the giant swimming pool was discontinued in 1967 when the Arizona Health Department required chlorination and lifeguards.

Eventually the enterprise began to crumble. The property was finally sold to an individual who offered health seminars and a place for naturopathic physicians to practice alternative therapies. It was renamed from "Indian Hot Springs" to "Healing Waters."

I visited Healing Waters to help with the repairs. A 70's hippie invasion was beginning to fade from the property. What I found was a small, tranquil group of skinny gypsies with nauseating skin infections in rags living communally off of melons from the sparse remnants of a garden, hardly able to lift a hammer or a shovel, bathing in the staph-contaminated mud and meditating every evening in the turret library on top of the old three-story hotel. Out on the grounds I stumbled on evidence of their transient quarters during concerts and other lengthy outdoor gatherings. I found parts of their primitive teepees in the rattlesnake-infested dirt, rancid torn sleeping bags, scattered clothes and open fecal latrines swarming with sulcus flies. The swimming pool was polluted with bacteria, debris, and algae but the hot springs kept flowing through it all. After some tree trimming and interior woodwork, like the water, I also continued on my journey. Under new ownership, it is again called "Indian Hot Springs" but beyond an occasional tour there is no public access to the sacred springs.

>‹‹‹‹(((O>   >‹‹‹‹(((O>   >‹‹‹‹(((O>

Nalu is a tribute to native shamans and natural healers everywhere. We will thoroughly explore the aquatic science within their art. No individual person or culture can honestly claim the origins of aquatic therapy and bodywork. They are as old as shamanism throughout the world. Today it is thought that aquatic exercise, aquatic therapy and rehabilitation, aquatic bodywork, water fitness, whichever you choose to call it, is still in its infancy. The fact is it is not a recent creation. It was discovered long ago and will be re-discovered again and again.

The Aquatic Exercise Association describes the Kravitz and Mayo (1997) compilation of about sixty abstracts briefly reviewing aquatic exercise research as "the most comprehensive review of aquatic research ever assembled." Most of the studies in the thin booklet concern running on treadmills in water, then measuring oxygen consumption, heart rate, blood pressure, energy expenditure, body composition, and flexibility after the aquatic activities. Therefore, the greatest part of the research was on

aerobic capacity after deep-water running. That was the sophistication of "modern" aquatic therapy in the year 2003. The numbers of articles in professional journals that skim through the usefulness of water is increasing, but most of the re-discovery is ahead.

Come out of the Healing Waters oasis now to the plateau and view the beauty of the vast horizon. In front of you, I introduce a modern-day shaman, Barbara Courtney, opening gateways of consciousness and the future of aquatic mind-bodywork; Alexander Georgeakopolous who captures the essence of today's aquatic bodywork; and the following chapters tying the art of aquatic exercise and bodywork to the science of current research as well as my own experience in this field.

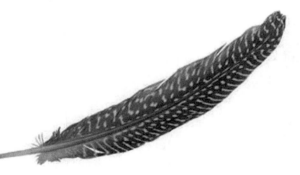

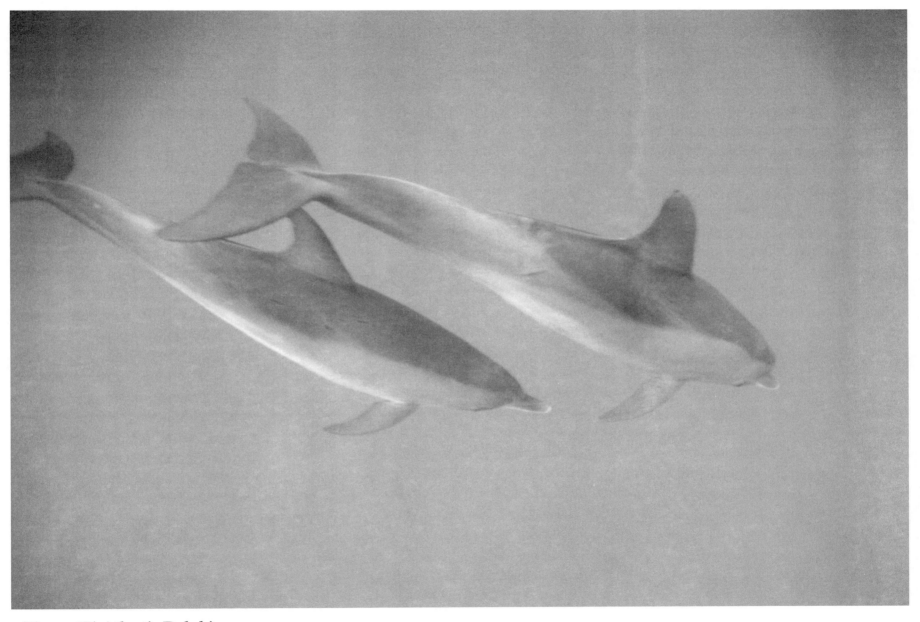

(Figure 2B) Atlantic Dolphins

Nalu: The Art and Science of Aquatic Fitness, Bodywork & Therapy

Biographical Photos of the Authors

Douglas Bedgood
holding early Aquatoners handmade
at the Cherokee Sheltered Workshop
in Western North Carolina

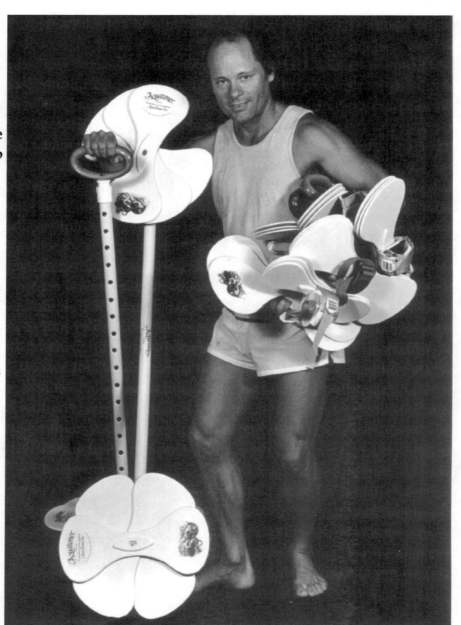

(Figure 3)

Nalu: The Art and Science of Aquatic Fitness, Bodywork & Therapy

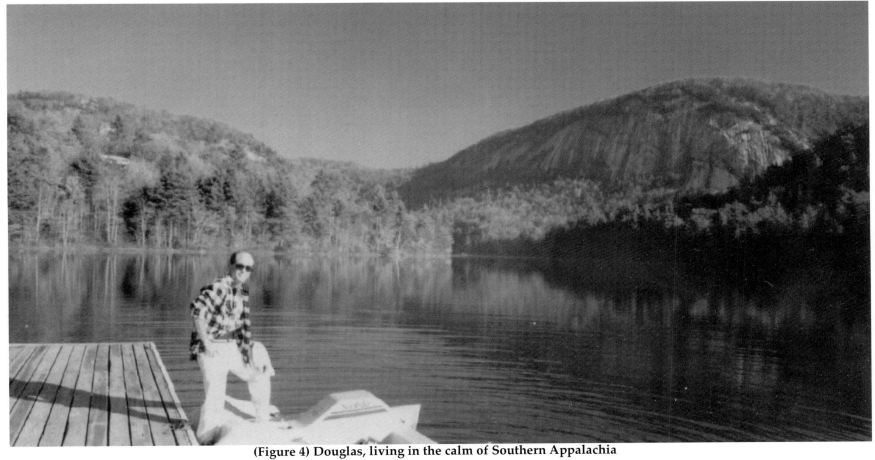

(Figure 4) Douglas, living in the calm of Southern Appalachia

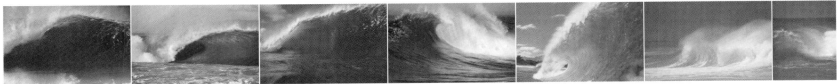

(Figure 5a) The thunderous roar of Hawaiian Nalu

Nalu: The Art and Science of Aquatic Fitness, Bodywork & Therapy

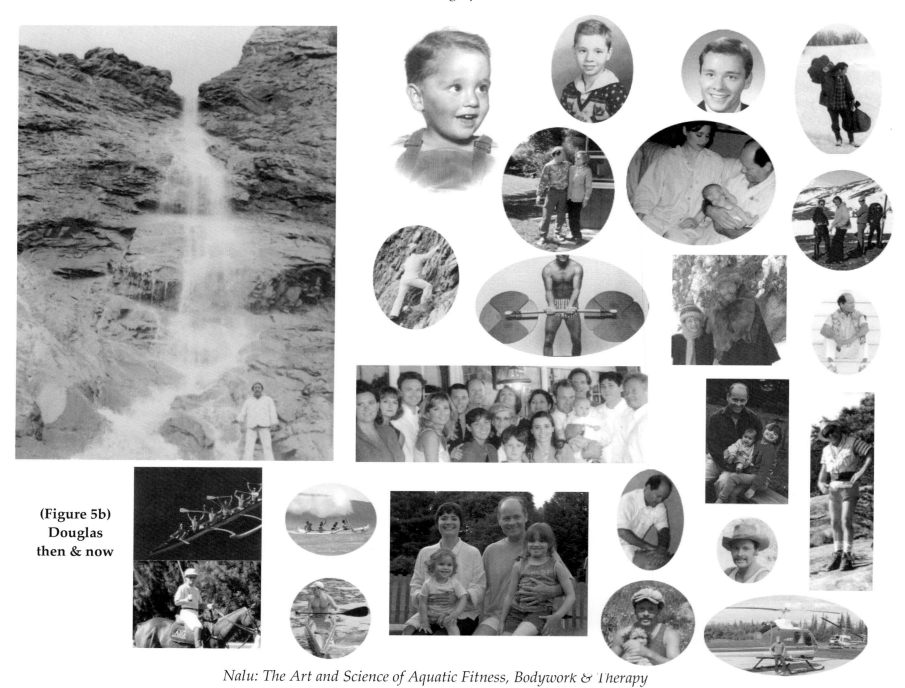

**(Figure 5b)
Douglas
then & now**

**(Figure 6)
Barbara Courtney**

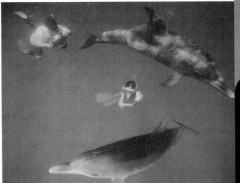

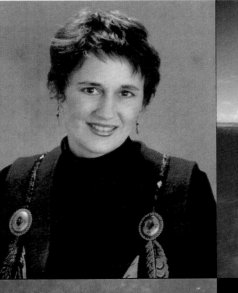

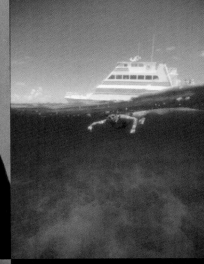

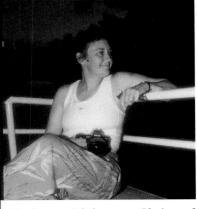

"I love swimming with wild dolphins and humpback whales. It's an incredible gift when they share their world with us."

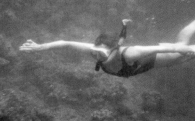

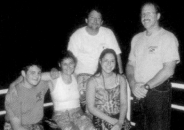

Barbara with her son Chris and fellow dolphin enthusiasts during an underwater photography course that was taught off the coast of Bimini.

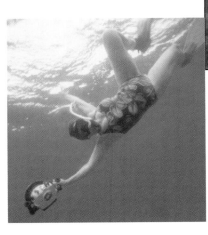

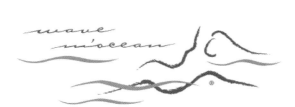

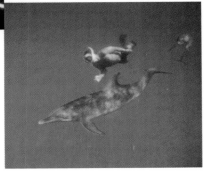

Nalu: The Art and Science of Aquatic Fitness, Bodywork & Therapy

(Figure 7)
Alexander Georgeakopoulos

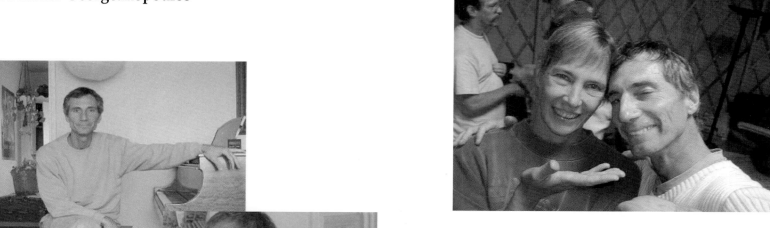

Alexander and Inika

Alexander and Theri

Alexander with a class

Color Photos of Aquatic Bodywork

Watsu: Harold Dull, the founder of Watsu, is shown in these four photographs applying some of Watsu's creative stretches. In the Dolphin Wave the receiver is undulated as could only be done in water.

(Figure 8)

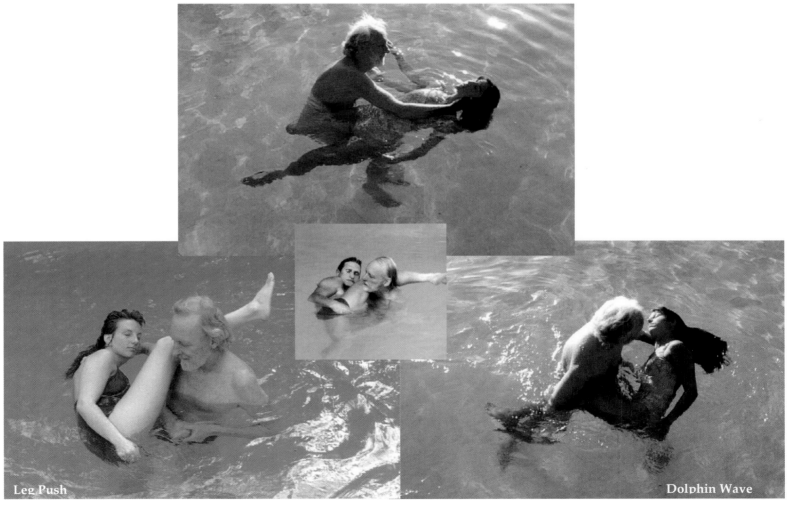

Nalu: The Art and Science of Aquatic Fitness, Bodywork & Therapy

(Figure 9)

A Watsu session always begins with the stillness of the "Water Breath Dance". The "Accordion," featuring repetitive bilateral hip and trunk flexion, is one of Watsu's most maternal moves. The "Near Leg Rotation" abducts both legs. The "Arm Leg Rock" alternately abducts the shoulder and flexes the hip.

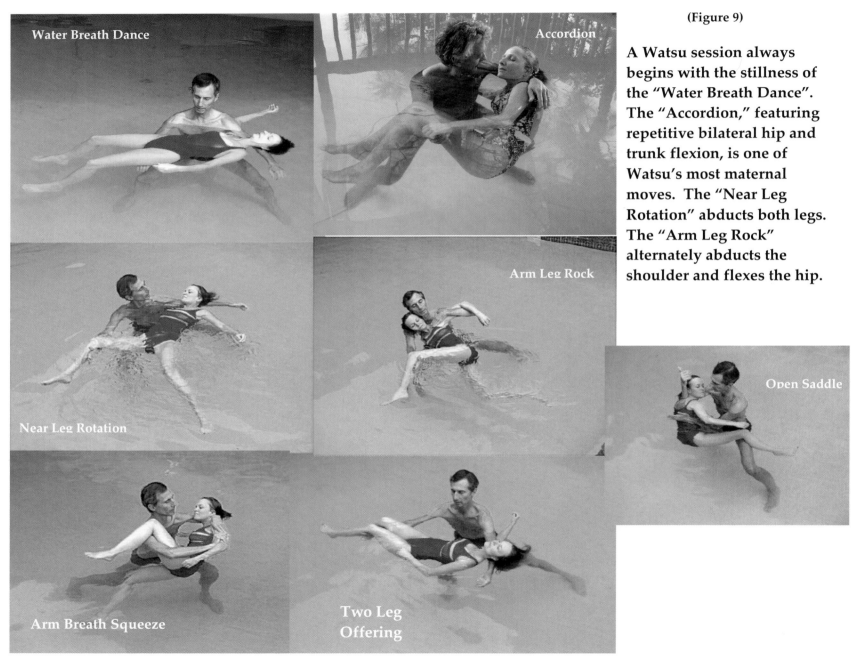

Water Breath Dance

Accordion

Near Leg Rotation

Arm Leg Rock

Open Saddle

Arm Breath Squeeze

Two Leg Offering

Nalu: The Art and Science of Aquatic Fitness, Bodywork & Therapy

(Figure 10)

WaterDance

Arjana Brunschwiler, one of WaterDance's founders, shows some of the underwater moves of her technique. The receiver enters a deep trance. The freedom, peace and dream-like quality of WaterDance are evident.

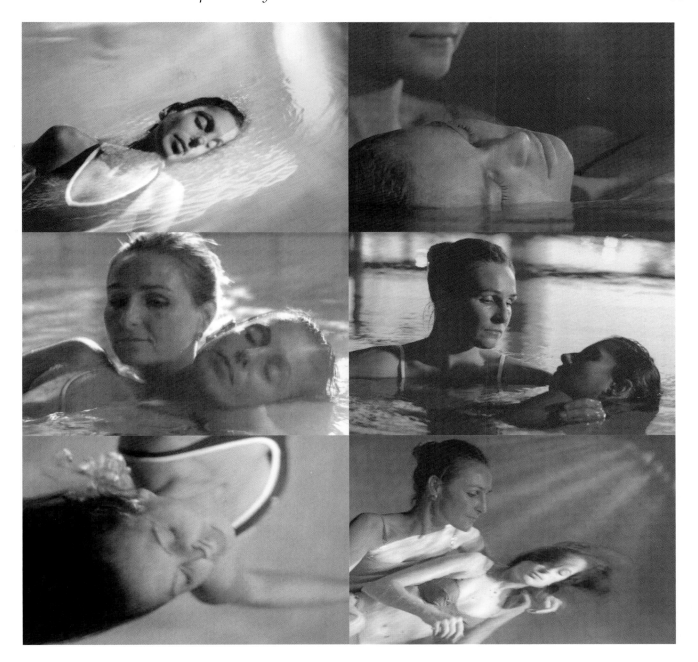

Nalu: The Art and Science of Aquatic Fitness, Bodywork & Therapy

Aquatic Bodywork

WaterDance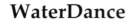

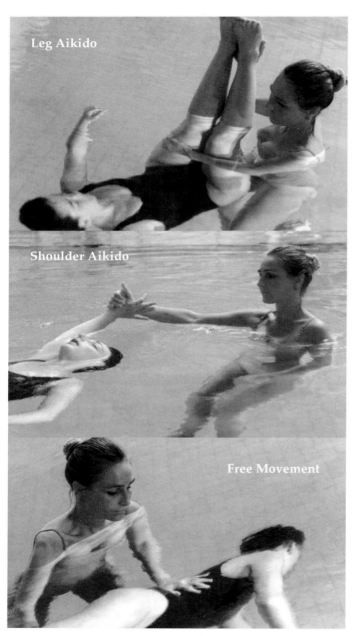

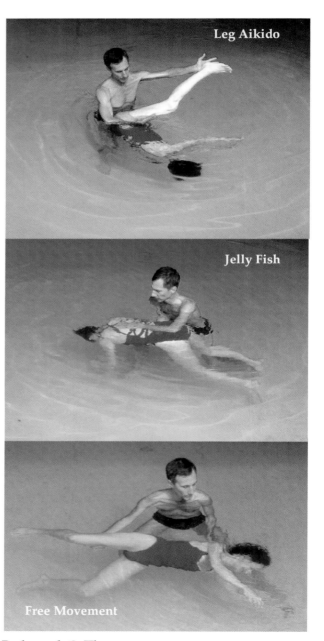

(Figure 12) **Healing Dance:** Co-author Alexander Georgeakopoulos demonstrates four moves from his technique, *The Healing Dance.* The "Whirlpool" is a fast, circling head traction. The "Vortex" is an exquisite arching stretch that turns in a curve.

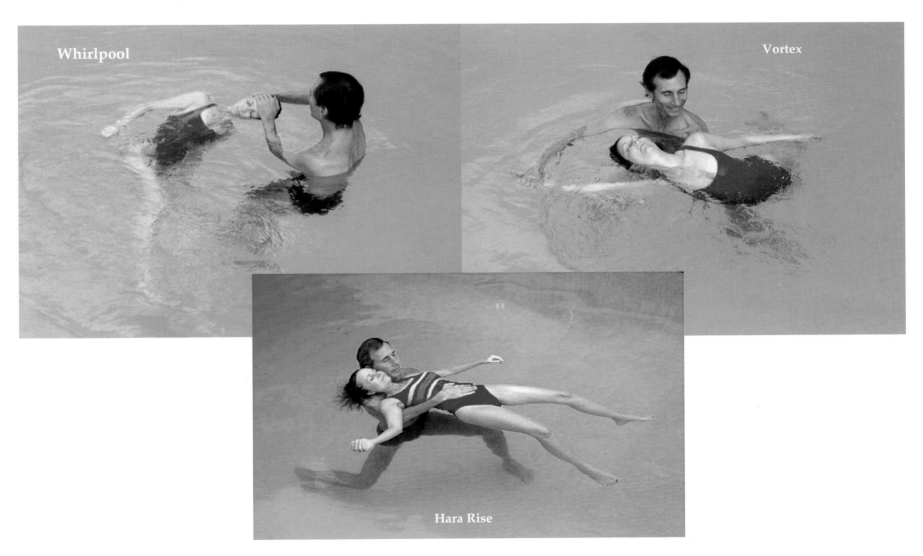

Nalu: The Art and Science of Aquatic Fitness, Bodywork & Therapy

Healing Dance

(Figure 13)
"Shins across Belly" offers a powerful
leverage to stretch the erectors. "Rib Walk"
is a strong stretch to the lateral trunk.

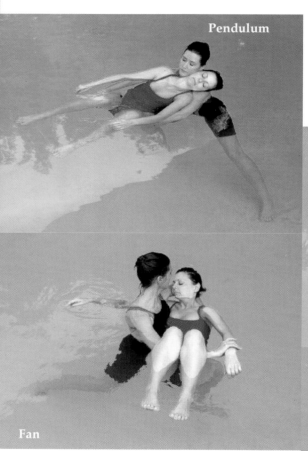

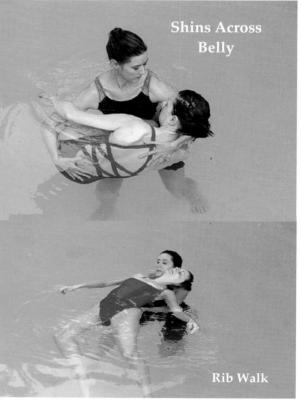

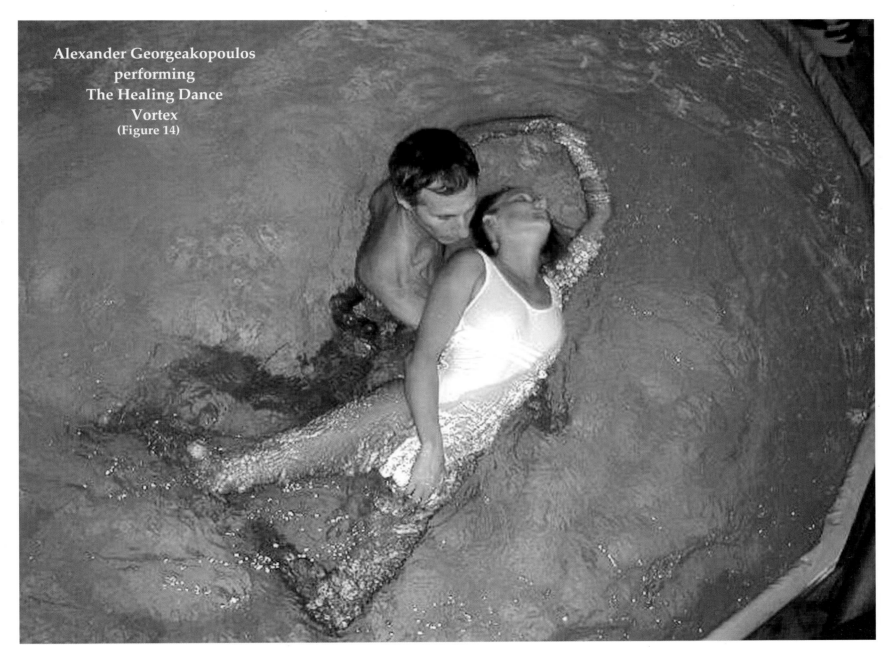

Alexander Georgeakopoulos
performing
The Healing Dance
Vortex
(Figure 14)

Nalu: The Art and Science of Aquatic Fitness, Bodywork & Therapy

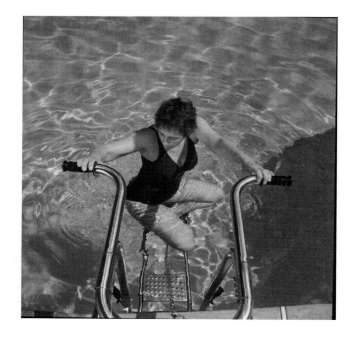

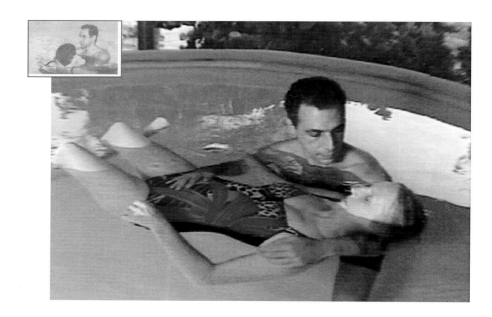

**Barbara Courtney, founder of
Wave M'ocean**   (Figure 15)

Mario Jahara, founder of the Jahara Technique™

(Figure 16)

The Founders of Aquatic Bodywork:

Healing Dance — Alexander Georgeakopoulos, California
Jahara Technique — Mario Jahara, Brazil
Wave M'ocean — Barbara Courtney
Watsu — Harold Dull, California
WaterDance — Arjana Brunschwiler & Peter Schroter, Switzerland

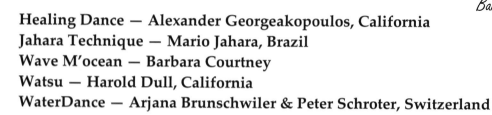

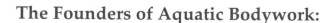

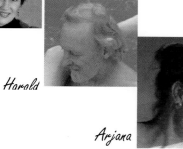

Alexander

Mario

Barbara

Harold

Arjana

(Figure 17)

Nalu: The Art and Science of Aquatic Fitness, Bodywork & Therapy

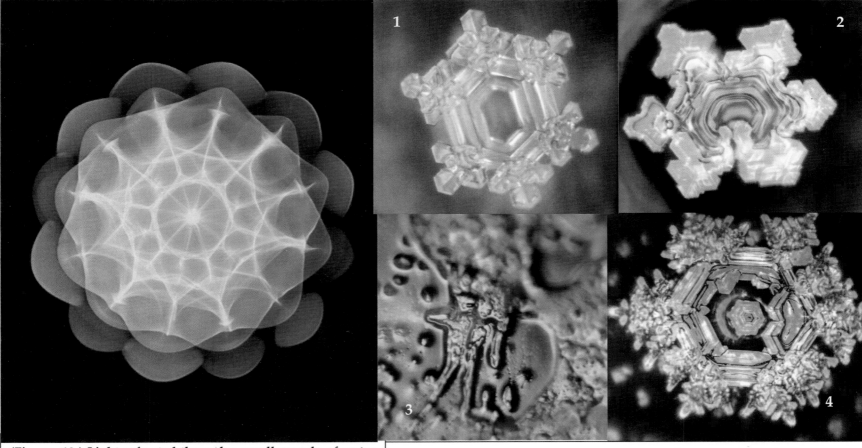

(Figure 18) Light refracted through a small sample of water contained within a circular ring on top of a lens that is being vibrated by audible sound frequencies. The light is projected from beneath the lens, illuminating the standing waves created by the sound, thus forming this beautifully symmetrical harmonic pattern.

From a series of experiments in Cymastics by Dr. Hans Jenny. Photo used by permission ©2001 MACROmedia www.cymaticsource.com

(Figure 19) Photographs and interpretations of water ice crystals by Masaru Emoto

1. Sample water crystal exposed to the word "wisdom."
2. Sample water crystal exposed to Mozart's "Symphony Number 40."
3. This sample was distorted, imploded and dispersed after exposure to expressions of violence.
4. Crystal sample after offering a prayer to water.

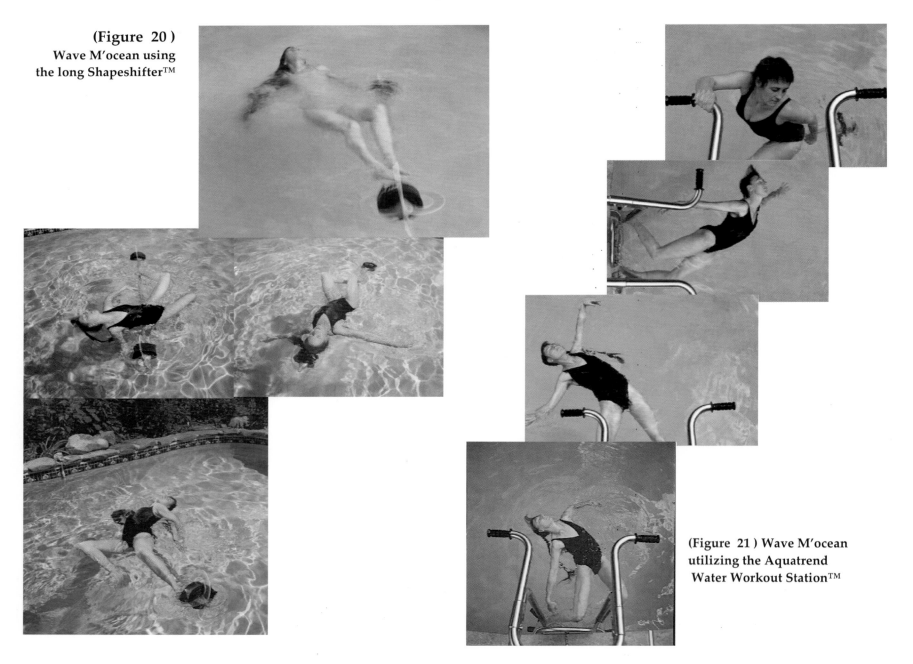

(Figure 20)
Wave M'ocean using
the long Shapeshifter™

(Figure 21) Wave M'ocean
utilizing the Aquatrend
Water Workout Station™

Nalu: The Art and Science of Aquatic Fitness, Bodywork & Therapy

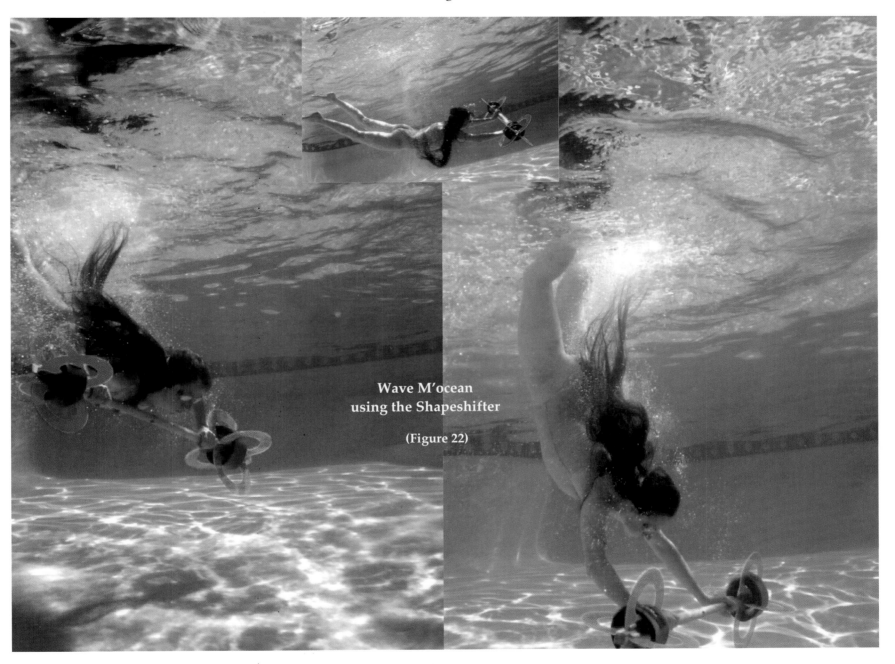

**Wave M'ocean
using the Shapeshifter**

(Figure 22)

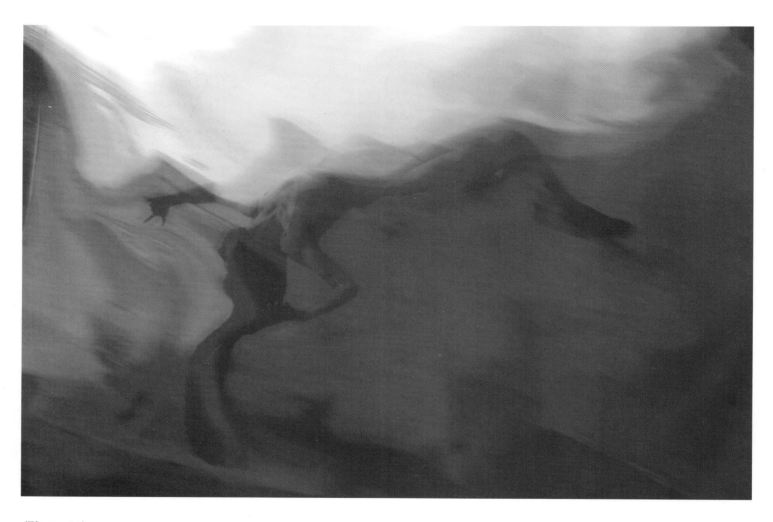

(Figure 23)
Wave M'ocean

Chapter 1
Healing Waters

By Barbara Courtney

"There is a place of healing within each of us, regardless of our spiritual lineage. To enter this realm of healing is to be elevated and forever changed."

Tom Kenyon

Dreamshifts

The foundation of the primarily water-based work that I call Wave M'ocean grew out of the somatic-imagery work that has evolved in my practice as a psychotherapist. This psychotherapeutic process, which I developed for my own use with clients, *Dreamshifts*, is one where a deepened state of focused awareness is created, providing a pathway into people's inner landscapes. Using this process, clients open to their own transformative abilities by entering into what I think of as a stream of consciousness of the five senses. This arena of imagery, sensation and guidance is an "experiential place" where people connect to an expanded consciousness, a heightened sensory awareness and a heart-centered desire to evolve.

I have been humbled by the power of simply allowing a client to be fully involved in a dreamlike state, exploring the language of their body and emotions. I believe that when a person is deeply connected in this way, they are accessing a higher order of intelligence. Some may say that this intelligence is a deep body-wisdom. Some may think we are accessing a stream of consciousness of our higher self or maybe our lower self. In any case, no matter how you look at it, we can say that through certain practices we can reach states of mind that bring us more into the present. Such states open us up experientially and we perceive our inner and outer worlds in new ways, such as matrixes of sensation and movement within an interconnected universe.

Activating the sense of magic is a spark that ignites the healing process. As young children, we have a natural curiosity and intimacy with everything around us. The boundaries between us and butterflies, flowers, animals, and tiny stones are almost fluid —almost nonexistent— because we are at one with nature and with the realm of dreams. Within this oneness, ecstasy comes easily. As our imaginations grow, we experience the power of dreams through fairy tales and myth. Our experience is one of knowing that dreams come true and that parallel worlds exist simultaneously. We can be anything we want at any time. All we have to do is dream it and it will happen. We can drift into another world and out again whenever we desire.

Then, at some point culture convinces us that we are not all ONE and that we must learn how to be separate from our surroundings from other people and even disconnected from people and even disconnected from ourselves. We sever ourselves from these rich dream states for our own survival in a culture that frowns upon daydreaming and fantasy. We are warned that to continue in these ways would be immature and maybe a sign that we don't have a grasp on reality.

Many waking dreams of my childhood were played out in a nature wonderland near my home. This magical place was created and nurtured by a kind and gentle neighbor, Mr. Taylor, who was completely in tune with nature's spirits. He lovingly cared for this land along with every inhabitant, be it plant, animal, insect or small girl. This was an enchanted little forest complete with a schoolhouse, wishing well, a living pond, squirrels who could communicate, humming birds sent from heaven, a wise sage and a magic tree. I could climb through the big entry hole in the magic tree and when I got to the other side, I could be anywhere and anyone I chose to be. I was able to return to what I knew was true - everything is ONE, and magic is just the way things are. I know now

that Mr. Taylor and his sacred space awakened my inherent ability to perceive reality beyond everyday life. I am eternally grateful to him and to nature for keeping these truths alive in me.

My work in client therapy sessions on land and in the water is a way of "paying forward" some of these gifts of connection and magic. I would like to pass on to others the opportunity to enter rich, imaginal realms because I know what is found there — our multidimensional selves. I believe these powerful expansive states are the keys to our ability to heal ourselves at every level— emotionally, physically and spiritually. This must be so, because I know that when a person has a powerful inner experience of connectedness to oneself and to the ALL, they are living the highest truths. From this vantage point, even if only for short glimpses, all is well and anything is possible. When we access those glimpses and nurture them into waking dreams of our creation, we are now swimming in the healing plenum of our bodies, hearts, minds and souls.

Wave M'ocean

In my work with clients, it has been clear that the more fully people can access and embrace an expanded state of consciousness during transformational work, the more profound and meaningful the transformation will be. Working in the water offers a unique opportunity for full involvement of every part of our being simultaneously. The aquatic submersion supports the unfolding expression of the language of the body through movement. The multidimensional self is set free from gravity and density, while at the same time the deep, internal, emotional body of the self responds to the water in a resonant way, creating permission to release. This environment offers the tremendous freedom, support and safety necessary to do powerful transformational work.

Aquatic classes in Wave M'ocean build a kind of container for a client to do transformative work. Here in the water, they open to their body's intra-communication and energy exchanges at many levels. Participants have a chance to integrate it all by closely tracking themselves, staying aware of what is needed next in their unfolding process. Water is mesmerizing, and I believe most people can enter into a waking dream state simply by immersing themselves. Because of water's tendency to alter their state, it is the most natural medium to do many healing practices.

Much in the same way that a shamanic journey allows us to go to other worlds of experience to heal, immersing ourselves in water with certain intentions allows us to shift perspectives. It is within this larger context of our own existence that we can draw from understandings, perspectives, sensory experiences and physiological opportunities that we didn't engage before. This act of "engaging" is what I think of as transforming. When we open to emotional, physiological and energetic information, we are most alive because we are fully participating in life's exchanges. At this level of intelligence, the event that we experience as healing is the emergence of our physiology's ability to self-organize.

Wave M'ocean is an educationally based, self-healing modality that I refer to as *active healing*. As a society, we are in great need of models for self-healing. We are experiencing a paradigm shift where we are releasing our victim relationship with illness, and we are beginning to seek and embrace self-empowerment on the healing journey. It is my belief from my own healing experiences and what I have witnessed, that true healing must come from within. It is from this premise that I offer the concept of active healing.

Conceptualizing active healing requires first turning ourselves upside down and shaking out the beliefs that a person or substance can heal us. Humans are the only beings on the planet that turn to outside intelligence to do the inside job of healing. The other creatures of the world rely on a body wisdom that is naturally set into motion when the need arises. Native American medicine men have connected those in need to this innate intelligence by calling upon the Medicine Bear to bring wisdom. Bears are animals known to use plants and herbs for self-healing. When they experience illness or injury, they instinctively seek what is needed to set their healing in motion. We too, have the circuitry for self-healing but it lays dormant due to thousands of years of "forgetting," sometimes referred to as evolution. In active healing, the practitioners and their medicines are more effectively looked upon as secondary to the internal and lifestyle changes that the illness has demanded of the client. This is empowering and helps us to heal ourselves. If we don't honor the constant flow of sensory and emotional information that runs through us, we are disconnecting from our bodies. Our already existing intra-communication system is incredibly powerful when we make the choice to tune in and participate in it. Getting to the place where we make this choice, however, is often difficult.

Why is it difficult to choose to tune in to our self? Wouldn't someone want to be self-empowered in his or her healing process? The problem here for many people has to do with belief systems. First of all, the medical model has laid down the dominant belief structures in our society. These belief structures are based on external authority when it comes to "managing our bodies" (industrializing our bodies). To give up our Western relationship to health, illness and the healing process would mean changing from a passive mode to an active mode. This involves releasing authoritarian beliefs about how healing happens and changing our relationship with ourselves. The dynamics of our current medical system encourage passivity at a time when we most need to be fully responsible and active. Healing is a process, not an event. In active healing, this process needs to come through the person who needs the healing. I believe that healing is *activated* when a person has a "love-based" (self- accepting) realization that they are ultimately the only one who can bring about true healing. Finding meaning in one's challenge, summoning the willingness to introduce change into what has been created or hosted and engaging in

change are the *activating forces* that communicate with cells.

As a culture or a "collective," we are in the middle of a paradigm shift where we are sorting out our beliefs about how we get sick and how we get well. However, our beliefs are so ingrained and feel so natural that we don't think of them as beliefs at all. We treat these beliefs as fact because the new awareness and perspectives are only just starting to emerge. The old paradigm is still the path of least resistance. Many people don't yet know where to begin when trying to understand their physical condition from any perspective other than traditional Western medicine. In the beginning, choosing to tune into our own wisdom and power to heal can create a conflict within us or with our doctor. However, when we release the disempowering paradigm, "I'll pay you to heal me; this is your responsibility, not mine," we reclaim our personal power and responsibility for healing. By releasing this belief we are accessing the truly powerful healer — ourselves.

Bringing awareness to the dynamics of beliefs is important because *beliefs themselves* are challenged and reinvented as we go through the process of healing. Self-healing modalities embrace this truth because it is necessary to shift beliefs in empowering ways if we choose to heal ourselves. We can look at cells as complex structures made of manifested thought form. For instance, when using qigong for self-healing, we embrace the idea that we can transform our cells with "holographic" information from the universe (energy). This energy re-patterns our cells. A shamanic-based example of exploring and shifting cellular "beliefs" is The Personal Totem Pole Process (Gallegos,1985). This guided self-healing practice involves transcending ordinary reality and belief systems so we can change behavioral, psychological and biological patterns. We can achieve this by integrating new awareness (beliefs). The fields of psycho-neuroimmunology and neuro-linguistic programming are also based on the premise that belief structures and cellular intelligence are inseparable. These bodies of work explore and reconfigure our complex mind-body-spirit intelligence.

Wave M'ocean is an exploration in self-healing. It provides a medium to connect with ourselves and to change the perceptual position of engaging with our physical and psychological experiences. By re-positioning ourselves or changing the context of our experience, we can open to new possibilities physically, psycho-logically and spiritually. The self-healing aspect is built on the premise that we can participate in the rich and intricate communication network that swims within us. This organic, constantly changing "intelligence" is accessed through the movement of thought "forms" and holds the secrets to our own mutability. The intention of using Wave M'ocean as a self-healing modality is to teach people how to attune to primary movement and process the experiences that are held in their bodies.

A useful tool for tuning into ourselves is to use our bodies, emotions and lives as mirrors. In other words, what we manifest in each of these arenas reflects something back to us about ourselves. If we are willing to listen to what our bodies, emotions and lives are telling us, active healing becomes simple, although not necessarily easy. Often we really don't want to hear what our bodies are saying. We can ask our back, "What is the problem that makes you give me all this pain?" Our back says, "Look at how you are not dealing with your boss at work. What do you expect?" This may not be an understanding that is easy to accept. We often discover that there is much resistance wrapped tightly around our worst problems. In the same way that tissue around an injury doesn't want to let go, we have great difficulty recognizing how we are *holding onto* a familiar psychological pattern.

Active healing in an aquatic setting really lends itself well to dealing with some of these issues. There is or can be an expectation that the client brings as much healing to the experience as the practitioner. This can be true even for a passive modality, such as Watsu or Jahara Technique, because an intention is set that communicates to the client, "I will bring you to the shores of your own healing. What you do with it internally can be very powerful. Your job is to let go, receive and track your own experience of opening to what is there for you." Wave M'ocean work and certain other modalities in the water allow a person to work through much of the resistance to tuning in. With Wave M'ocean work I think this is true because it is really a process that builds on trusting yourself while learning to let go of internal holding.

On an energetic level, psycho-therapeutic work and bodywork are about the reconfiguration of patterned information and exchanges within the person. In both instances, we introduce resources that can potentially melt away old structures and hold an "environment" where the individual allows new information into his or her system and processes it according to body wisdom.

It was my participation in Continuum Movement trainings that stirred me to think of the human body as an environment. Continuum Movement, founded in 1967, is a unique field of movement education that nourishes the inherent wisdom in our bodies. The pioneer of this work, Emilie Conrad, taught me that water is a resonant medium. Emilie teaches innovative ways of introducing sound, breath and movement to create resonance with the fluid in our bodies. Her model for movement education is based in part on the insight that we increase our biological adaptability by activating our "fluid body." In other words, breath, sound and movement are forms of "information" that nourish our bodies. They inform our movement and our state of mind. I became particularly interested in how the fluid in our bodies resonates with the water in the pool. Water is a messenger of fluidity to our bodies and lives. In Wave M'ocean work, I consider the water to be the container that holds the therapeutic process. When we are in the aquatic realm and feel relaxed, we are resonating with a state of mind, a state of existence that the water "knows." Here we sense and know things we can't articulate

because they are experiences beyond ordinary reality.

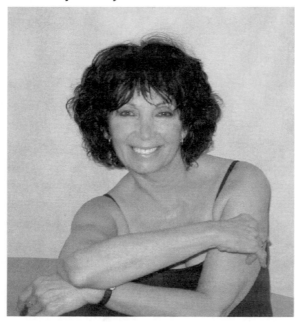

(Figure 24)   Emilie Conrad, founder of Continuum Movement

Creating an internal state that sets the stage for healing is another means for *taking responsibility*. In Wave M'ocean, all healing is self-healing in that a creative process emerges from the open and receptive internal environment that the client creates. By being aware of how *energy follows*

attention, the client focuses on the natural state of wholeness and engages in aquatic movement from that point of awareness. Movement is explored within the understanding that *we are mutable creatures*. As we engage in primary movement, we remember that being mutable is related to our ability to evolve. We practice certain deepening experiences using breath, sound, primal movement and expanded states of consciousness. Our intention is to access the forgotten body-based intelligence associated with mutability.

Wave M'ocean is process-oriented movement. The process is about being present, allowing the integration of emotions, body awareness and movement. The practice is to allow whatever wants to express, heal and evolve. Often this plays out very simply but powerfully, as it did with a client who discovered she could reconnect with lost aspects of herself. As we worked with slow fluid movement, she discovered a curious feeling that she was drawn to. The movement was making the curious feeling more present. Certain movements, as resources, enabled her to remember something at the body level. What her body was remembering was what it felt like to be innocent and free as she was when she was young, before she was sexually abused. As the movement unfolded, the memory of her innocence revealed itself in freer and freer movements. She began to cry as she reclaimed what had been taken. As we stayed with the process, the movements later evolved into something stronger and her body seemed to be calling in self-empowerment. This session allowed her to complete emotions and movement sequences that were waiting decades to come through.

Participants in Wave M'ocean workshops are supported to explore whatever movements, sounds and emotions are unfolding. This occurs within a structure of certain intentions and points of reference. The intentions may be anything from imbued thought forms in the water to invoking a quality of a particular animal into their movement and heart. The points of reference may be equipment or a certain way to perceive or join movement. This all serves to move clients away from over- stabilized movement and identities. When rigid movement patterns fall away, a process of unwinding starts to occur. This can be experienced as being in a trance with their movement. It can feel ecstatic. They can feel as if they have found the stillness in their movement. All of these experiences are akin to entering portals of awareness where inspiration and healing can unfold.

The Six Awareness Portals of Wave M'ocean

An awareness portal is a perception that, when embraced, leads to self-discovery. Each portal acts as a bridge to an "expanded presence" with a particular way of being and perceiving. In Wave M'ocean we invite ourselves to bring our attention to the portals of *movement, sound, breath, sense, dream and elemental consciousness* to call forth the multidimensional self. Each portal has its own context of perception that connects us with our world and ourselves in a unique way. Within the varying contexts of these awareness portals, we are invited to unify three realms of experience: witnessing, feeling and engaging. Uniting these three elements allows us to know a "dynamic wholeness." When the unification occurs, the whole becomes greater than the sum of the parts and a deeper dimension of self becomes available. If we are able to stay attuned to the dynamic wholeness created at a portal we can ride a wave of awareness that allows our experience to go beyond the ordinary and we can dive deeply into self-empowerment. I am not referring to power culturally defined as force, but instead to a powerful presence of self that is witnessed, felt and expressed. Immersed in the water, we are encouraged to evolve within this dynamic wholeness. Here, we find much opportunity to bring dormant potential and desire into discovery and expression.

Movement Awareness Portal

The movement awareness portal is of primary importance in water-based therapy. It is found within our ability to alter ordinary perception of movement by shifting orientation. Once we have found this ability, we can create an expanded experience of movement from many different perspectives. This portal is about discovering the many ways we can release static land-based movement patterns and explore other possibilities, such as *evolutionary movement, somatic resourcing, fluid resonance and dorsal orientation.* When we create a receptive internal environment we can become exquisitely focused on a movement process. By engaging with movement as a "witness who collaborates" we are allowing the body's communication to become conscious and thereby initiate a vital integrative process.

I refer to *evolutionary movement* as movement that emerges from an experiential connection to the animal circuitry within us. The experience of ourselves as animals is one we have actively abandoned as a condition for living in our culture. Ironically, we need to come home to this primordial aspect of ourselves because it is the reptilian brain that knows about survival. For thousands of years most cultures have worked very hard to detach from animal nature and become civilized. Only now, through the work of Peter Levine (1997), Emilie Conrad, Susan Harper and others are we coming to realize that we have thrown the baby out with the bath water.

One of the unfortunate results of disconnecting from our true nature is that we have lost touch with the ability to heal ourselves. We have "forgotten" the inherent permission that we once had as animals to allow our bodies the natural physiological responses as we interact with our world. We are mostly unaware that we interfere with the processing of emotions, events and trauma. When we inhibit the authentic unfolding of these reactions to prevent social discomfort for others and ourselves, we interfere with the "software" needed to process and resolve these experiences. Censorship of our animal innocence and power leaves us split off from ourselves. Peter Levine defines this as "disassociation from our organismic intelligence" (Levine, 1997). Ironically, the organismic intelligence that we have disassociated from is what we seek to connect with when we go to various kinds of therapy hoping to unearth our authenticity. Evolutionary movement helps us reconnect with impulses, movements and even raw emotions that we have been cut off from as a result of cultural conditioning. Finding our way back to "wildness," our ability to respond, is fundamental to reacquainting ourselves with our self-healing capacity.

An exercise as simple as exploring the movement of a jellyfish can acquaint you with your biomorphic capacity. Simply put floatation around your waist and then bring awareness to your belly as the center of movement. New possibilities come into play when the movement becomes curiosity-oriented as opposed to goal-oriented. Merging with the jellyfish will spontaneously initiate unfamiliar but interesting movement such as pulsing movements from your center outward. When moving laterally, you are stimulating more primitive aquatic circuitry. Your center of gravity, your "center point," is constantly shifting. Feel how your jellyfish center point pushes you out laterally and then contracts inward. This wave motion wakes up your nervous system and if you pay close attention, you will notice how you begin to let go into the rhythm of movement. There is a sense that the body is behaving *more* intelligently than during controlled movements. You have invited yourself into primal fluid process. If you observe aquatic creatures you will notice that there is much evidence that the flow of survival intelligence seems to travel through the same channels as seeking pleasure, stimulation and nourish-ment. Experiment with opening this same channel and follow the flow of pleasure as a way of connecting with primal intelligence. Engaging in these reshaped perceptions leads to a change in the "shape" of movement that is created. The core organization of your movement will align with the movement of the jellyfish. Give yourself permission to feel safe and free while you explore the emerging movement. The hydrostatic pressure supports your ability to stay present in your body while integrating movement with awareness.

I believe evolutionary movement can be a vehicle for transformation because it allows us to leave social conditioning behind and reclaim vital movement. Transformation can only come from a wholeness that includes our primal nature. Evolution occurs thanks to an organism's capacity to register and process change – to rearrange itself. This is what enlivens us and ultimately increases what Emilie Conrad calls our "probability of existence" both at the individual level and as a species. Primal aquatic movement engages lower order circuitry that stimulates our adaptability and healing. This *is* evolution in the sense that we are "remembering" how to be mutable. When we embrace both our primal restorative capacity and our human ability to consciously participate in change, we have set the stage for our personal evolution.

Somatic resourcing refers to our ability to arrive at a felt sense of support. It occurs when we find and allow movements, thoughts, memories, sensations and physiological states that lead to competency, self-soothing, empowerment and authentic expression. These "resourced states" support us in orchestrating transformation. In biology we learn that the organism is always seeking nourishment. Likewise, we seek somatic nourishment such as movement in order to experience the vitality of who we are. This in turn opens up the reservoir of healing potential that lies within. Water, of course, is a basic, readily available somatic resource for clients during Wave M'ocean classes and sessions. There is a reciprocal relationship between sensing and moving. Clients internalize the felt sense of containment and wave motion from the external body (water in the pool) and can manifest these qualities internally, integrating them into self-awareness and movement. The internalized sense of being held combined with the freedom to move (wave motion) is reflected outwardly, creating a reciprocal loop of movement, receptivity and integration. In the context of this circular dialogue, clients dive deeper into their movement resources and the orientations that feed their physiology and strengthen their sense of self. Slowing down the movement with awareness will help them to stay present and assimilate an exchange that wouldn't otherwise occur.

Sourcing one's movement from the solar plexus puts the "heart and gut intelligence" in charge of the experience. The heart and the gut are two powerful centers of authentic expression. To experiment with this, source your movement from those centers by rooting your arms and legs in your solar plexus. Start by noticing wave motion in the solar plexus area. Allow the movement of "legness" to be sourced from this wave motion and spread downward into your pelvis and upward into your chest.

Your arms and legs receive and interpret movement from this heart and gut-centered core self. Ask yourself, What am I able to reclaim here? What would it be like if my heart moved my legs? What would it be like if my gut moved my arms? What movements bring competency or a sense of personal power? What dormant qualities are emerging? Are there any surprises? Stay open to the answers and allow the stream of body consciousness to support and orchestrate the integration of heart, gut and movement. Amplify the movements and feelings if that helps you stay with the flow of resourceful expression. This full experience serves as a somatic resource to activate the electrical connections between freedom and personal power in our body. Whenever we go inside to access states of pure and free-flowing personal power, we will always go to the places where this somatic information is stored – our navel and our diaphragm. Doing this consciously can be quite transforming.

Fundamental to Wave M'ocean is the concept of resonance or attunement to that which vitalizes us. Our movement can resonate with an idea, intent, feeling, emotion or an element such as water, and this attunement defines how movement is occurring. Engaging in *fluid resonance* is the practice of identifying and embracing the external fluidity and then becoming aware of the interior fluidity. The water we are immersed in acts as a cue to our "aqueous body" and a conversation begins. We can invite the awareness of internal wave motion by imagining that the dynamics of fluid movement on the outside of our skin are also occurring throughout the fluid systems on the inside of our skin. This can feel like something is moving us from the inside, instead of the water moving us from the outside.

Resonance is a gift that keeps on giving, which is why it is such an important concept in Wave M'ocean. In my view, resonance actually creates a rippling effect or a wave motion throughout all aspects of our human experience and is even reflected in our life. As a therapist, I have observed that when one aspect of our being can participate in perceptual attunement then other aspects of the self begin relating to that attunement. What follows is an example of this wave-like movement of perception as fluid resonance transforms the experience of self.

The first level of resonance most often occurs at the cognitive level where we attune to an *idea* such as "I am made of water just like the water in this pool. Through resonance, I can activate fluidity in my own body." This awareness reverberates into the realm of *felt sense*: "I can feel oceanic tides inside my own body stretching and massaging me." The rippling of awareness continues into *movement*. As we experience fluidity as an intelligence with which we can consciously move in concert, we might have the thought, "I can *create* these tides, and it feels powerful. The tides stretch me from the inside out and it make me feel like I can go beyond ordinary limitations." This empowered fluid resonance state communicates with our *emotional*

body, teaching us about the ebb and flow of the receptive - expressive tides: "I can allow the natural flow of *feelings* in the same way that I have been able to feel the tides of movement in my body." At the outer ripples of fluid resonance we attune to the *flow of life*: "I am aware of an adaptability in me that is like water in the river flowing around the rocks." As we work with fluid resonance in this way with clients they can find resources in cultivating a greater sense of wholeness.

An axiom in Continuum Movement is that the context of our movement defines the quality of our movement. The post-industrial human body has become over-stabilized in the sense that we have habituated patterns of forward, upright movement while slipping away from the body awareness and the biological flexibility available within the human organism (Conrad, 1997). One way that we have reduced adaptability and narrowed the repertoire of movement is through our frontal orientation. We are used to greeting, receiving and interacting with the

world frontally and from our limbs rather than our core. The movement patterns that we are "over-identified" with such as linear, repetitive movements are entrenched conditioned patterns. A mechanized, task oriented relationship to our bodies has restricted our approach to exercise and healing. In the quest to expand movement possibilities, we can dive into the aquatic realm to "remember" multi-directional movement and shed the patterns of movement identity. Here, we can release the need to have a definitive front and back, and the center of our movement can be everywhere.

In the practice of *dorsal orientation* we engage in a perceptual shift in order to release the frontal orientation, freeing up innovative movement, promoting neuromuscular integration and heightened awareness of the body in space. The intention here is to orient ourselves to our backbones or ancestral dorsal fins. Although humans don't actually have fins, I believe that we do have energetic memory of our ancient form and that it is still possible to become both receptive and mobilized from a posterior, or dorsal perspective. Exploring dorsal orientation expands our perceptual field so that we can wake up from the familiar into the ancestral experience. In the practice of dorsal orientation, I ask students to reverse the mode by which they interact with their environment and drop down into a deeper way of sensing. Participants focus their awareness allowing the tops of their heads to lead the way or allowing their backs to sense and express how they want to move. This is helpful in releasing the spine and initiating the undulating movements known to aquatic life. Dorsal orientation opens people up to a 360-degree awareness of freedom and support that never lets them down as long as they trust that it is there. Once established, the dorsal awareness can be amplified and explored.

Using aquatic equipment as a resource

Creating reference points to leverage traction or to maintain a connection to a point of stability while engaged in fluid movements is key to Wave M'ocean. Equipment can help us initiate movement from different areas of the body. The *Shapeshifter* (Figure 185, page 344) was devised in an effort to simultaneously provide fluidity and stability. This copolyester and wood aquatic device is useful in supporting both fluid movement and the need for "contact stability." The Shapeshifter provides a stabilizing point of reference, even though it is moving in the water with you. Contact stability refers to the use of a point around which the movement organizes. Having contact with the point stabilizes core movement. This is similar to having a dance partner where there is a point-counterpoint relationship. At the psychological level there is much opportunity for expression and integration by being in a flowing relationship with both self and environment simultaneously. A kind of trance state of flow begins to

develop, drawing us deeper into our personal rhythms and out again into expressive movement. Used in this way, the Shapeshifter can become a physical reference for a perceptual shift, fostering a sense of freedom and creativity.

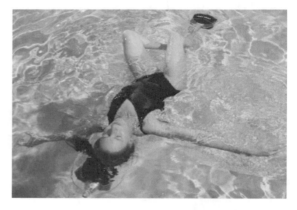

(Figure 25) Using the Shapeshifter for contact stability.

Another piece of equipment that is a valuable resource for Wave M'ocean movement is the *Aquatrend Water Workout Station* (Figure 186, page 345). This equipment fits into a ladder receptacle at the edge of the pool providing stability while the body is free to open and undulate. I instruct clients to build a "movement scaffolding" using their body in partnership with the equipment. The contact points where body and equipment meet at any given moment are opportunities for leverage so that movement information is driven back into the core and out again. The body is undulating in a constant flow of metamorphosis and the contact points keep shifting. This allows the body to create internal traction for deep movement. A syncopated rhythm of momentum can be created, as one stays fully present with the primal movement flow and the point/counterpoint relationship. The constant shifting of angles and pace of movement bring a surprising agility and sense of exhilaration. The Aquatrend Water Workout Station has been a wonderful resource because it enables the possibility for the asymmetrical, spreading, stretching movements that lead into the body's natural wave motion. These oscillating movements release rigid patterning and liberate the expressive body.

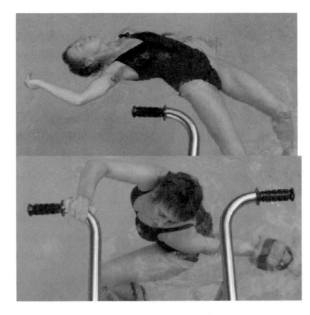

(Figure 26) Creating internal traction on the Aquatrend

Sound Awareness Portal

Quantum physics has now been able to confirm for us what the ancients knew: all matter is essentially vibrating energy. Sound is also vibrating energy albeit at a higher frequency than the human body. To prepare to enter the sound awareness portal, we embrace the vibrating energy that comprises our bodies as organized consciousness that is vibrating at a low rate and appearing to be a solid mass. We merge sound and intention to create an intelligence that rides the waves of vibrating matter. This wave of intelligence— what we experience as sound from our voices — is actually encoded vibrational information that interfaces with the vibrational patterns of our human organism. This interfacing, or vibrational rapport, is what I am calling resonance. Resonant healing occurs when the body recognizes the encoded information in sound and comes into congruence with it. A great resource for more detailed information about the dance between sound and matter is Hans Jenny's groundbreaking book, *Cymatics (1967).* Hans Jenny gives us a visual understanding of how matter shifts vibrational patterns as it comes into relationship with various tones and frequencies. In Jenny's book and in videos of his work, we can literally witness the movement of sound through the medium of matter. As the tone changes, so does the visual configuration of the vibrating matter, creating geometric patterns of astonishing beauty and complexity (Fig.18, page 41).

We enter the sound awareness portal by bringing our conscious awareness to the creation and movement of sound vibration. Here we participate in resonant healing by absorbing vibrational nourishment, something intrinsic to us from our earliest experiences. To appreciate the wisdom and significance of bringing sound into the water as a healing resource, it is helpful to remember where we come from experientially. Our earliest sensory experiences as a fetus in the womb are of sound and vibration. We floated weightlessly in body temperature amniotic fluid experiencing sound vibration and sensation as our primary sensory experiences. From the fourteenth week of gestation the inner ear, developing from the eighth cranial nerve, began to charge the brain as it received and processed sound. The fluid in our ears pressed against our eardrums, amplifying this rich sonic world where sound travels 5x faster than through air. In utero this "underwater" sound and movement served as an impetus to the development of our nervous system. The blissful floating in fluid and the symphony of sound patterns that we experienced in utero are deeply embedded in our subconscious for the rest of our lives. I believe we can re-activate this receptive and formative fetal experience by recreating the associated sensory stimulation and, hence, brainwave states that are conducive to expanded consciousness and healing.

Human beings have been using sound to expand awareness, access deeper states of consciousness and heal the body for thousands of years. In Wave M'ocean we reawaken the prenatal reality by participating in the dynamic interplay of consciousness, sound and movement. There are four perceptual relationships with sound that influence this dynamic interplay. These are the aware states of *witnessing, receiving, engaging and expansion*.

Our experience as a *witness* is a passive one where we behold the phenomenon of sound. With water and vibration merged, we are held in a truly reflective environment that amplifies our ability to witness sound. The hydrostatic pressure and the "dreaminess" of the underwater world help induce an altered state where we can witness at a deep level. To open witness awareness, float comfortably with your ears submerged. Breathe deeply and relax. Imagine that you have traveled to the dimension of sound, where you discover that you can interpret experiences through hearing and feeling. Sound is a way you can be with yourself and your surroundings. Your cognitive mind drifts away and there is a focus on the sound of your breathing and your body. The sound of your breath just *is*. Notice how the water is amplifying the sound. Drop into the rhythm alone. How do the sound and rhythm cue your physical body and emotional body? Are you noticing any shifts in awareness as a result?

Receiving is opening to the sound and feeling its movement. Our language doesn't have a term for feeling sound, but we need one here. I use "sound sensing" when describing how we resonate with the quality of the sound and allow it to translate into a felt sense. When we are relaxed and focused we can notice sensations that are associated with sound. Sound sensing is allowing oneself to absorb sound in the brain, tissue and bones and feeling the movement of sound throughout the body. We may feel it as vibration, warmth, or as wave motion. We can also notice the continued sensation of the sound after the sound has stopped and the movement related to the sound continues. Sound sensing and movement are very intertwined with emotion. Try sound sensing your heartbeat while floating with your ears submerged. You will find a renewed sense of being present in the merged realm of sound and sensation. Notice how you feel about yourself and your world as you are immersed and held in the subtle sounds of your heart and breath. What emotions are there? What movement comes from

this? You will find that the ability to feel the movement of sound is amplified because your ears are submerged. Sound sensing is reminiscent of pre-birth early sensory experiences in the nurturing environment of water and sound. It opens your receptivity to emerging primal movements that your organism had before social conditioning. I believe we are more receptive to sound and its healing qualities when we are in the water, possibly because the medium of delivery (water) is the same substance that our bodies are made of — just as it was in utero.

Engaging is the co-creative relationship we have with the movement of sound. When we engage with sound there is no separation between creation and evolution. We must go beneath the cognitive experience of sound to access the vibrating self. We are engaging co-creatively when we allow a transfer of information (transformation) between the wave-like self and the wave movement of sound. Therefore, we are experiencing ourselves as self-

transforming vibrating organisms by consciously engaging in the creation of sound. Here we discover our innate ability to use sound to initiate flow and change in our mind and body. Toning, for example, is a way to use our body and voice together as a transforming instrument. Toning is the empowerment of the breath by adding the dimension of sound vibration. Many traditions over the span of human existence have engaged in toning and chanting for transformational purposes. The Wave M'ocean practice of vibrating breath with sound and intention is used as a vehicle to awaken a deeper consciousness. This simple act truly shifts awareness and is an invitation for body, mind and spirit to come into alignment. If one is toning from a balanced place inside, it is a fundamental tone that can set off resonance in other octaves, bringing the body into harmony. Changing tones and pitches sends information to different parts of the body, as well as offering shapes of sound and movement patterns throughout the body.

We can now measure the effects of toning on our physiology through biofeedback, PET scans, (Positron Emission Tomography), CAT scans (Computed Axial Tomography) and through the eyes of people who read auras. We know that changes in brainwaves and energy fields begin to occur within 20 to 40 seconds of toning. Changes in tonality orchestrate blood flow and neural connections that we know are related to consciousness (Campbell, 1990). This becomes evident in Wave M'ocean when we experience changes in our state of awareness and our perceptions begin to shift. All of these changes are highly conducive to healing.

Toning underwater is very soothing to the nervous system. Choose a low frequency sound such as "ohm." Ohm is known as the subtle vibration of creation. When ohm is toned with mindfulness, your awareness will gently expand inwardly and will go to more and more subtle levels. From this subtle perspective you can more readily recognize peace, happiness and bliss. Try this by comfortably floating in the water; you may use whatever floatation you prefer, as long as your ears are submerged. Begin toning and notice the inward expansion of awareness. Play with the sensory experience of the sound traveling through your body. Bypass ordinary reality and become the sound. Journey with the sound into images and movement. Take time between breaths to feel the sound continue to move even as there is no sound being created. Notice that your body may make movements to direct the sound waves to a particular location.

You may also engage with visual perception of sound by tracking the vibration moving through an area of the body. Allow it to bathe the bones and connective tissue in light and you can, through visualization, watch the light travel up the tubular dural sheath that surrounds the spinal cord, aligning the vertebra as it goes. The results can be profound because the body-spirit-mind organism as a whole is involved in the healing at the subtle levels of light, sound and consciousness simultaneous with the denser level of felt sense. This is co-creative transformation using sound and intention at the fundamental level and it activates the healing process.

The body, water and sound are all energetic systems that are in constant interaction with each other. How marvelous it is that we happen to be made primarily of water, and we came equipped with sounding instruments (voices) that can vibrate that water, sending vibrational information to all parts of our being simultaneously. When we are toning or making low frequency sounds, using our body as an instrument, the vibrational information entrains the brain to slow its function, and therefore brings us into an altered state of consciousness (expanded consciousness). Sound vibration creates a bridge so we can find ourselves—or at least an aspect of ourselves—that we want to connect with, such as our primal selves. The aquatic setting supports this opportunity to go deeper into our primal selves because immersion triggers our organism to "remember" biologically based movement from our ancient past. Our ancestors who successfully evolved were co-creating themselves in harmony with the forces of nature. We too, can work co-creatively with sound to wake up our cells to the memory of evolution, facilitating healing.

We move into a relationship of *expansion* with sound when we create a field of vibration by toning while feeling connected to self and the environment. Expansion is a process of going deeper and deeper into more subtle awareness. The subtler our awareness becomes, the closer we get to ONENESS. Expansion leads us to unified consciousness where we feel connected to everything. When we are immersed in water and sound, a sense of unity can be experienced at a sensory level. Here, there are no spaces between our smaller human body and expanded body. Everything is one interactive organism. From this vantage point, introducing sound creates a unified field of vibration — a force field that allows us to shift consciousness. The exchanges that can take place have to do with letting the sound inform the movement. It can

feel like the sound is a shared phenomenon occurring on both sides of a permeable membrane. The sound creates a permeable interface between the inner and outer worlds of vibrating water. The interface is opened. There are no barriers — there's no resistance. There is only one body of vibrating consciousness. This is empowerment. In this context of expansion it is possible to use intention to raise the frequency of the vibration by engaging in "coherent emotion" or the emotions that assist us in feeling whole. Emotions are currents of energy with different frequencies (Kenyon, 1996). Fear, for instance has a low frequency and love vibrates at a higher frequency. Merging a high frequency emotion with toning creates a wave of intelligence with which our whole being will want to resonate.

Through expanded sensory awareness it is possible for the experience of one sense to evoke a second perception through another sense portal. For instance, often in my therapy practice when a client is journeying in a deep state, they will

have the expanded sensory experience whereby they discover their "fourth dimension of sensing." They might share with me "I see color patterns when I tone that sound." or "My body becomes very cold as I visualize this memory."

Here is a quote from an individual who *sees* sound very clearly during his ordinary reality:

"When I hear musical sounds, I also see colors. Musical instruments each produce their own particular color. When I hear a piano, I see a specific shade of blue. Tenor saxophone? You've got a floating ball of a hundred coiling snakes made of purple neon tubing ... with some musical colors I can stick my hand right into them and move them around. Like the sky-blue mist I see when I hear a piano: it will swirl like smoke, as if its being affected by my hand, but I don't feel anything." (Day, 2003).

This person's experiences are examples of what author Gary Zukav (1989) refers to as the evolution of the five-sensory personality to the multi-sensory personality. He suggests that as a species we are evolving into an expanded dimension of experience and ability. This dimension has a higher frequency range than what we have been vibrating at. As a result, we are beginning to use our sensory apparatus in new and expanded ways, drawing in more perceptual information through our senses than we have in the past. Water makes us more receptive to experiencing our expanded sensory perceptions. When we return to the womb-like state and feel unified with our world, we move into a deeper level of our being. It is at this deeper level that we discover our intuitive and perceptual abilities.

Breath Awareness Portal

Breath is intimately connected with all aspects of being. There are five ways we can experience breath that are important to mention here: breath as the *conveyor of life force,* as an *alchemical facilitator,* as *movement,* as a *portal to our aquatic past* and as *portal to our aquatic future.* Experiencing these reference points as we explore breath in the aquatic setting can prove to be fulfilling, empowering and

transforming. Each of these ways of approaching breath affects our sense of self within our environment and opens up new pathways of creativity and movement.

All spiritual healing traditions agree that breath is life. Our ability to be alive is intertwined with an energy referred to in the yogic tradition as prana or in the Chinese healing tradition as chi. Self healing practices in these and other traditions use the breath to activate and increase the level of *life force* flowing through the various bodies (physical, emotional, and etheric). "When a human body breathes air into the lungs, the prana within the etheric counterpart of this air is taken into the etheric counterpart of the body and is then transformed into the various energies that one uses in everyday life: mental energy, emotional energy and physical energy. The oxygen which is taken into the blood via the lungs of course plays a part in metabolism, but it is only a minor role compared to the importance of the intake of prana." (Jasmuheen, 2000).

According to ancient Eastern and Aboriginal traditions, the free movement of breath infused with awareness and sometimes with specific intentions releases energy blocks in the physical and emotional bodies. In Wave M'ocean work, we can bring our attention to breath as *life force* and experience energy in motion. Here, we seek to promote the fluidity of energy, movement and emotions. With our attention focused on the flow of breath, movement and emotions, we initiate a body level understanding of the movement of energy. The awareness of breath as life force itself changes our experience of breathing immediately and can awaken the healing process. Immersing ourselves in water during or following breath work accentuates the movement of life energy because the water communicates fluidity at the organic level. The movement of our breath will assume the fluid quality of water through the phenomenon of resonance.

Sometimes we play with water and various breaths according to the movement of the water we are in. For instance, the forceful, "energetically charged" movement of water in a spa is matched well with the rapid, pulsing rhythms of yogic "breath of fire." It is difficult to effectively communicate certain breaths in text, so I suggest that you have fun using breaths that you know and try matching them with an environment you would like to resonate with. You may be at a serene lake, near the ocean where there are powerful waves, or in a warm pool. You can resonate with these states by choosing a breath that attunes you to the energy, and then use your awareness to track the movement in your physical and emotional body. In this way you are using breath as a link to life force at the organic level. By amplifying the flow of breath and life force, you may create an increased supply of healing energy, which might evidence itself as improved circulation, feeling more present, clearer thinking, a feeling of body, mind and spirit being more integrated or just feeling more alive.

As a connecting and integrative force between body, soul and the infinite,

breath is an *alchemical facilitator*. By alchemical facilitation, I am referring to our ability to combine breath and consciousness to create a subtle but powerful breath phenomenon. When the aware state links breath to tissue, bone, and circulating fluids throughout the body, an alchemical process is initiated. Shifting from the terrestrial to aquatic context adds another dimension, which I refer to as *alchemical compression*. This idea is based on truths that were shared with me by shaman healer Elan O'Brien. She enlightened me as to the alchemical interaction of pressure, water, consciousness and the human body. I came to understand how to drop down into my consciousness using breath, and experience the feeling of atmospheric pressure. Here, we create increased pressure on all body and consciousness systems each time we release our breath and drop into a deeper awareness of self and unity. Elan teaches that these perceptions assist in the creation of homeostasis. As the depth increases, so does the pressure on our cells, thereby affecting the permeability of

cells and improving intercellular communication.

What follows is a depth breathing experience that can bring about alchemical compression. Experimenting with it will introduce you to the shifts that occur with depth pressure. To prepare for depth breathing in the water you must be willing to allow perceptual shifts to connect you to inner depth and a sense of unity. The one alchemical property that needs to be present at all times is the commitment to hold unconditional love, which facilitates the process of transformation. I am referring to an unconditional love that is not an emotion, but rather a high resonance state of participating in your experience without resistance or judgment.

Begin by floating on your back with light neck support and light ankle floatation strips (or if that is not comfortable this can also be done vertically with waist floatation). Free your mind by focusing on your breath and entering a meditative state. It is very important to take the time to become deeply relaxed. Inhale, allowing the breath to expand your belly and lower back, applying pressure against the water. With the exhale, reverse the pressure and allow yourself to fully imagine and feel yourself dropping a few feet deeper in the water (your physical body floats, so you can breathe easily, however your energetic bodies will go on the depth journey). Keep in mind that the thought of allowing yourself to go deeper will bring on the total experience if you are willing to let go into the pressure and can maintain your focus. Each time you exhale, feel yourself drop and notice the increased pressure at the new depth. Rely on your senses to tell you how rapidly you are dropping and how deep you are. How do your physical and emotional bodies respond? Find your rhythm taking a gentle, soulful breath, pausing and letting go into an exhale while you drop. In the pause that follows, feel your depth. Allow the compression to calm you. Here, pressure and unconditional love are the keys to a deeper level of consciousness. Breath facilitates our ability to drop into our depths where

barriers to subtle awareness are softened and we can exchange consciousness with all life forms. Keep allowing yourself to drop deeper with each exhale until you feel as if you have stopped dropping. Remain at the depth where you stopped, asking yourself what stopped me? How am I feeling? Was there a particular thought or concern that was coming in when I stopped; or was it a sensation? Witness the feeling, thought, concern or sensation without merging or judging. Hold it in the context of unconditional love; experience it all as energy and notice what happens. If appropriate, continue to the next depth, journeying to a deeper sense of integration. Depth breathing is a vehicle of expanded consciousness that is rooted in organic reality and can awaken the healing process.

Breath is intimately connected with *movement*. In fact, breath *is* movement within the physical and emotional bodies. Being with this truth in the aquatic setting, we find we can attune to how breath creates movement very easily. In the water, we are more able

to have the physical freedom and lightness of body to breathe with every part of our bodies, the way babies do. When a baby breathes, its belly, back, arms and legs move with every breath. This is natural, but as we become conditioned by trauma and a mechanized world, we limit the movement of breath to our chests. In the water, it becomes natural again to relearn how to allow breath into our belly, sides and whole of our backs. Emotionally, we are assisted to return to the natural state of a baby. A baby's emotions and breath flow in perfect synchrony, without censorship or restriction. The water gives us the opportunity to unlearn the tightening of our chests used in the suppression of emotions. We can free ourselves from these frozen patterns, allowing fluidity in breath, body and emotions "by varying breath, thereby introducing new movement… All movement is initiated or stifled by the scope or limitation of the breath. When we free the breath from habitual patterns, we can initiate altered brain states and likewise, altered movement experience" (Conrad, 1997). Emilie Conrad's work has revealed that when we use breath and sound together we can facilitate variations in tissue mass, allowing the release of dense holding patterns. We alternate a soft, expansive breath like the yogic "oujai" breath (pronounced oo-jyi) with a vibrating breath, such as "ohm."

In this fluid movement of breath exploration, it is helpful to support yourself with the use of hand buoys. Start with the gentle breath of oujai, which has a soft "H" sound in the throat. The mouth is closed and relaxed, while inhalation and exhalation flow very quietly and slowly through the nose. Rock yourself vertically with breath in a oneness of breath and water. You will rise during inhalation and fall during exhalation. As you bob up and down with the movement of your breath, you become your breath in a super-sensory way. You will feel your breath move you and sense your movement as breath. Here, all movement is the movement of breath. In the water we move ourselves and our environment simultaneously with the intake and release of breath. It is a

powerful way to experience oneness and feel breath in the form of movement. Play with this for a few minutes, and then alternate with the vibrating breath of ohm. Tune into your etheric field to sense a different kind of movement. Allow your body to interpret this ohm breath-movement. Notice how in the water, breath and movement are happening symbiotically everywhere at the same time. One cannot separate breath, movement and the ebb and flow of the water. As you alternate these two experiences, you are quieting your left-brain and becoming more present with your experiential capabilities. What is especially powerful is that you are out of ordinary context in two ways: novel breathing and movement, along with freedom from gravity. This allows you physically and emotionally to shift out of entrenched patterns and be with the rhythms of the present moment.

Breath is the key to the nervous system and mirrors our emotional state. Whatever is going on in the system is reflected in the breath. The movement of emotions happens in

tandem with the movement of breath. In Wave M'ocean we find we have the ability to use breath to affect the fluidity of emotional states. There is a breath used in Continuum called "hu," (pronounced who) which is reminiscent of panting. I like to offer this in water with the intention of reconnecting the breath/emotion link we were born with. Using this panting breath with loose, expressive mouth and face, we traverse a myriad of emotions in a spontaneous flow before we ever have a chance to attach a story to what we are experiencing. The result is the simple return to emotional fluidity. As animals, we weren't built to attach a story to every emotion. However, as conditioned humans, that's exactly what we do. Doing this breath in the water and allowing the spontaneous associated movement returns us to our original fluid state. As a premise for healing, it is important to remember that it is physiologically difficult or maybe impossible to experience the breathing pattern of one state while maintaining a different state. For instance, it would be difficult to maintain a state of fear while practicing a breathing pattern that is an expression of relaxation and openness. We can set certain breath-movement rhythms designed to introduce new physiological information into a stuck dysfunctional system. We can use the rhythms of breath to entrain the mind and body—to slow it down, to open awareness, to focus and introduce choice to our organism. Instead of letting the emotional state determine the breath, we reverse the process. Then we can re-organize ourselves around the new breath-movement state, where the breath informs the movement.

How we engage with breath can become a *portal to our aquatic past*. Humans as fetuses experience aerobic cellular respiration in the womb. In this way we are not far afield from all of our aquatic cousins. Beginning at birth, however, pulmonary respiration and weight begin to shape our movement and our bodies. Unlike cetaceans, our breath is involuntary—we don't have to remember to breathe, or even be conscious in order for breathing to continue. However,

because man is a descendant of aquatic creatures, we still have the capacity and inclination to influence our involuntary breathing when we are in the aquatic world. It is possible to return to a sense of embryonic respiration if we can create the proper internal and external fluid environment. One must be in a very quiet, warm aquatic space where there is a sense of safety about relaxing. One's internal environment is serene and receptive. A horizontal floating position is assumed. Here, we let go into soft, natural diaphragmatic breathing where the belly and lower back expand gently upon the inhale and relax upon the exhale. The breathing is so subtle and quiet that it is as if one is not engaging in pulmonary breathing, but instead has returned to the womb. It is a totally unifying experience where eventually the border between oneself and the water blurs. "All is well" in a symbiotic oneness with the fluid environment. The water or our larger self "breathes us" and moves in unison with us in a kind of wave motion -- one unified breath. There is no separation, no perceptible breath.

The focus is on feeling a symbiotic circular exchange.

Let us now connect to a watery respiration that goes back even further than our embryonic experience. By returning to our aquatic origins to explore breath, we access our cellular memory of breath in the ocean's depths. Pioneers in the field of movement, such as Emilie Conrad, and in the field of breath-hold diving, such as Jacques Mayol, have taught us that what we think of as evolution is really a process that is present within our human form. We have memories of our past forms and perceptions at the cellular level. Both Conrad and Mayol have investigated the evolutionary process, each in very different ways. They have conveyed through their lives and work evidence that we have dormant physiological links to our ancient aquatic past, and that we can activate some degree of cellular and/or energetic memory of various past life forms. There are several breathing techniques that help us get in touch with this memory experientially, enabling us to become more flexible and even to heal ourselves. There are slow, full bodied breaths that engage the sense of cutaneous respiration whereby gases are exchanged through the skin, such as the respiration of a frog. There are breaths that activate the ancient circuitry for respiration through gills. Combining a lateralizing breath (such the oujai breath in the yogic tradition) with the imagery of spreading and contracting laterally moves into the aquatic primordial experience (most of these breaths are difficult to describe without demonstration). One exercise that is simple to play with is a buoyancy breath. Here, we focus our consciousness in our gut and open up our inner space to receive and hold the level of oxygen we need according to the level of buoyancy we want. Imagine there is a small balloon-like air bladder in your gut that inflates to control your buoyancy. Inhale and feel it inflate and check your buoyancy. Imagine you can control your buoyancy as you breathe naturally by simply visualizing your bladder of air, as if you were a fish, inflating and deflating as you wish to go up and down. These breaths seem to activate a memory of sorts, which can feel enlivening, satisfying and even eerily familiar.

If we expand our human (pulmonary) respiration into conscious breath, suspendeding intentional respiration, we can approximate dolphin breathing. Conscious breath is a way of breathing that helps us call upon the dolphin within us. The idea that we are related to cetaceans (whales, seals, porpoises, dolphins) is supported by the lifetime work of researcher and breath-hold diver, Jacques Mayol. In his book, *Homo Delphinus, The Dolphin within Man (1999)*, Mayol explores the aquatic origins of man and the potential for mankind to awaken the dormant dolphin within. He postulates that the circuitry of cetaceans lives deep within our human form. Mayol sought to awaken the dormant dolphin within by studying the physiology of cetaceans, learning to slow his own respiration and improving the oxygenation of his lungs. Through the methods he used, Mayol was able to complete several record-setting dives, including his historic 100-meter (330 ft) deep breath hold dive in 1976. With appropriate breath work and movements, Mayol learned to become dolphin-like, living in harmony with dolphins his entire life.

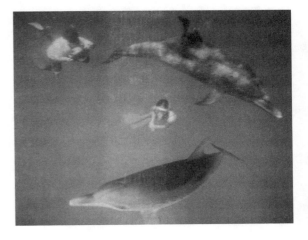

(Figure 27)
There is a growing interest in the human – dolphin connection.

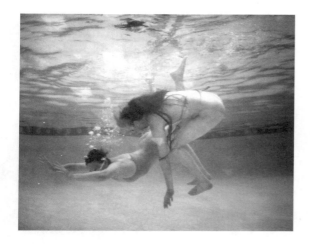

(Figure 28)
Free dance underwater with a
dive and sip rhythm

established, the feeling is reminiscent of ecstatic trance dancing. Something shifts and pleasure emerges; emotional channels open up. Could this be a cetacean secret to well being?

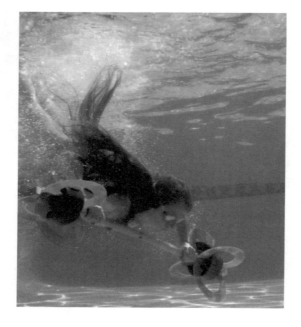

(Figure 29)
Dive and sip with Shapeshifter

In Wave M'ocean, we introduce the joy of breath-movement rhythms activating dormant cetacean potential, such as "dive and sip." Exploring the many ways to dive down, using the Shapeshifter as a movement counterpoint, we sip air as our heads break through the surface, and in one continuous rhythm we are undulating back into the water. Once a rhythm is

In addition to Jacques Mayol's research with cetacean breath and Emilie Conrad's exploration of primordial breath, there are still others who are exploring the breath of

other life forms as a *portal to our aquatic future* and our own mutability. What does all this mean to the future of human aquatic breath? There are some people who believe we are entering an evolutionary expansion of breath, and that this expansion is directly related to our ability to resonate with oceanic life. A pioneer in the exploration of exchanges with other life forms in support of our own evolutionary process is shaman Elan O'Brien. Elan has been guided to act as a conduit in the human dialogue with plants of the deep ocean and with cetaceans. She co-creatively prepares essences that hold vibrational information to be used for this purpose. One such essence is instrumental in transforming the breath of the cells, and thereby assists our evolutionary process.

While Elan and I were together on a dolphin encounter trip, we watched as a pod of dolphins passed a string of seaweed from one to the next. I was aware of a sense of ritual and honoring of this blessing of the sea. Then, humans and cetaceans watched together as Elan was gifted this seaweed treasure by one of the dolphins. Later, when she received her vision from the plant it was in the image of a tree-like form, with the purpose of sharing information with the intrinsic consciousness of the cells. She was instructed to prepare an essence to be named "Sacred Breath of the Divine" which is to serve in our evolutionary process. "It supports an evolutionary crossover point that allows a fuller, more integrated expression of breath derived out of our water based forms, then evolving to include an internal respiration similar to that of a tree. It is like the breath of a tree being brought through the oceans, akin to the tree of life being activated in our human cells." We will explore more about Elan's work in my upcoming book, *Aquatic Resonant Healing*.

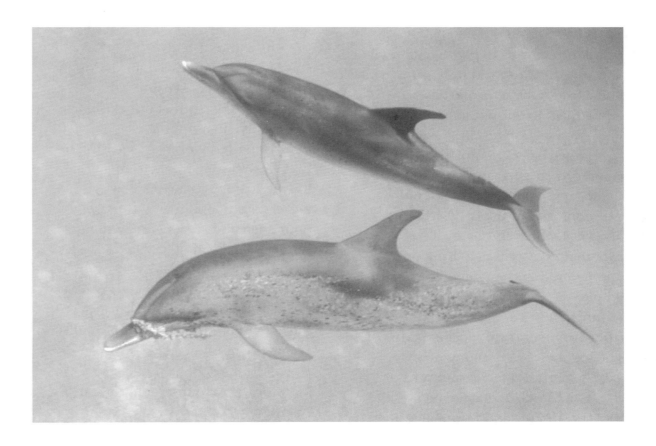

(Figure 30)
Dolphin swimming with seaweed
on its nose before gifting it to Elan

Sense Awareness Portal

It is natural for us to perceive, interact and process the world fully through our senses, where the portals of relatedness to our world are found. However, as humans in Western culture we have attempted to compartmentalize our ways of perceiving. To a large extent, our emotions, sensations, physical selves and existential selves are all experienced as separate from one another, rather than integrated into a whole self. Consequently, we attempt to function in a state of disconnect from our instinctual sensing body. The resistance to thinking of or experiencing ourselves as animals results in a lack of engagement with innate receptive and responsive capabilities. The primitive body system is the home of our most valuable resources for processing feelings and experiences and in relating our deep internal world with the outer realms of experience.

Wave M'ocean offers four points of entry into the portal of sense awareness. They are *orienting,* *embodiment, attunement* and *sensory flow.* In each, we find new ways to be present with our body's consciousness and wisdom. Through the exploration of sensing, we experience the truth of our existence: that we live in a completely interconnected world. As we discover that we are inseparable from all that touches us, we come to a new understanding of how we are nourished and we emerge with new resources in healing.

As biological organisms, we learn to thrive, survive and seek pleasure with the help of our innate *orienting* ability. Plants orient to the sun and sources of water. Deer orient to subtle sounds to monitor their environment for danger. As humans, we also are always orienting to something because we are hardwired to be aware of our environment and to interact with our world through our senses. As infants, we orient to the breast for nourishment and pleasure. Young children might orient to the sound of an approaching ice cream truck. There are ways in which cultural conditioning causes us to create a static system of orienting. For instance, as a therapist I sometimes see people who have become rigid in orienting to their "story," to their family or other group identity. People in psychiatric hospitals are oriented to an idiosyncratic set of phenomena. We can become stabilized in our habitual orientation to unhelpful referents. In the context of the sense awareness portal, we can look at the healing process as the opening of possibilities for new kinds of orienting and perceiving which feed our natural ability to be flexible and adaptive. The aquatic setting can rejuvenate our responsiveness to our bodies and environment. In Wave M'ocean classes, we transmute our cognitive orientation into "witness status." This frees us to engage in inquiry and amplification of body-based orientation. We observe and explore sensations, movement patterns, sounds and breaths that invite new behaviors, imagery and feeling states to add richness to our internal experience.

The earth's pull on the body significantly changes upon immersion in water and we lose our usual orientation. This helps to release the static patterns we use to locate and stabilize ourselves with linear movement on land. We can begin to reinvent movement. I believe that by orienting in space while we are in the water, we access the primitive spectrum of our adaptive capabilities. I base this idea on the Continuum work of Emilie Conrad who teaches that novel movement experiences, coupled with varied relationships to gravity engage the primitive brain in the movement experience. This affects the way movement is occurring, helping people reconnect with their abilities to resource themselves.

The martial arts of Tai Chi and Qigong are ancient Chinese self-healing movement practices. Both employ novel movement and multi-directional awareness as part of a gestalt that include specific ways of orienting and grounding oneself. As far back as two thousand years ago, qigong masters in ancient mystery schools appear to have merged the primitive brain with higher consciousness to create a powerful

healing dynamic. By moving consciousness into a state of open awareness and focusing on a spherical field of chi around their body, they practiced movement that was often torqued (movement occurring in unusual angles) and novel (spreading, multi-directional movement) compared to ordinary functional linear movement. One of my Qigong teachers, Master Fu, the founder of the Er Mei Sudden Enlightenment School in China, illuminated this movement and orientation dynamic for me. In his Qigong style "Wu-Chi in Motion," one holds an expanded field of awareness while practicing slow but spontaneous Qigong movements. At the same time, one constantly changes the perceptual relationship to gravity by shifting the referent point from where movement begins. Sometimes movement occurs in relationship to walls or by allowing the body to buoyantly reach upwards while on the floor. The expanded field of awareness allows the muscles and body systems to fire differently than they would within a narrower field of awareness. This practice of expanded awareness during movement in all

directions, such as practiced in Wu-chi in Motion and in Continuum Movement, allows the body to have the sensory experience of being infused with and moved by the chi field. In these practices, movement rides the waves of energy and consciousness. I include these practices of novel movement, expanded awareness and a freer relationship with gravity in Wave M'ocean to introduce new ways of orienting. In this context, we find new shapes in our movement, new ways of orienting ourselves in space and of feeling grounded.

Embodiment is the incorporation of multi-sensory information into the structure of the whole self. It is the result of organizing the breadth of our experience. The open and present state of consciousness that facilitates embodiment brings the perceptions of the body, mind and spirit into congruence. In Wave M'ocean, we integrate our ability to self-observe with the capacity to feel and do. When we are alive in our senses while in a witnessing state of mind, we enter a gateway to our inner space and our deeper self. An empowered presence emerges when we witness ourselves living through our senses and exercising our capacity to respond. Exploring embodiment in the aquatic setting awakens our responsiveness because the water opens a new dimension of movement as the expressed language of the body. The messages carried by sensations and movements tell us where and how we want to open or unwind our body. In Wave M'ocean, sensing these messages is how we interact with body intelligence at a deep level. I encourage clients to observe, feel and express the sensations of their movement process as a pathway to embodiment and personal power.

Attunement is the sensing of relationship. Whether it is attunement to spirit or attunement to our organismic circuitry, our sensory system is the pathway of entry. As the portal for relationship, sensing is our way of bridging the inner with the outer world. We are wired for attunement and contact, but through conditioning, humans have learned to

live in a world of symbols as opposed to genuine contact with their inner and outer world. Why do we avoid our birthright to participate in the pulse of life? Admittedly, it is contact that brings about our deepest wounding, yet it is also contact that gives birth to our deepest healing. As a therapist, I believe that the only way out of a problem is through the same doorway we came in. In the aquatic setting, it is contact with oneself that unearths authenticity. Contact with other participants, the therapist and the water bring support to the healing process. When we experience violation, hurt or trauma in our lives, we often disassociate from the pain, and if so, we do not complete the experience at the sensory level. This is because we may want to avoid what created the pain. We may stop attuning to contact, including the contact that nourishes our healing.

To re-introduce contact in a safe way, I encourage people to find and "live in" the internal resources of breath, movement, posturing and imagery. The necessary external resources are water, equipment and a trained

therapist. With this in place, the client can retrieve their self-empowerment and exit the holding pattern of trauma and loss. What does such a session look like in the water? Each is unique. The therapist holds the container for the client to explore ways to move back into attunement with self and the world. This involves starting with embodiment and finding ways to feel supported. The therapist assists the client to inquire at a sensory level, "How am I receiving support?" and to deepen into the sense of feeling supported and how it translates to emotion, movement and internal postural expression. The work involves an ongoing process of inquiry and reflection, which might evolve into the question, "What would the breath expression of that feeling of being supported be?" When aspects of the trauma are awakened, the client is supported to stay emotionally and physically resourced. I find that clients can quickly attune through their skin to a sense of physical resource.

Skin is the external layer of our central nervous system and is our largest sensory organ. It is a gateway through which we receive nourishment from our world. Sensory information that enters this gateway is translated to our physical, emotional, relational and spiritual aspects of being. Skin is the edge where "me" and "not me" meet. It is the surface of who we are and it transmits and receives information. Tactile sensation is one way we bring the external world inside. Body-worker Deane Juhan characterized the skin as the surface of the brain (Juan, 1987):

All tissues and organs of the body develop from three primitive layers of cells that make up the early embryo: The endoderm produces the internal organs, the mesoderm produces the connective tissues, the bones, and the skeletal muscles, while the ectoderm produces both the skin and the nervous system. Skin and brain develop from exactly the same primitive cells. Depending on how you look at it, the skin is the outer surface of the brain, or the brain is the deepest layer of the skin. Surface and innermost core spring from the same mother tissue, and throughout the life of the organism they function as a single unit, divisible only by dissection or analytical abstraction…

The implications for activating a healing state through tactile attunement become intriguing within the context of Juhan's perspective. Clients can resource themselves through the skin when received into the yielding but supportive fluid viscosity. They attune to various textures (of moving and still water) and temperatures while their own movements and sounds nourish them. In this rich plenum, they can respond to sensory input in an unrestricted way. This sensory attunement leads to a relaxation response, which opens the potential for healing.

In Wave M'ocean, we attune to three forms of contact movement. In all three, the sensory attunement to relationship occurs within a point/counterpoint movement dynamic. This refers to the relationship of exchanges occurring between two points, one or both of which may be moving. Our sense of self in relationship varies greatly depending on the responsiveness of our counterpoint. In the first form, *"dropped movement,"* we follow our sensations and emotions into movement using the Aquatrend Water Workout Station (Figure 186, p. 345). This counterpoint drives our focus and energy inward because we are not receiving movement input from it. This sense of self in relationship is what is often referred to in the martial arts as "dropped." It is as though attention drops inside and is less involved in awareness of the counterpoint, which acts a stabilizer and supports the movement. This dropped state allows us to tune into the depth of movement within.

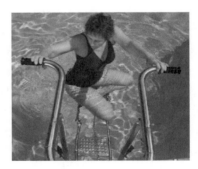

(Figure 31)
Dropped Movement

The second form of contact movement is *"fulcrum movement."* Here, we use the Shapeshifter as a fluid lever (Figure 20, p.42). This constantly shifting counterpoint provides just enough stability to bring form to our movement. Our awareness is receptive and inclusive. This means we incorporate the dynamics of the Shapeshifter's movement into our own. Water flows through the Shapeshifter so it can stay in fluid relationship with the undulating body.

The third form of contact movement is *"partnered movement."* Here, we sense ourselves and relationship through movement exchanges between two people. Whether we attune to relationship through one-pointed contact, as in back to back, or through a constantly shifting contact, we attune to a sense of *one* organism, pushing and pulling within itself, constantly redefining its equilibrium. The state of awareness is simultaneously dropped and merged with one's partner. We are fully present with our self, inclusive of our partner and minimally inclusive of

the world beyond the partnership. We attune to rhythms of movement and breath as the dance evolves, focusing on what emerges in each moment. When both participants stay present with what is being created through the contact, they find synchrony and communication. There is the invisible field where the attunement is felt within the physical, emotional and spiritual bodies. The benefit of contact-movement with a partner is that it introduces new movement that they don't have in their repertoire, helping them disengage from unhelpful, over-stabilized movement patterns. While each person will attune to the field of movement in a unique way, they are constantly in relationship. As the movements of the partners are communicated into the collective body, there is a novel and primal sense of affiliation. It is fun and engaging to work this way. Like all water mammals, we love to play!

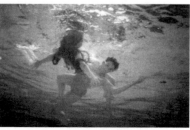

**(Figure 32)
Partnered
Movement**

Sensory flow is the opening of one's awareness of and participation in our inner sensory and emotional landscape. If the environment is right, we slide into a river that streams through the landscape and we trust it to lead us into a meaningful expression of ourselves. Working with individuals in the water initiates fluidity, which informs the sensory flow naturally and allows the outer layers of identity drop away.

In the aquatic setting, the center of sensory flow is the belly or gut. The belly is a center for digestion on many levels— not only do we digest food in our belly, but also our emotions. When we feel the connections and emotions of love, it is "delicious." When we feel anxious, we get that "gut-wrenching feeling." Reactions to people or experiences are often first felt in our belly, such as in a "gut reaction" having an "appetite" for a person or activity that we enjoy. We can also find our ways of knowing from gut signals, such as when there is a felt sense of desire or a "hunch" coming from the belly area. Trauma is often stored in this part of the body, causing us to contract the abdominal wall to hold in bottled up emotions. In the search for authenticity, we often find that our personal power is sparked here, as when we have a "fire in the belly" signifying that the true self is fueling us. The digestive fires are also akin to the fires of transformation, and in shamanic work these fires are accessed to transmute one's perception of an experience.

The portrayal of a jellyfish as a pulsing brain-mouth-belly is an interesting overlay for aquatic clients to experience sensory flow. In developing Wave M'ocean, I began to ask people to orient to their bellies, or "gut brain," to access their responsiveness, their ways of digesting and feeling emotions. As a result, they found new ways of knowing, connecting with personal power and with their self-transforming fires. Bridging back to this primitive, simple existence seems to help people orient to the ancient circuitry of the gut's way of knowing and feeling. The following exercise is meant to familiarize participants with this orientation in aquatic movement and to explore sensory flow originating from the gut-brain.

Begin by visualizing a jellyfish. Take your time to get to know it, watch how it moves in your mind's eye. Find the pulsation of the jellyfish that emerges from your center. Imagine your brain, digestion, emotional capacity and center of movement are one. Merge this felt-sense imagery into your human body so your torso becomes your gut body and your limbs receive movement from it. (Some people use floatation around the waist, which is helpful to amplify the felt sense of the gut-body.) Begin to connect with the felt sense of a jellyfish whose purpose and activity center on taking in nourishment, digesting what is needed and releasing the rest. Explore how it feels physically and emotionally. What is your sense of self in relationship to your environment?

Expanding the sensory flow is about slowing down and feeling, making room to receive the inner experience. Flow is what we experience when we are enjoying something. We simply forget our identity and our usual orientations. As jellyfish, allow your spine and limbs to interpret undulations originating in the belly. What do you feel through the lens of gut perception? How do you propel yourself through the water? Activate all movement from the gut-brain. What are the "gut feelings" that are expressed in the movement? Track sensations in the digestive tissues. The felt sense in this region and the resulting movement bring the subconscious into the realm of sensory awareness. Create wave motion in your gut body by finding the naturally occurring pulsation. Imagine the pulsation loosening the holding patterns within the gut wall. Using audible breath, connect the sensations of the pulsing and the emotional states. Allow the abdominal walls to open, releasing limiting beliefs and initiating empowering movement. This sets the stage to re-organize around the emerging authenticity.

Dream Awareness Portal

I believe that one of the most powerful ways to experience our "dreaming body" is in the water. The concept of a dreaming body is common to healing practices in many indigenous cultures where people live in balanced connection with the earth and spirit realms. To initiate the dreaming body, a shaman or medicine man contacts a larger context of reality through expanded consciousness and sensory awareness. This is referred to as "journeying." In some tribal practices, the shaman will interact with figures, such as an animal or an element (e.g., fire or water) or a spirit, such as the Sun God. The shaman may bring back some form of understanding or helpful information from the journey to a person or community being healed. In other tribal practices, the shaman embodies an animal, referred to as "shapeshifting." The shaman takes on a quality that the animal possesses to solve a problem. For instance, he may embody the energy of a snake that sheds its skin to invoke transformational powers. In some

Native American traditions, the shaman sponsors the journey of the one to be healed. In this practice, the journeyer is helped in a variety of ways to alter his consciousness. This may include chanting, drumming and mind-altering herbal preparations. The shaman is present while the journeyer travels deep inside an inner landscape to participate in what may be likened to a lucid dream.

As I became familiar with shamanic work, it was natural to enter my dreaming body by merging with something – an animal, an energy, a feeling or a sound. In developing Wave M'ocean, I found a portal to dream awareness while in the water and discovered multi-sensory imagery. The dreaming body experiences animated impressions through senses, memories or spiritual elation. The impressions translate into explorations, expressing a variety of perceptual states. Aquatic journeying provides a platform for a fuller kinesthetic expression of a dream reality. The ability to maintain a visceral connection to the changes occurring throughout the journey is

what allows the transformational process to flow and integrate. Dream awareness generates a flow of sensory information to the brain, body and spirit that isn't ordinarily engendered. The new sensory input can be used for transformation, empowerment or pleasure. When we dream in our sleep, we are fully engaged in a different dimension of awareness than in our waking life. Water helps us stay connected to ourselves while we are in a dreamlike state because we feel contained, reminiscent of embryonic bliss. We're in constant contact with a world of novelty. Our body feels freer than usual. Our relationship with gravity is ever changing. This is a kinesthetic reminder that we are in a non-ordinary context, helping to hold the state of expanded awareness. All of these factors make it easier to focus on full presence in the body. We are living in the moment instead of attending to the cognitive chatter that tends to consume our lives. Here, we engage in dreamlike states of *offering and receiving movement*. It is through these point/counterpoint exchanges, that we are able to experience new perspectives of movement and integrate them. Similar exchanges can also take place with water, movement equipment, and other people. How we inhabit the dreaming body depends on what we are connecting with. If we embrace the essence of an animal, for instance, the associated sensory impressions translate into movements. By merging with an animal that comes to us in a journey, we access the felt sensory existence of that creature. As we recognize and attend to the felt sense, an animated experience of self and environment emerges. The water and certain aquatic equipment offer support to stay connected to the animal-self and we take on its sensing ability. As the animal expresses itself through us, its ways of orienting, attuning and breathing become more apparent in our movement and breath. We can explore how they are supported in their world and their unique relationship to gravity and buoyancy dynamics. Ultimately, we are learning about ourselves. If we take the time to experience the emerging awareness, we will have set the stage for a new repertoire of responses and we will

integrate changes in our movements, orientation, behavior, reactions and feelings. The dreaming body is a messenger from our emotional core and our biological intelligence. Tending to these core expressions helps us to claim personal truth. Just like the shaman who can slip out of ordinary perceptual boundaries and enter into a heightened receptivity to the larger field of experience, we all have had glimpses of another reality. Most of us can recall passing through perceptual boundaries in our dreams.

 The other night, in a sleeping dream, a mystical red and black bird appeared outside my window. It took my breath away as it landed and instantly transformed into a celestial cat of enigmatic beauty. I was filled with awe and reverence for this being's knowing of the great mystery. The living magic within me was awakened in a powerful way as I connected to this creature. Often in Wave M'ocean work, I ask a client to bring a dream like this into the water. This kind of awakening to a powerful or magical experience can often be a

bridge for a client to connect to an aspect of themselves, such as their passions and their own healing process. While working with clients in the water, I encourage them to merge with a figure from their dream and discover how it expresses itself through body posturing. These changes translate into physical, psychological and spiritual shifts that occur as part of the whole experience.

It is well established that when one engages in imagery experiences a host of physiologic changes take place. In her book, *Molecules of Emotion*, Candice Pert (1997) demonstrates how there is a dynamic information network within us connecting the emotions, the brain and the functioning of every system of the body right down to the cellular level. In my work on land and in water, I help people connect with their bio-morphous circuitry, by helping them merge their human identity with creatures that come to them in shamanic journeys or in their dreams. In the example of my dream, I can take the experience of merging with the bird into the environment of the water. By being with my dream in the water, I have the opportunity to realize that I appreciate this magical creature because it is a reflection of me. Releasing the rational mind, I embody the magical bird and sense its essence within my physical self. When I imagine flying, I am connecting with an urge that is primal, awakening my own physiological expression of flight in the water. By embracing the ancestral memory, I find freedom of the heart on the emotional level and discover the physical self-empowerment of flying through the water. In this experience, my spiritual self knows that I can be anything (I can morph into a cat). The work of Candace Pert and others supports the idea that each of these experiences has a physiologic component. As I take time during my aquatic journey to explore each of these qualities, I discover new movement in my chest as my heart and wings open. I propel myself from a different source of movement and I fly through the liquid sky according to the will of the mystical bird. In Wave M'ocean, each person is supported to relax their cognitive

mind while they engage in a journey that is like a lucid dream. The immersion in water acts as a kinesthetic reminder that they are allowing their usual orientations to be set aside while they give their attention to journeying into the dreaming body. From the depth of self, they invite images, breaths, sounds and sensations to be their guides. The watery environment helps them to stay connected to their dreaming body by stimulating a heightened sensitivity to somatic signals, symptoms, movement impulses and emotional flow. As with any journeying practice, being fully present with what is felt while staying connected to the imagery experience allows the inner healing process to unfold. Giving expression and movement to what is emerging opens the portal to an enlivened sense of self.

Inhabiting the dreaming body does not require a trip to the Peruvian jungle. So much of what is fun in life can be derived from our natural shamanistic tendencies. Whenever we are focused on an activity like dancing or playing monster games

with our children, we are in an altered state of consciousness. My goal is to help people recognize their own ability to shift consciousness and journey in the water by moving through a perceptual lens. Throughout the journey, there is a reverence for powerful and unseen forces and a willingness to "dialogue" with "irrational" desires or messages. The dialogue unfolds by allowing a stream of impulses to flow. I encourage people to let go of organizing their movement in familiar ways. Clients amplify the movements of what an animal presents in the journey, such as their power, innocence, or even how they are wounded. This facilitates the client's flow of psycho-physiological states. Utilizing the therapist as a resource, clients work through and integrate the body's expression of states such as grief, trauma or vulnerability. Simultaneously, they maintain contact with the support and freedom available to them within the larger dreamscape. Awareness is as fluid as water and can settle into any aspect of the dreamscape to bring back information to the journeyer.

Likewise, the creative energy in the dreamscape can flow through the body in a purposeful way when clients surrender to the flow of dream consciousness. I ask clients to find the breaths and rhythms of movement that correspond to the creature they are embodying. In the water, it is possible to enact dreamlike realities, such as becoming a creature that undulates, swims, flies, swings from the treetops, pulsates, slithers or has qualities that free it from gravity. There is freedom of movement as in no other arena. It is my belief that our bodies, psyches and spirits are nurtured by acting out the dream, allowing critical aspects of the self to be discovered and embraced.

The work I have described in this dream awareness portal has ancient origins and modern applications. Psychoanalyst Carl Jung introduced shamanic-like imagery work to the psychoanalytic community between the years of 1913 and 1916. His therapeutic technique of "active imagination" embraced the idea that we can engage with impulses, images and the resulting expressive body movements, giving form to our personal healing process. Jung describes a typology of the senses wherein "motor imagination" facilitates the creation of a dance out of a motif (Chodorow, 1997). The "motif," as it presents itself in Wave M'ocean, consists of sensory and imagery impressions. Marie-Louis von Franz reports that Jung once told her that symbolic enactment of the body is more therapeutically efficient than ordinary active imagination, but he could not say why (von Franz, 1980). Jungian analyst Arnold Mindell developed the concept of active imagination to specifically include the awakening of the inner shaman, or the dreaming body (Mindell, 1993).

There are vestiges of the shamanic dreaming body practice that are found in some dance and movement therapies, biofeedback techniques and hypnosis. While I believe that they all contribute great value, I favor those therapies that retain the sense of magic that has been so vital to indigenous people for thousands of years. The magic of the active imagination taps into wisdom from many sources, sparking a healing alchemy. Magic in the primordial sense is the experience of existing in a world made up of multiple intelligences. In Wave M'ocean, a vital intelligence that we interact with is the water. This interaction begins with the perceptual shift of approaching our world believing, as indigenous people do, that everything is alive and possesses its own form of intelligence. This changes our experience of being in the pool to resemble a shamanic-based view of journeying. From this perspective, the water has its own capacity to be in relationship to us. It has its own power to take up space, push its way against you, open its doorway of spaciousness to you, and even communicate with you through resonance (which we will discuss in the next portal). Interacting with all the animated intelligence that emerges in the journey is a way for people to be present in their dreamscape and create a theater of the imagination in a fluid environment.

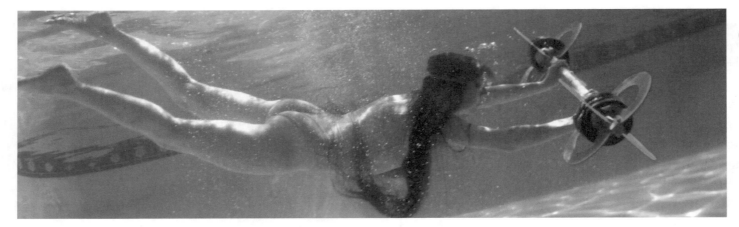

(Figure 33)

Elemental Consciousness Portal

From the perspective of this portal, water is alive and provides an opportunity for us to connect to expanded consciousness. The experiential connection to the consciousness of water lies within the perception that everything is ONE. The idea of a unified field from which everything manifests is the crux where quantum physics and Eastern spiritual philosophies meet. This quantum physics term, unified field, refers to the unification of all the forces of nature. At the most subtle levels, these forces comprise a unified

field of pure energy before manifesting into form. This is true for us and for water. At the most subtle level, our existence is a unified field of what quantum physics would call energy and what Eastern spiritual philosophy would call consciousness. Everything that exists in subtle reality and in physical reality is the vibration of organized consciousness. Unified field theory dares us to return to our ancient tribal understanding that everything is connected and alive just as Native Americans relate to trees or rivers as spirits. In the elemental consciousness portal, human consciousness expands. This happens through the practice of recognizing that water is a metaphor for *fluid*

consciousness, engaging in a *co-creative process* and allowing a *transfer of intelligence.*

Many spiritual and meditative practices use water as a metaphor to teach about *fluid consciousness,* a desired and balanced state of being. Eastern spiritual meditation practices help people to "still" their minds like the depths of the ocean, release attachments, and be fluid with the changing present moment. People are taught to let water inform them in allowing an ever-evolving expression of self. Waves are a visual example of fluid consciousness. Thoughts occur on the surface and they cycle in and out of awareness. These waves of thought are observed as they arise and subside. Healing movement practices, such as Continuum Movement, teach us to let our fluid body move us according to its biological intelligence. The aquatic setting provides an ideal environment to experience the fluid structure of our conscious mind and body. Here, the water supports us in concrete and subtle ways.

Consciousness itself is truly a fluid structure. Because it is not tangible, it is helpful to merge consciousness with a material aspect of reality. We create metaphors to mirror something formless (as water mirrors consciousness) so we can interact with it and learn about ourselves. For example, artwork is a structure through which formless ideas can be expressed, such as the concepts of inspiration or desperation. The artistic interpretation of these concepts brings them into a dimension where we perceive them concretely and can sense our own response vividly. When the fluid systems in our body resonate with a larger body of water that we are immersed in, the body can recognize itself as consciousness

because it has the capacity to inter-relate with the fluid consciousness of the whole. We can create an easy to understand experiential example of the unified field by being aware that the water in our body is the same intelligence as the living consciousness we are immersed in (the pool, pond, ocean, bathtub). This is *reflection* with the potential for us to realize our own fluid consciousness.

A good practice to introduce a client to fluid consciousness is meditative in nature, but it is the *body* that meditates. I guide participants to oscillate between being the depth of the ocean and being the waves. As surface waves, participants create the sounds and movements of waves and they experience the interrelationship with everything that is happening on the surface (waves, sounds, people, equipment). This is followed with deep, quiet breath-hold dives where they experience the stillness within a slow-motion trance movement. Being able to easily move between these two states mirrors fluid consciousness because fluid consciousness effortlessly ebbs and flows between

expanded and ordinary awareness. Practicing it on the physical level with attentiveness facilitates the integrative process of the conscious body.

The *co-creative process* also begins with the realization that the consciousness of your being is the same consciousness as the water. This is a simple intention to connect you to the unified field where co-creation can occur. In your mind you can begin to sense that you have an essence that understands the nature and fluidity of water because you are mostly water. To support your deepening into this experiential understanding, you allow yourself to be supported and informed by the water that holds you.

I turn to Huna knowledge to better understand the initiation of the co-creative process. Huna knowledge is the ancient Hawaiian spiritual philosophy still practiced and taught by Kahunas today. I have great respect for Huna, especially because of what it offers to the practice of embodiment. I studied the Huna knowledge of Ho'oponopono with Kahuna Haleakala and received teachings on reaching higher states of consciousness through the care taking of the "low self." According to Huna knowledge there are three levels of existence: the "high self"(Aumakua) which embodies the super conscious mind, the "middle self" (Uhane) embodying functional awareness and the "low self"(Unihipili) embodying elemental consciousness. The aquatic setting provides a wonderful opportunity to explore body consciousness because it is a playground for the low self. This is the part of us that is child-like in its pure innocence and resonates with the nature spirit. Huna knowledge tells us we must go through the portal of the low self (Unihipili) and experience our "subconscious mind" (which is connected to the "subconscious mind of the planet") to reach the Aumakua (high self). In other words, it is necessary to connect to the natural world in an innocent and playful way to reach expanded consciousness. Our Unihipili or elemental consciousness must be present in the moment with faith, trust and playfulness to facilitate the potential for co-creation. Elemental

consciousness is a literal consciousness that experiences everything exactly as it occurs. Thoughts, feelings, and sensations are not censored. Similarly, water does not censor. It reflects back to us exactly what we put into it (sound, intention, movement, essences, color, light, temperature and even pollution). This reflective nature is an alchemical ingredient in the aquatic work I am introducing to you now.

"Elemental dreaming" is a collective journey in the water where people explore the inter-related mysteries of imagination, consciousness and water. I began to offer aquatic elemental journeys in workshops as an outgrowth of my experiences with Continuum teacher, Susan Harper. Susan has innovated a land-based transformational group experience called "Dreamtime," where she creates a context for a communal dream to unfold. I decided to experiment with it in the water. Instead of *having* a dream on the *inside* of our being, the consciousness of the water holds the dream awareness for the group. Participants can then

immerse themselves inside the dream that the water holds. When they place themselves inside a dream, ordinary reality dissolves in the water, and they experience and interact with the water's dream. Elemental dreaming is a group process that facilitates "the formless" coming into expression through the alchemy of co-creation.

Before diving into the dream, participants connect with images and experiences from a group journey. The collective journey is given over to the conscious field in the pool to hold all aspects of the journey simultaneously. Participants are witnesses to unique aspects of the dream and the dream as a whole. The pool becomes a conscious womb that is a container of collective creation.

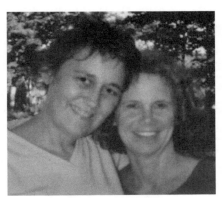

(Figure 34A)
Barbara with Susan Harper

Although much of the experience of these collective dreams defies description, what follows is a portrayal of the archetypal elements that emerged in one group's aquatic elemental dream. In this experience, each participant had the chance to enact or witness each element. There were five elements to the dream. The first dream element that was put into the water was the masculine archetypal God of the ocean, representing an aspect of personal power. The embodiment of this element created huge powerful waves that rocked the entire pool along with rhythmic whooshing sounds. The polarity element to the personal power was unity consciousness. Baring witness to unity consciousness took the form of starting out as an ice cube that melted into the water and flowed with the huge, powerful waves. Witnesses had powerful experiences of dissolving the small, non-fluid self into an experience of an expansive fluidity or "no self." One person reported the sense that they could be everywhere in the pool at the same time. Some people found that once they were dissolved, they had a transformational experience with the waves of personal power that were coming from the other end of the pool. Letting go of having a body allowed the waves to wash through. There were the archetypal elements of giving and receiving. A "shaman of the winged heart" served others by taking their hearts into flight. First, she gathered "flight ability" into her heart. Then she took on the receiver's heart and brought it on a flight through the liquid sky to teach their heart about flying. The receiver's heart was then returned through an embrace. The last element was the embodiment of playfulness through the essence of a sea otter. The sea otter emulated innocence and pleasure seeking as it traveled throughout the pool, witnessing, rolling in circles, undulating, playing and sometimes causing mischief. Like a child, the sea otter focused his curiosity on everything that was going on around him. As the participants in this group discovered, magic is a spark for self-transformation. As they deepened into elemental consciousness and their connection to Unihipili, they found magical doorways to their subconscious mind and the spirits of the earth. They were grateful to the water for dreaming about them.

The interfacing of human and elemental consciousness is a co-creative process that results in a *transfer of intelligence* through resonance. The natural world consists of many interconnected fields of energy. These fields are conscious because they respond with intelligence to changes in and around them, including human energetic information. Water, as a field of intelligence expresses itself both in the physical realm and the subtle energy realm. As such, we can have healing exchanges with water through physical and subtle energy contact. We interact with water at the physical level by drinking it, swimming or bathing in it, and even going sailing in it. Water expresses its unique form of intelligence by responding to movement, temperature, pollution, context and its innate tendency to create homeostasis. The motion of water serves us to create inherent balance.

We enjoy subtle energy exchanges with water by listening to water, sitting near it, watching it and resonating with it. When we resonate with it, typically we are receiving information in the form of vibration. Water has the capacity to reflect organic intelligence, such as a plant essence. Water can also reflect human consciousness. Its crystalline structure changes in response to thoughts, intentions, prayers, symbols, words and sound. Like the artist who brings the formless into form, water creates impressions of these subtle energies. Thanks to the visionary work of researcher Masaru Emoto (2002), the ancient understanding of water as

alive and responsive is re-emerging. As the president of IHM General Research Institute in Japan he has embarked on a quest to understand water's relationship to consciousness and its ability to receive, store and reflect information. His work explores water's crystalline structure in relationship to sound, emotion, intention and environmental factors. Masaru Emoto presents striking photographs of water crystals after exposure to the healing effects of coherent love-based intentions (Figure 19, page 41). Water that was mistreated by negative intentions had the appearance of disorder and lost its magnificent patterning. Water that was imprinted by love, gratitude and prayer showed complex symmetrical beauty and the brilliance of a diamond. In hundreds of experiments the crystals transformed as he introduced varying forms of toxic or positive information. He also found that the simple imprinting of a word or symbol could alter water. This research poses interesting ideas and questions about the relationship between consciousness and water. It raises the possibility that if human

thoughts can alter the crystalline structure of water, perhaps thoughts can change the world within and around us.

While we all have the potential for self-healing, the perceptions and experiences that create an internal healing environment are different for each individual. Therefore, in practice, the experiential structures of all the portals become interwoven. The varied perceptual contexts that we swim in lead us to self-discovery. The journey begins with the realization that the true healing waters are *within* and are set into motion when we immerse ourselves. In the water's embrace, we physically experience what our spiritual self knows — we are held within a dynamic wholeness, fluidity is our intrinsic nature and freedom is the heart's desire.

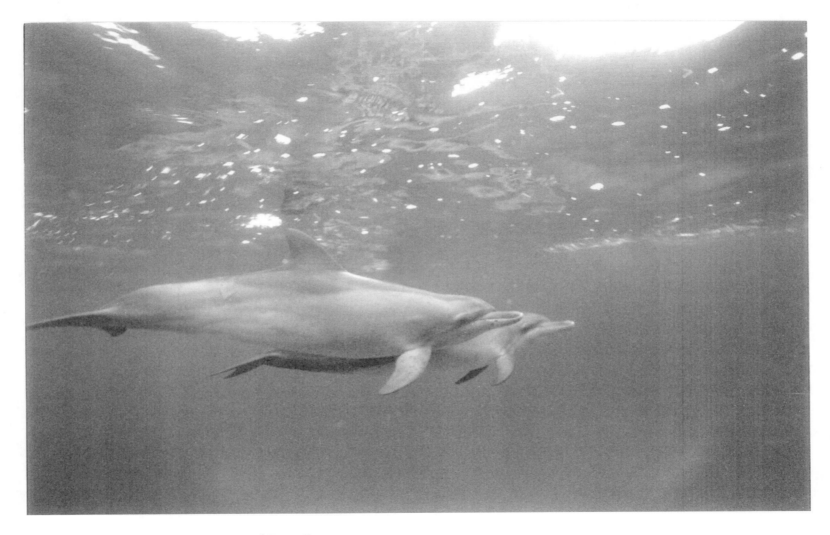

(Figure 34B) "The Resonance of Love"

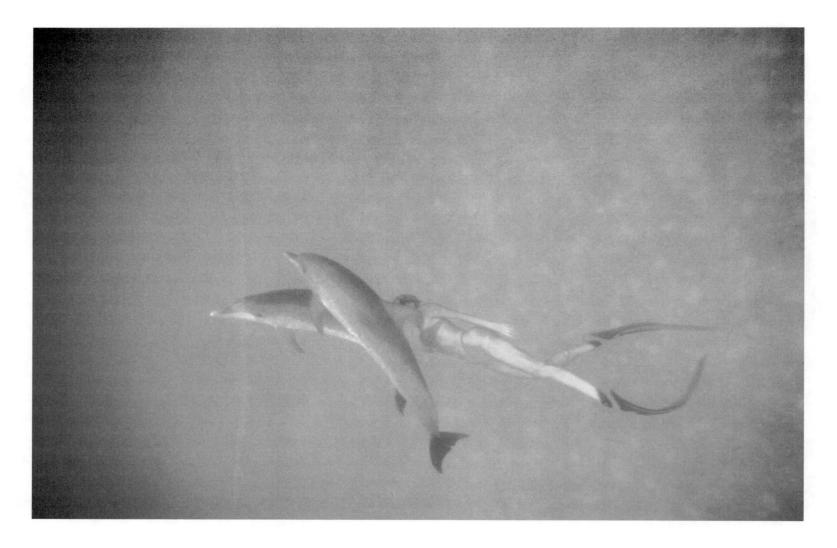

(Figure 34C) "Inter-species Wave M'ocean"

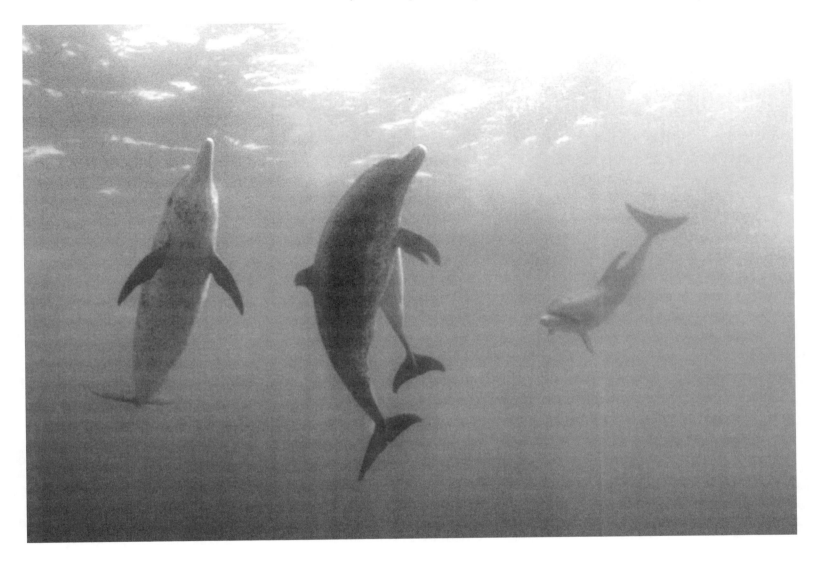

(Figure 34D) " Dolphin Dreamtime"

Chapter 2
Aquatic Bodywork

by Alexander
  Georgeakopoulos

*Nothing in the world
is as soft and yielding as water.
Yet for dissolving the hard and inflexible,
nothing can surpass it.*
        from verse 78 of The Tao
        Te Ching of Lao-tzu

Introduction

Throughout the ages people have been entering hot springs, lakes, rivers, and seas to recuperate from life's stresses. We turn to water for the refreshing swim and the soothing bath; we relish its slippery resistance and buoyant support. Water circulates ubiquitously through the skies, across the continents and in the oceans. It flows through the body's fluid systems and fills our cells. And yet, for all its familiarity, water holds many mysteries. It has been the object of much research in recent decades, as evidenced by the development of several sophisticated treatment technologies (Mikesell, 1985). Through a variety of agencies water can be purified, oxygenated and energized and thus induced to form molecular microclusters more easily absorbed into the cells. Such water has been shown to precipitate chemical toxins and heavy metals out of the body. Applications go far beyond human health: in agriculture, to increase crop yields and resistance to disease and pests; in the environment to restore polluted lakes and rivers; and in industry to treat effluent water.

Along with this greater interest in the nature of water, our relation to it is evolving. Spas and water parks are burgeoning; hydrotherapy, water sports and many forms of aquatic exercise are gaining in popularity. Water birthing, baby swimming classes (Odent, 1995), and underwater music concerts known as liquid sound are spreading. Belonging to this growth in new water activities has been the advent of water-based healing modalities. In the 1980's and 90's there arose in this country and in Europe what is known today as *aquatic bodywork*. It differs from other forms of aquatic rehabilitation previously practiced, such as the Bad Ragaz Ring Method and the Halliwick Method, in that its first focus is not clinical. Instead, aquatic bodywork is holistic, appealing to the whole person—body, heart and spirit.

This chapter will first enumerate the effects of warm water immersion during aquatic sessions and then take a look at the fascinating ways in which the human body is adapted to water. Next, the unique state of passive motion seen in aquatic bodywork will be described. After this, we will familiarize ourselves with the body's hydrodynamics when passively moved by an aquatic practitioner. Then all the forces at play in generating movement in water will be explained. We will explore four major modalities of aquatic bodywork: Watsu, WaterDance, Healing Dance and the

Jahara Technique™. An examination of the body mechanics and basics of support employed by aquatic practitioners will follow. Finally the effects and applications of these modalities will be presented.

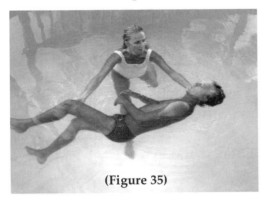

(Figure 35)

The Swing is one of Watsu's gentle and spacious rocks that follows the tempo of the receiver's body.

The Body in Warm Water

Warm water is a very friendly medium indeed. Sessions of aquatic bodywork are conducted in water heated to 35° C (95°F), that 'just right' temperature that warms the body without being too hot. At this temperature, just a little warmer than the skin, one can remain comfortably immersed for an hour or longer. A trio of water's physical properties-- heat, pressure and buoyancy -- elicit a range of healthy reactions in the body's structure and physiology.

The beneficial effects of heat are as follows:

1) Promotes muscular relaxation.

2) Increases body temperature when water temperature is higher than skin temperature. Also, as skin temperature increases, cutaneous vasodilation occurs. (Bates and Hanson, 1996)

3) Causes loss of sense of body shape and boundary when water temperature approximates skin temperature.

4) Reduces pain sensitivity. The warmth 'distracts' the pain, with sensory input that travels on nerve fibers larger, faster, and with a greater conductivity than the pain fibers. (Kessler, 1983)

5) Decreases muscle spasm.

6) Prepares connective tissue for stretching.

7) Increases peripheral circulation in temperatures greater than 34°C (93°F). (Hall, 1990)

Water's hydrostatic pressure produces these results:

1) Helps stabilize unstable joints, making aquatic bodywork quite safe for injured participants when administered conservatively.

2) Provides more resistance to the expansion of the ribcage and abdomen in breathing, thereby strengthening the diaphragm and intercostal muscles.

3) Compresses all soft tissues, enhancing lymphatic return even with minimal water depth immersion.

4) Aids venous return in the legs. A body immersed to a depth of 48 inches is subjected to a force equal to 88.9 mm Hg, slightly greater than diastolic blood pressure. This is the force that aids the resolution of edema. Giving aquatic bodywork is good for the practitioner's legs!

5) Displaces approximately 700 cm³ of blood from the extremities and abdominal vessels into the great veins of the thorax and into the heart on immersion to the neck. This causes a significant increase in right atrial pressure, stroke volume, and cardiac output, resulting in bradycardia, the slowing down of the heart rate. This is the dive reflex. There is an effect on systemic vascular resistance, which drops dramatically, and on muscle circulation, which increases several – fold. (For more information and research, go to the Pathways to Energy section in Chapter 3, *Contractile Physiology in the Pool).*

6) Increases intra-thoracic blood volume.

The buoyancy of water results in the following responses:

1) Muscular relaxation. With gravity counterbalanced, our muscles are freed from their continual work of holding us up, and become completely relaxed.

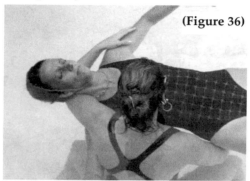

(Figure 36)

Melting into the warm water in First Position, Watsu's basic position of support.

2) Loss of muscle tone. According to James McMillan, the developer of the Halliwick Method, muscle tone is influenced by proprioceptive input stimulated by gravity. In other words, tone is a function of weight. After the effects of weight (gravitational force) have been neutralized by 15 minutes of immersion, a person's tone automatically decreases. This change in tone lasts for up to 1.5 hours after leaving the pool. (Ruoti, 1996)

3) Joint decompression. As muscles relax and joints are relieved of their weight-bearing function, they decompress. Movement becomes

freer and with less pain in the case of injuries. The need for splinting and guarding decreases.

4) Sense of lightness. The receiver notices that she is easily supported and moved by the practitioner, and feels light. (For consistency in this article, the term practitioner will be designated as he; his counterpart, the receiver, will be designated as she.) This is usually a positive experience, sometimes evoking associations with childhood and infancy.

5) Reduced oxygen requirements. Igor Tcharkovsky, the pioneer Russian researcher into water birth, has established that in the nearly weightless state achieved in water, the body's oxygen requirements are dramatically lowered, making possible the accelerated growth of premature babies (his own, for example). Relating this to aquatic bodywork, there is a tendency for the respiratory rate to decrease, leading to the onset of a calm, trance-like state.

The Water Body

It is hardly a surprise that warm water immersion is so agreeable when the body itself is 70% water. It is literally in its element. Furthermore, an intriguing array of anatomical and physiological features, some not seen in other primates, adapt our bodies to water. Taken as a whole, they give convincing support to what has become known as the Aquatic Ape Theory (AAT), which proposes that Homo sapiens sapiens (that's us) diverged from other primate populations as a result of a change in the environment, such as a sudden incursion of the seacoast. (Morgan, 1994) Consider the following:

1) Human infants possess instinctive swimming and breath-holding reflexes operative until the age of four months, after which the neocortex re-learns these functions.

2) The previously described human dive reflex, a set of cardiovascular responses to immersion, allows the body to conserve heat, maintain blood pressure and remain underwater longer than it could otherwise.

3) The nose is conveniently situated in a buoyant structure, the head. The sinuses, air-filled cavities in the bones of the face, give the head its lightness. The length of the nose and the downward facing direction of the nostrils allow humans to swim face down and headfirst. Located as it is in the middle of the face, the nose also allows a supine floating position in water.

4) The larynx of the newborn connects directly to the soft palate, making it possible to breathe and nurse at the same time. Then, during infancy, the larynx descends, giving the capacity to breathe either through the nose or the mouth, a useful design option for creatures wanting to swim.

5) Humans possess voluntary breath control, also a practical feature for swimmers.

6) The arm and leg muscles are strongest in the locomotor motions employed in swimming: elbow flexion, arm extension, and hip and knee extension.

7) Although it has an embarrassing tendency to 'prune' from dehydration, the skin is waterproof and safely permits prolonged immersion.

8) The sometimes ample layer of body fat humans possess, in contrast to other primates and in common with aquatic mammals, both insulates and gives added buoyancy in the water.

*A*bout the insulating value of fat, some events that illustrate this point occurred one chilly, rainy winter at Harbin Hot Springs, where I lived between 1989 and 1996. Without the sun to heat it, the outdoor swimming pool had become quite cold. Two of Harbin's stalwarts challenged each other to see who could survive the most laps. One was the veteran of several rigorous vision quests, a survivalist who could live off the land for weeks. He dove in first, barely completing three laps before his body became too stiff to move. He pulled himself out and headed straight for the sauna. The other, also a rugged outdoorsman held out a little longer by an effort of will before giving up and likewise retreating to the warmth of the sauna to recover. The Great Contest had a victor. Word of the outcome spread through the community.

Later that week, from my viewpoint by the stove in the kitchen overlooking the pool, I saw a guest ponderously making her way to the pool—a woman of average height, but weighing perhaps 300 pounds, most of which was fat. She donned her bathing cap and began swimming laps in the freezing water with an ineffective but steady stroke. Half an hour and dozens of laps later she was still swimming. She emerged finally and made her way back to her room to dress for lunch after what was for her a routine workout.

>=((((O>   >=((((O>   >=((((O>

Morgan also cites other features that differentiate humans from other primates and link us to aquatic mammals. These include a) a relatively low body temperature; b) the ability to form tears; c) face-to-face orgasmic sexual behavior; d) large brain size; and e) low cell count combined with high hemoglobin levels in our blood composition. Indeed, the Aquatic Ape Theory is a worthwhile topic to explore, especially for anyone who feels a kinship with dolphins and whales.

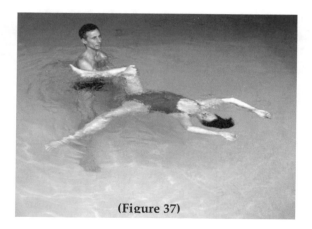

(Figure 37)

Wag the Dog is an underwater movement of great freedom from Healing Dance.

The
Passive Body

In this universe we are all passengers. Every one of us has a ticket to Planet Earth. This attraction spins on its axis and orbits devotedly around the sun. The solar system is set on its own course in a spiraling galaxy that in turn has an adventurous trajectory through the Vastness. It's a wild ride, measured in miles per second. Thus no matter how self-propelling we may seem to be, backpacking up Mount Whitney or attempting to samba in a Rio nightclub, we are at all times being given a ride through space. The universe carries us.

As a species, we are fascinated by everything that conveys us effortlessly through space that puts the wind in our face and sends the landscape racing by. Whether sailing, skydiving or driving our SUV's, people love speed. And we don't mind putting a little effort into pursuits such as roller blading, skiing and bicycling so long as a long power glide is the payoff.

There is an even more profound pleasure in allowing another person to carry and move us, for then associations from childhood and infancy come into play. Perhaps our father swung us in circles by the wrists or carried us on his shoulders; our mother surely rocked us in her arms, and even before that in her womb. Jean Liedloff, in her 1985 book, *The Continuum Concept, In Search of Happiness Lost*, concludes that the human infant has an innate need and expectation to be carried and held in contact with its parents for the first several months of life. She bases this conclusion on her observations of the successful child rearing practices of indigenous South American tribes. A child raised in these cultures is carried through the day by its parents as they clean, prepare food, and socialize. At night, instead of being confined to a crib in a separate room, it sleeps next to them. The child ends this phase of its own volition, in short order learning to walk, run and become thoroughly independent. Few people in modern Western society have the benefit of such an upbringing. As if to confirm Ms. Liedloff's hypothesis, many receivers of aquatic sessions feel a sadness and reluctance to place their feet on the pool bottom at the finish. They report that the experience of being effortlessly carried was so delicious and not nearly long enough!

In giving over responsibility for our body and allowing another to carry and move us, there is a tendency, perhaps an instinct, to become receptively, contentedly passive. This combination of motion and passivity is the underlying phenomenon of aquatic bodywork. The practitioner carries and bestows various therapeutic movements upon his client, who receives them openly and passively. The feedback of her nervous system is of comfort and effortlessness, a veritable kinesthetic re-education, leading to the release of habitual tension. It would seem that when effort and restriction corrupt movement, the remedy is simply to get a fresh impression. Consider how after witnessing a ballet performance the audience emerges from the theatre energized, with a lighter step. The effect is more immediate and personal in aquatic bodywork. The key to this response is trust. The receiver can let go and surrender when she feels safe in the arms of an aquatic practitioner.

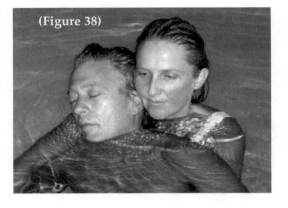

(Figure 38)

The Head Cradle offers a nurturing, restful moment in the Basic Flow of Watsu.

In aquatic bodywork not only the receiver's physical body, but also her feeling self is sensitively 'carried,' leading to even deeper levels of surrender. Could it be that our very soul longs to be cared for, to find a safe haven, symbolic of returning home and being enfolded in the Creator's arms?

The Hydrodynamic Body

The human body is designed primarily for bipedal terrestrial locomotion and secondarily for aquatic locomotion. Clearly, its shape is not as adapted to moving through water as that of aquatic creatures. People haven't the fins, scales and highly deformable, streamlined bodies of fishes. Man will never dart through the water with the startling velocity of a dolphin that Kevin Costner seemed to achieve in the film, *Water World*. Not having cone-shaped heads, we lack the ideal fusiform hydrodynamics of a shark's body (cylindrical and tapered at both ends). Even so, our body shape facilitates the flow of water around it when immersed. The roundness of the head and shoulders and the cylindrical, elongated tapering of the torso, arms and legs aid the water in flowing past. A person can swim like a fish without the use of his arms in what is called axial locomotion with the dolphin kick or fin swimming. More common is appendicular locomotion using the arms and legs. In this mode, the broad, paddle-like surfaces of the hands and feet catch the water for efficient propulsion. In the final analysis, the human body is relatively well adapted to move in water.

When swimming, the body is self-propelling and self-organizing. Isometric muscular stabilization maintains body shape, while concentric muscular contraction produces movement at the joints. A passively surrendered body in water behaves according to quite different principles. It demonstrates a clear preference to be pulled rather than pushed, or if you will, persuaded rather than coerced. In sessions of aquatic bodywork, stretches and tractions pull the body through the water, leading each movement. Suspended in near weightlessness, the body takes on a length and languor, following in a leisurely manner the guidance from the practitioner's hands. It needs more time to comply with these elongations than if it were on land, as it moves within the heightened viscosity of water. The impetus to move must pass through each joint, subject to the flexibility of ligaments, fascia and muscles, and to the range of motion of each intermediate joint in the chain.

In terrestrial locomotion, weight is transmitted through bones to create force against the earth. In passive aquatic motion, the flexibility of the soft tissues entraining each other is operative. Most of the pulling aquatic stretches have what is referred to as a 'soft end feel,' meaning that neural feedback in the soft tissues, rather than bone impacting bone, determine the upper limit of the stretch. Consequently, the receiver has more awareness of lengthening in the soft tissues, and the bones seem to disappear from awareness as they so rarely participate in the sensory equation.

When a passive movement is hydrodynamic, the body becomes streamlined by water resistance. This is an indicator that a movement is, in fact, hydrodynamic. The body is designed to swim headfirst. The passive body, not surprisingly then, is most streamlined when pulled by the head. The arms and legs conform to the currents passing over the skin and streamline in toward the longitudinal axis of the trunk. Aquatic bodywork has several such headfirst moves, both at the water's surface and underwater.

The second hydrodynamic movement that streamlines the body occurs when it is pulled feet first, but only when they are held together. The legs act as a single leg, the feet like the point of a spear, and the arms are pushed up over the head. Organized in this way, the body streamlines and offers minimal resistance. Subaquatic techniques feature such pulls of the body by the feet with the head submerged.

The third hydrodynamic movement of the body is the wave. Whether waved from the chest or pulled by the head, arms or feet, the body retains its symmetry. When the trunk is waving in lateral flexion or flexing and extending, the body follows the practitioner's pull with little resistance, so long as the amplitude of the wave remains small. This is to say that the more the wave is pulled

rather than swung across, the more hydrodynamic the movement will be.

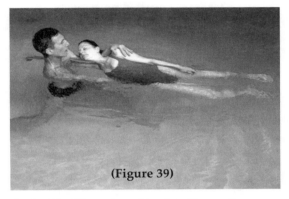

(Figure 39)

In the Hip Wave from Healing Dance the receiver rounds and arches through the water.

Spirals are a fourth hydrodynamic movement of the passive body. They may be thought of as integrating lateral flexion waves with flexion-extension waves. Simply walking backwards and circling the receiver's chest, hips or feet, creates spiral movement.

The passive body streamlines in a fifth way when revolved about its

longitudinal axis. The roundness of the skull and the cylindrical form of the neck, torso and limbs suit the body to roll both on land and when suspended in water. The body rolls compliantly in water, especially when the legs and torso align and traction is given from the head or feet.

Circling spins may be executed with the body arched or rounded in the horizontal plane or as somersaults in the vertical plane. Guided from the head or arms, or led by the feet in the opposite direction, spins constitute a sixth hydrodynamic category of passive motion.

Figure Eights with the back flexed form the seventh category of hydrodynamic movement. They take advantage of the roundness of the back always leading into the movement. When the practitioner walks backwards in an eight-shaped pattern the body becomes even more streamlined, since this reduces the angle at which the water encounters the back.

The Sources of Aquatic Movement

The physics of movement in aquatic bodywork involves an interplay of forces. Aquatic movement arises from four sources: the practitioner, the receiver's body, gravity, and the physical nature of water. The receiver's body becomes the visible, physical resolution of an ongoing, moment-to-moment equation where various forces intersect. Let's enumerate and explore them in action.

1) The *practitioner* is but one source of movement among several. What he supplies, however, is considerable; only the water is as active a partner. He raises and lowers the receiver vertically. He moves her laterally in arcs at the surface and in rolls on the longitudinal axis. He generates waves through the body and guides it through spirals, figure eights, somersaults, releases, catches, stretches, and tractions. Did I leave anything out?

2) The *receiver's breath* generates movement as it modulates the body's specific gravity. With each inhalation and exhalation it causes the chest and hips to rise and sink. The breath links into the dance between the buoyant force and gravity, temporarily favoring one and then the other. In subaquatic moves, the extent to which the lungs are filled determines the ease with which the receiver can be submerged and surfaced, and whether she will ascend, descend or suspend when released.

3) The *dance between the center of buoyancy (COB) and the center of gravity (COG)* is always active in the water, whether the receiver is breathing or holding her breath. The COB resides in the mid-chest. With the residual volume of air in the lungs that is never expelled, combined with air that is inhaled, the COB is the lightest part of the body. The COG, on the other hand, lies in the region of the pelvis, slightly higher in men than in women due to their heavier upper body musculature. In water, the COG wants to sink down beneath the COB

and the COB wants to float above the COG. The two are constantly on the move in opposite but complementary directions. In other words, the chest wants to float and the hips tend to drift downward.

4) The *elastic recoil of muscle tissue and ligaments* from stretched length to resting length creates movement. Muscle tissue is unique in the body for its capacity to contract, but like other tissues, it can also be stretched. Once a stretch is finished the fibers within the belly of a muscle return to what is called their "resting length." During a stretch they exert resistance and after a stretch they generate movement during the recoil. (For more information and research, go to The Series Elastic Element section in Chapter 4, *Mobility*).

5) *Gravity* is fully operative in water. Water, like any other substance on or near the earth, is subject to the earth's gravitational pull. If it were not, there would be no pools or seas, no contained water. So it is natural for water, as a liquid, to humbly seek out the low places, falling from clouds to earth, descending in streams and rivers to the seas. Our personal experience of gravity in water, though, is colored by the buoyant force, which creates a sensation of near weightlessness. Think of water as a low gravity, high pressure/viscosity environment. (For more information on gravity go to Gravity in Chapter 12, *Floating into Therapy*; and for research go to Response to Strain Rate, The Integrity of Osteons, Effects of Aging on Bone, and The Ascension of Density in Chapter 7, *Bone Density and Aquatic Exercise*).

6) The *buoyant force* exists as a result of gravity acting upon water. In a body of liquid water, the molecules closer to the surface weigh down upon those deeper down. A pressure is created that increases with depth and pushes any submerged object upward with a force equal to the weight of the water displaced (Archimede's principle). Buoyancy is the single most significant factor in making aquatic bodywork possible. It relieves the practitioner of the task of supporting over 95% of the receiver's weight, for

a human being weighs approximately the same as an equal volume of water, men a little more and women a little less, on average. (It is actually more tiring to hold one's arms out in front of the body on land than to support a receiver in them in the water—for more information go to Buoyancy in Chapter 12, *Floating into Therapy*).

7 In the context of physics, *inertia* is defined by the *American Heritage Dictionary* in three ways: a) the tendency of a body in motion to resist acceleration; b) the tendency of a body in motion to stay in motion in a straight line unless acted on by an outside force; and c) the tendency of a body at rest to remain at rest. It seems bodies like to keep doing whatever they are doing. Sir Isaac wasn't referring specifically to the human body when he formulated his law, but it applies. In simpler English he is talking about resistance to **a)** speeding up, **b)** changing directions or stopping, and **c)** getting going. In all three senses, inertia plays a role in aquatic movement. The first mentioned form of inertia is overcome to create an exhilarating surge for an

already moving receiver. The second form of inertia is what sustains the glide after releases and is responsible for the follow through of the body after other movements are completed. Whenever we change directions or bring movement to a stop we must overcome this second manifestation of inertia. Resting inertia is more easily overcome in water than on land, as there is less weight to surmount. Here we are speaking of initiating movement from still positions.

8) Before continuing, we will need to define some terms and concepts. As a liquid, water has a certain viscosity or thickness, imparting to it resistance to movement greater than that of air, but less than that of say, molasses. The hydrogen bond attractive forces between H_2O molecules cause them to cohere to each other and to adhere to most immersed objects. These same weak molecular bonds are responsible for the phenomenon of surface tension, where the water's surface layer behaves like a stretched elastic membrane, allowing small insects to skit across it.

Water, then, with its cohesion, viscosity, adhesion and surface tension resists movement of fully or partially submerged objects (or persons). This opposition is termed *drag*, and water generates twelve times more drag than air. Drag is considered a negligible influence in terrestrial locomotion (unless you happen to be walking into a gale). Drag is generated upon a still object within flowing water or, as in aquatic bodywork, against a moving object within still water. In either case, water flows around submerged objects in parallel layers. When these layers do not mix together, as happens at lower speeds, we have streamline or laminar flow, a defining feature of the Jahara Technique (page 104) with its slow tempos. At higher speeds, the streamlined layers start mixing together to create turbulent flow. The turbulence appears in the form of eddies and vortices. An eddy is a circular current contrary to the direction of the main flow; a vortex is a spiral motion of fluid. For more details on hydrodynamics, see Capter 11, *The Kinetics of Water*.

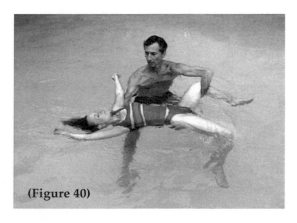

(Figure 40)

In this Watsu move, the Hip Tug, the receiver's far arm and leg are stretched by drag as the practitioner turns in a circle.

Okay, let's relate all this to aquatic bodywork. To start, surface tension is a negligible source of drag in movements on the vertical plane, but figures to a degree that can be felt in horizontal movements breaking the surface. Tractioning the receiver by the head at the surface brings a hydrodynamic force into play, as the water below our diagonally inclined partner pushes her up toward the surface and streamlines the limbs in toward the body's longitudinal axis. Tractioned quickly enough, the body would hydroplane right out of the water, as a water-skier who has lost his skis and persistently holds onto

the pull line well understands. More significantly, the submerged portions of both the receiver and the practitioner generate drag. This is not necessarily undesirable in aquatic bodywork. Moves from all four techniques, but especially from Watsu, take advantage of drag to create and intensify moving stretches.

Moving on to the phenomenon of turbulence, it has several aspects in aquatic bodywork. On the energetic and esoteric levels turbulence is 'friendly.' In stimulating the touch receptors of the epidermis, it contributes to the sensory overload supportive of trance states. Additionally, it may have a cleansing effect on the part of the aura radiating from the skin known in oriental medical theory as "defensive chi." Another possibility is that in wave movements traveling through the pool the unidirectional brushing motion of turbulence helps to channel energy downstream out of the body. Excluding still positions, nearly all the movements of aquatic bodywork, whether hydrodynamic or not, are fast enough to create turbulent flow.

Hydrodynamic force is utilized in transition moments in aquatic bodywork. In a typical transition, the hand supporting the pelvis or legs shifts to a new position, leaving the legs at risk to sink toward the bottom. This loss of support can be unsettling and stressful to the lower back, creating a condition of lumbar hyperextension. To prevent this from happening, the practitioner quickly tractions the head with his other arm and turns in place. Hydrodynamic force on the underside of the receiver's inclined body pushes it up toward the surface, to maintain the spine and legs in a safe alignment and bring the knees within grasping range.

Origins and Principles of Aquatic Bodywork

Watsu is the first-born, the mother of aquatic bodywork. WaterDance, Healing Dance and Jahara Technique all trace some roots back to Watsu. Watsu was first taught in the early 1980's in the United States and by the mid nineties had entered mainstream consciousness as luxury spas included

it in their menus and American physical therapists began treating their patients with it. WaterDance, the original subaquatic technique, originated in Europe and was first taught in 1987, incorporating some of Watsu's surface moves into its opening sequence. Healing Dance entered the scene in 1993 and Jahara Technique in 1995. Both Healing Dance and Jahara Technique began as variants of Watsu before defining themselves further. Several other similar techniques, such as Aqua-Healing, Aqua Wellness and Aqua Relaxing, also came into existence at this time, primarily in Germany and to a large extent derived from Watsu and WaterDance.

The impulse to care for each other is intrinsically human. If we have any doubt as to the authenticity of such an impulse, we need only look to young children to believe that kindness is in our nature. And who has not seen children at the seashore take each other in their arms, carefully floating each other in the course of play? In the context of our humanity, aquatic bodywork is so natural, so inevitable,

that it must have surfaced in other forms at other times and is only now being rediscovered. The stage has been set for this widespread re-emergence by the general availability of warm water pools and by the acceptance in several modern societies of nurturing contact in public and therapeutic settings. These therapies have arrived once again out of the collective unconscious and as is the way with inventions, are starting to percolate up everywhere at once. I have met aquatic 'primitives,' untrained in any technique, who say they have been doing similar work on their own for years.

These new techniques comprise the aquatic counterpart to other 20th century land-based modalities, such as Zen Shiatsu, Trager Work, Rolfing, and circulatory massage. Firstly and most fundamentally, they all share a holistic viewpoint affirming the unity of body and psyche, touching the person via the body. They relate to the body's structure, physiology and energy in a scientific manner and to the inner person with sensitivity and compassion. In a synthesis of Zen philosophy and enlightened New Age thought, they view the bodymind as a living system fully equipped to heal itself, and needing only the safe space provided by the practitioner to do so. This implies a trust of natural processes arising during a treatment. Demonstrating an attitude of nonviolence and empathy is essential to gaining the trust of the receiver's wounded self. Watsu, WaterDance, Healing Dance and Jahara Technique each take this approach in a unique direction, but the foundation is the same. In the profession, a practitioner who relates in this way is said to possess the quality of *presence*, as in, "She has a lot of presence," or "He is very present." It is the very heart of aquatic bodywork.

An additional factor lends great power to aquatic bodywork, and that is its similarity to the prenatal state. The pool water is warm like amniotic fluid. The rocking movements in the sessions suggest those experienced by the fetus as its mother breathes and ambulates. The state of open passivity evoked in receivers is that of the fetus. The muffled, omni-directional quality

of sound when the ears are immersed in the pool matches the way the fetus hears. (The greater speed at which sound travels through water than through air reduces the time lag between ears by which sound direction is sensed.) The enveloping presence of a nurturing being is common to both settings. Finally, some of the positions of aquatic bodywork fold up the receiver, knees to chest, mimicking the fetal position before birth.

David Sawyer, whose previous background lies in shock and trauma therapy, prenatal psychology, and in developmental movement, is exploring this facet of aquatic bodywork. The approach he has been teaching since the late 1990's, called Prenatal Journey, provides the water community with deeper psychological insight into the receiver's process in water as well as the tools to support it. (Sawyer, 1999)

Watsu

The birth of Watsu was serendipitous. Harold Dull, one of the poets of the 1960's San Francisco Renaissance, had become interested in Zen Shiatsu and studied it from Reuho Yamada and Wataru Ohashi in the United States and from their master, Shizuto Masunaga, in Japan. In the early 1980's Dull began to lead workshops in Zen Shiatsu at Harbin Hot Springs in northern California. In off-hours, experimenting with Zen Shiatsu's stretches in the warm water of the pools, he received feedback that the work was more effective than on land. What he came to call Watsu (combining the two words, Water and Shiatsu) took shape over the ensuing years. Watsu is renowned not only for its creative stretches, but also for its nurturing maternal quality. Its gentle rocking movements and still cradling positions convey receivers to the peace and simplicity of their earliest childhood and prenatal states (Dull, 1993). Elaine Marie, one of Watsu's greatest teachers, in particular honored this feminine aspect in her own adaptation of the work.

Watsu is characterized by flow, one movement blending smoothly into the next, with still pauses at intervals for integration. When the physical body is sustained in a movement flow, the feelings also tend to come into flow. Emotional blockages come up into awareness and are gently resolved, one after the other.

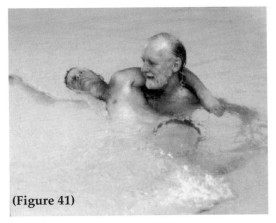

(Figure 41)

Harold Dull, the founder of Watsu.

Watsu is a purely surface technique with no completely submerged movements. It utilizes the stances of Tai Chi, with the practitioner shifting his weight, but rarely taking steps. The breath is as integral to the technique of Watsu as it is to Zen Shiatsu. By breathing with the receiver, the practitioner is better able to empathetically attune to her. The practitioner breathes from his hara (abdomen) and relaxes, moving in rhythm to the receiver's breath. From the beginning, emphasis is placed on adapting the moves to the receiver and to one's own physique. At its most advanced level, Watsu abandons its practice sequence and becomes free flow, a creative ongoing dance in which the practitioner follows movement impulses arising in the receiver and in himself.

WaterDance

WaterDance (also known as WATA or "Wassertanzen" in German) is the original subaquatic technique. It was first taught in 1987 in Europe and from 1993 in the United States. WaterDance arose out of the loveplay of Peter Schröter, a degreed psychologist, and Arjana Brunschwiler, whose background lay in dance, yoga, tantra and healing. It is on the one hand a powerful therapeutic instrument, and on the other a form of energy work and bodywork (Schröter, 1996).

WaterDance sessions begin with the receiver being cradled and stretched at the water's surface. Then, wearing a noseclip, she is gently taken entirely underwater at intervals for gradually longer dives. Once freed from the bounds of head support and gravity, the receiver's body can be waved, rolled, spun in circles and taken through somersaults in the three-dimensionality of the underwater world. The joy and delight of Peter and Arjana's initial explorations continue to imprint the work.

Just as Watsu could be characterized as having a maternal nature, WaterDance embodies a strong masculine or Father energy. The movements are large and often dynamic; at times the receiver is completely released and allowed to coast through the water. Still inverted positions are particularly evocative. The human dive reflex is fully activated in WaterDance, enabling receivers to effortlessly remain underwater for 45 seconds to a minute on average; two-minute and longer dives are not unusual. Receivers frequently report they feel so at home underwater that they don't want to come up. According to Indian yogic tradition, when the breath stops so does thinking, and when the mind is thus stilled the Truth emerges. This phenomenon of kumbhaka frequently occurs in WaterDance sessions, accompanied by a state of literal bliss in which the receiver surfaces with smiles and laughter. Spontaneous meditation and visions can also arise from the stopped breath state of kumbhaka.

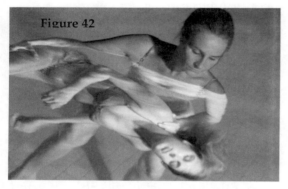

Arjana, one of the WaterDance founders.

WaterDance employs some of the spiraling patterns and leverages of Aikido in its body mechanics. It is a traveling technique; the practitioner walks in circles, figure eights and wave patterns. It is an advanced technique requiring a level of focus

only possible when basic support skills have become second nature. The practitioner learns to read the breath impeccably, signaling and submerging at exactly the right moment, remaining fully attentive to his receiver underwater, and then surfacing. WaterDance is the Zen Lexus of aquatic bodywork. Completely without intention or massage elements, and utilizing underwater movement alone, it produces astonishing physical releases, deep states of relaxation and psychological transformation. Kumbhaka!

Healing Dance

In 1990, while a resident at Harbin Hot Springs, I studied Watsu from its founder, Harold Dull. Following the course I began experimenting and improvising in the Harbin warm pool, influenced by my background in dance, by my experience as a practitioner of Trager Work, and by the qualities of water itself. After studying WaterDance in 1993 from Arjana Brunschwiler, a new spaciousness and three-

dimensionality appeared in my experimental moves. By then, I had created a side branch of Watsu, something flowing, dancing, and, if the truth be told, somewhat flamboyant. Healing Dance, as the technique I innovated is now called, has had to refine itself down from the sheer joy of movement to discover its full therapeutic potential. Since 1999 Inika Sati Spence has collaborated closely with me in defining and growing the work into a distinct technique. Theri Thomas joined the roster of teachers of Healing Dance in 2003, having already made significant contributions to its development.

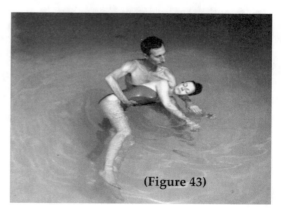

(Figure 43)

The Hara Hug is a positional sanctuary belonging to Healing Dance.

Healing Dance has many aspects, all based on the healing power of movement. The practitioner establishes an empathetic connection with the receiver and is trained to mirror any incipient moves. Like an orchestra conductor, he establishes a rhythmic field at the beginning of the session through his breath, movement and state of mind. He looks for the rhythm of awareness in each moment that allows the receiver to feel the psychological reverberations of the movement in her being. Movement is understood as medicine and carefully dosed, intermixed with restful pauses in quiet positional sanctuaries to allow for integration of its effects. The practitioner 'dances' the receiver, who has an experience of grace and beauty, sometimes leading to deeper emotional releases. Healing Dance could be understood as silent music, consisting of rhythmic impulses of pressure, touch and movement played upon the body's sensory system. The dance is between the subliminal message within each movement and the receiver's subconscious mind. That which has slowed down or ceased to move

within the psyche is inspired to awaken into playful participation. Thus, the healing comes from within (Georgeakopoulos, 1998).

Healing Dance is taught in two surface classes and two subaquatic ones. The subaquatic training Continuity makes the transition into and out of the underwater kingdom more fluid, so that there is less surprise at the 'border crossing.' It is about creating bridges for people. These bridges consist of a continuity of rhythm, movement, shape and body position. When these elements are first established at the surface, the receiver experiences a less radical change at the moment of submerging. The artificial division between surface and depth dissolves. Crossing back over the bridge in the opposite direction, that is, surfacing with this continuity, likewise lessens the division in the receiver's mind between above and below. The gifts from below are then conveyed to the surface without loss, similar to the dream recall technique in which the sleeper remains still in the position of

awakening in order better to remember her dream.

The other subaquatic training, Shape and Space, pays special attention to the creation of pure and spacious underwater movements. A beautiful and exciting repertoire of dives conveys the receiver across the length and breadth of the pool. In addition, Shape and Space explores the art of adaptation, improvisation, and facilitation of the interactive receiver.

Healing Dance's wide variety of original techniques reflects how water and the body naturally move together. Blocked energies are opened up by more than thirty hydrodynamic waves and spirals, as well as various spatial mandalas in the form of spins, figure 8's and releases, freeing and re-animating the body. Healing Dance takes advantage of the full three-dimensionality of the water with broad dynamic movements. A variety of advanced body mechanics techniques such as moving by example, creative imbalance and traveling through the pool help to create not only bigger movements, but subtler and more sensitive ones. The essence of Healing Dance is flow, freedom and lightness. As the vocabulary of movements expands, students become more confident improvising and better responding to the needs of the receiver.

Jahara Technique

The Jahara Technique is the genius of Mario Jahara, a Brazilian-born author and teacher of Zen Shiatsu, now living in the United States. Mario had studied the other three techniques and was working as an aquatic therapist at Two Bunch Palms Spa and Resort in southern California. He recognized the need to develop an approach that was less stressful and more comfortable for the practitioner regardless of the receiver's size or weight. He developed several ways to invisibly integrate the use of the 'Third Arm' flotation device (those Styrofoam noodles used for pool recreation) to help move and support the weight of the receiver.

The Jahara Technique utilizes precise body mechanics and support of the receiver to create a constant traveling motion in the direction of the head. This steady, gentle traction aligns itself with the natural joint decompression in the spine occurring during immersion. The motion is kept at a slow, relaxing speed. A greater sense of expansion, an opening and self-releasing of the mental and physical body occurs. Emphasis is placed on releasing the atlanto-axial joint, allowing the head to roll freely side-to-side.

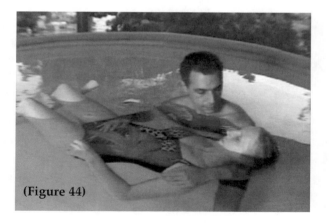

(Figure 44)

Mario Jahara, the founder of the Jahara Technique.

The Jahara Technique is rooted in the understanding of the fundamental elements of body mechanics and the physical properties of water. The practitioner moves in such a way as to remain aligned and grounded, while imparting a uniform momentum to the receiver, thus minimizing his presence. Circling footwork patterns are designed to create the illusion for the receiver of traveling in a straight line. The practitioner lets the water's tempo slow him down, avoiding turbulence. A variety of techniques are employed suitable to every body type, including long, gentle stretches, massage and accupressure. Through having a sound understanding of concepts and principles and a strong technical foundation, the practitioner can work without effort, relying on skill rather than physical strength.

In addition to two trainings of surface work, the Jahara Technique's third level teaches underwater moves. Instead of using a noseclip as in other techniques, the practitioner uses his fingers to softly close off the nostrils. In this level emphasis is also given to the creative exploration of transitioning movements to join all together in a continuous flow.

A Shiatsu class specifically designed for aquatic therapists is the fourth training offered within the Jahara Technique. This course focuses on awareness of the points and meridians and on developing a gentle but firm touch as required for the transposition of the techniques of Zen Shiatsu into the water (Jahara, 1997).

From the viewpoint of the receiver during a Jahara treatment, there is a sense of timelessness. The water washes constantly past without turbulence. There is no awareness of direction or the practitioner's location. A meditative expansion into stillness occurs. One leaves the pool feeling light and refreshed.

Levering the Body in Water

The verb, lever, derives from the Latin *levare*, to lighten, to lift up. I use it to describe how the giver effectively supports and guides the receiver's entire body in movement. A lever is a one or two-handed grip whereby this leverage, or power of action, is made possible. In Watsu and the Jahara technique, where the receiver is held is more or less uniform. Support will nearly always be from beneath the atlanto-occipital joint and the sacrum or the backs of the knees. Variations are minor, for the practitioner cooperates with the buoyant force, supporting from underneath to keep the receiver at the surface. In Healing Dance, in addition to supporting the receiver from underneath, the practitioner uses a greater range of holds, conducting her up and down in figure eights, waves, and spirals through the water's three dimensions. WaterDance and the subaquatic moves of Healing Dance use an even greater variety of leverages that must be adapted to each individual depending on her specific gravity and the amount of air in her lungs. The practitioner works not only *with* buoyancy, but at times he works *against* it, finding holds on the upper side of the body from which to guide the receiver downward. This occurs not only when submerging, but sometimes to maintain partner underwater, and even when surfacing if the receiver happens to be ultra-buoyant. Let's consider now the various parts of the body as places from which to lever.

Levering the Head

Tractioning the head in the crook of the elbow is used extensively in all four techniques, both to refresh the neck and to neutralize hyper-extension. Experienced practitioners integrate traction into all their moves. It is "the spice that seasons the movement." Combined with turning in place, tractioning the head is frequently used as a transition move that utilizes hydrodynamic force to keep the receiver close to the surface while the other hand shifts.

The Head Wave from Healing Dance is a move that levers the head. In it, the practitioner holds the head with both hands and walks diagonally backwards. The rest of the spine then waves freely with maximum articulation such as achieved in submerged WaterDance moves like the Footsnake.

Rotate the head and the body will follow, though not with the same alacrity and control as when initiating rotation from the knees or feet. The explanation lies in the nearly 90° range of motion in lateral rotation possessed by the cervicals taken as a whole. The head rotation must translate down through this range of motion in the neck before it will engage the torso. Needless to say, this must be done gently.

Levering the Spine

The spine may be levered from the lumbar up to the thoracic, but the cervical portion, the neck, is obviously off limits as a grip site. Where we hold the spine leaves the rest of the body inferior to the point of support free to move, so our grip serves as a 'point of articulation.' The greatest effect is on the joint immediately inferior, one bone of which is stabilized, the other free to move. Thus the practitioner can consciously change his grip to focus on different intervertebral joints. The more superior it is, the more of the body is free to wave. A wave sequences down through the remaining intervertebral,

pelvic and leg joints. Waves may be generated on the horizontal or vertical plane creating either lateral flexion or flexion-extension through the vertebral column. Body spirals can be created from any grip employed on the spine for waves by circling the grip and walking backwards.

Levering the Arms

The shallowness of the glenoid fossa and the extreme mobility of the scapula give the shoulder the greatest range of motion of any joint in the body. These same two factors also reduce the effectiveness of levering the body from an arm. Only when one or both of the arms are pulled are the results fairly predictable.

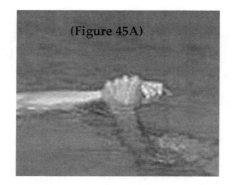

(Figure 45A)

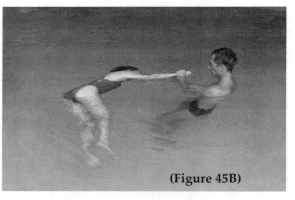

(Figure 45B)

The receiver is pulled by the arms through the water in the Waltz from WaterDance.

Levering the Knees

He who controls the knees, controls the body, for levering under the knees gives an efficient and immediate control of the pelvis owing to the security with which the head of the femur is held in the hip socket. This comes from two anatomical features: the depth of the hip socket and the strength of the hip ligaments. Pelvic movements, in turn, are rapidly translated through the torso via the tightly bound intervertebral joints.

Levering the Whole Leg

While the arms can only be pulled, the legs can be pulled or pushed, owing to the depth of the hip socket, the strength of the hip ligaments surrounding it, and the manner in which the knee locks into "home position" in hyperextension. The ample range of motion that the leg possesses works conversely when levering the body via the leg. The torso can be moved through full arches, roundings and rolls guided from a single leg. Whether a leg is pushed or pulled, the torso must follow; the depth and stability of the hip socket allow of no argument. Call it 'imperative guidance,' if you wish. The body must follow, and gladly, with all the eagerness of a would-be assailant leaping for the ground when Steven Segal catches his little finger just right. Of course, in aquatic bodywork, the motivation of pain has no place in enlisting compliance! The soft tissues are stretched, not stressed, in the leverages.

Levering Both Feet

When the legs are maintained straight, a powerful leverage is possible holding both feet at the same time. Pulling, pushing, rolling and releasing the body from a grip on the feet are all utilized in aquatic bodywork. Owing to the length of the lever arm (the entire leg), the practitioner must exert himself to produce a large movement.

Releases

Releases are the elastic recoil of the torso or legs after a stretch. A momentary sensation of heightened freedom is created and then sustained as the released part of the body remains free and in motion. Releases of another kind are utilized in submerging and surfacing the body. The entire body is launched out of the practitioner's grasp into an even more delicious moment of freedom. Observing the trajectory of the body, he must be ready to 'catch' the receiver again before she starts to sink. In the Healing Dance surfacing move, Shoot 'em Past, for example, the challenge is to impart enough velocity so that there is an excitement, a flying, and enough momentum to reach the surface before the catch.

The movements of aquatic bodywork may be categorized as follows:

1) Purely Hydrodynamic Moves

These movements are characterized by one of the seven hydrodynamic alignments (head first, feet first, waves, spirals, spins, figure eights and rolls). They are fishlike, occasioning little drag, or resistance to motion. The body is not challenged; it is at ease and naturally surrenders. Hydrodynamic force automatically organizes and streamlines the body position.

2) Hybrid Moves

These moves demonstrate a mixture of hydrodynamic and non-hydrodynamic qualities in varying degrees. Drag is intentionally exploited to stretch parts of the body left floating freely. To the extent that the head or feet are tractioned, the moves become more hydrodynamic.

3) Non-hydrodynamic moves

These movements do not conform to how the body most effortlessly moves and is moved through water. They are characterized by significant drag. It doesn't mean they don't feel good; they can be delicious to receive.

4) Bodywork in water

These are not full-body movements as much as bodywork performed in water. Suspended in the supportive medium of warm water, the receiver is 'shiatsued,' massaged and stretched.

5) Still positions

Still positions provide an essential counterpoint and balance to the movements of aquatic bodywork. They are incorporated at intervals into the sequence used in any session.

Body Mechanics for the Aquatic Practitioner

Thus far we have looked at the interrelations between water and the receiver's body. Let's consider now the technique of the practitioner, his body mechanics, as he supports and moves his receiver through the water.

Correct body mechanics serve both practitioner and receiver. With a good technical foundation, a practitioner is able to support sensitively and effectively, move flowingly, and relax. Giving sessions is enjoyable. Under these conditions, a receiver is more likely to have an experience that is pleasurable, nurturing, effective as bodywork, and spacious for inner exploration.

Knowledge of body mechanics reduces or prevents muscular soreness and injury when a receiver is particularly heavy in the water or cumbersome to work with. Tall men with long arms have an easier time with the aquatic techniques than short

buoyant women who sometimes struggle to stay grounded on the pool bottom. Yet, the judicious use of floats on receivers and weights around her own ankles enables even a petite women to practice aquatic bodywork successfully and offer her unique presence and quality of compassion.

Some physiques are more prone to injury than others, being more mutable and less substantial. Those of a sturdier build, born to the profession, with greater vitality and stamina will not need to pay as much attention to how they execute moves, to pacing, or to adjusting to heavy or large clients. Nevertheless, understanding how to economize on energy and honor the body will extend an active, injury-free career.

For the bodyworker, injuries are often part of the path by which honoring of self and refining of approach are learned. Many of my colleagues have related how physical troubles arising through massage became their teacher, directing them into gentler, more energy-oriented modalities.

Bodyworkers are drawn into aquatic bodywork for precisely this reason. It is kinder to the practitioner, less demanding to the hands, arms and back. When practiced unintelligently though, without using proper body mechanics or compensating for one's limitations or adapting the work to the client, it can be injurious.

The practitioner's movement most resembles a blend of Tai Chi, Aikido and partner dancing. The stances and the slow and deliberate tempos are derived from the Chinese martial art of Tai Chi. Other spiraling footwork patterns and leverages applied to the limbs are inspired by Aikido.

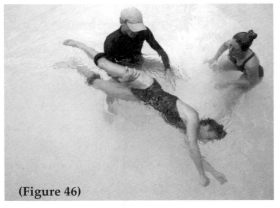

(Figure 46)

The Thigh Aikido from WaterDance uses the spiraling body mechanics of Aikido.

The changing, intertwining relationship between the practitioner's body and that of his receiver is reminiscent of partner dancing. The first four of the following eleven actions in body mechanics have much in common with Tai Chi. Let's have a look.

1) Standing up, sinking down

The most basic stance of aquatic bodywork has the feet about two shoulder widths apart, toes pointing laterally forward. The knees bend out over the feet and the hips drop down as the spine ascends vertical to the pelvis. This is the horse stance of Tai Chi, only wider. The buoyancy of water makes this wider stance possible without the added effort it would cost the practitioner on land. He and the receiver share a common center of gravity that is quite high and often lying outside of either body. A top-heavy and unstable structure is the outcome. This extra broad base then, gives the added stability needed to move the receiver at the practitioner's chest level in the water.

Buoyancy is the key factor affecting body mechanics in water. Buoyancy's drawback is reduced groundedness while its blessing is the ease with which it allows the practitioner to support another person. When bending the knees and immersing up to the neck, the body is lighter, gaining buoyancy. Standing up in the water, the body gains weight. Standing up or working in shallow water increases groundedness on the pool bottom and hence the leverage to move. Sinking low or working in deep water produces the opposite effect. A tall man in shallow water is much less disadvantaged than a short woman in deep water. He must take uncomfortably wide stances or kneel, even. Our short woman in deep water, however, can only put on ankle weights and keep it simple.

*A*lthough it may seem obvious that short-statured women would be at a disadvantage using these actions, they are often the ones who, through determination and resourcefulness, excel above their taller, stronger colleagues. A story to illustrate took place in 1993 during Arjana's first WaterDance training held in the United States. It was summer at Harbin Hot Springs and there were twelve of us in the class. The pool in which we were training was far from ideal. In addition to being too small, it had a sudden drop off in the middle, deepening from three and half feet to five feet in only two steps. We were learning the move called the Footsnake. The object was to traverse the pool, holding the feet only, while swinging our submerged receiver side to side. For most of us, crossing the deep zone was difficult but not impossible. One of the participants, though, stood less than five feet tall. Her first attempt had been unsuccessful. Submerged up to her crown and with no firm footing on the bottom, she could make no headway. She left the pool area and returned a few minutes later with a creative solution. Wearing ankle weights, a snorkel and mask, she was ready to try again. This time the crossing was successful (though at one point the zig-zagging tip of her snorkel was all I could see of her).

>≺((((O>   >≺(((((O>   >≺(((((O>

The experienced practitioner tends to work low in water. One who works in this 'crocodile style' expends less energy in maintaining his own posture or in supporting out-of-the-water limbs that don't belong to him.

2) Weight transfers

The weight transfer is a push off from one leg to the other. Leverage is dependent upon the feet having traction on the pool bottom. The push provides initial acceleration overcoming inertia. Once movement begins the practitioner acquires momentum. As the weight transfer finishes and establishes equilibrium on the second leg, the knee bends to absorb force. Overcoming inertia to change directions if a back and forth movement is used, the return weight transfer begins.

The initial push is on a downward diagonal, producing a lateral displacement of the body in the opposite direction. The leg communicates its force to the pelvis. The trunk rides across above the pelvis. Muscles of the torso contract isometrically to keep it balanced over the pelvis against the displacing factor of water resistance. The stabilizing contraction of the torso also creates a coherent platform for the shoulder girdle and arms to support and move the receiver.

3) Hip rotations

Often a weight transfer combines with pelvic rotation. The pelvis rotates in toward the femur of the leg receiving the weight. Rather like a bullfighter turning with a cape, the movement may then continue to create a longer arc. When we generate movement from the legs and hips in this way the arms and back are not overburdened. The arms remain directly in front of the shoulders and the ribcage and pelvis move as a unit, always facing in the same direction. This is the 'Tai Chi trunk.' Without it, the spine twists, which is destabilizing to vertebral alignment and straining to the back muscles.

Gravity is fully operative in water. The buoyant force in water counters gravity. (It is an outcome of gravity, actually, a result of water pressure increasing with depth.) Holding objects or people up in water is easier than on land, but moving them laterally is more difficult—the objects encounter the greater viscosity water has than that of air. The power to move a partner sideways through the water comes from shifting the weight from leg to leg, rotating the pelvis and stabilizing the back and arms.

4) Steps
A weight shift often broadens into a step, either to the front, side or back. The step is taken softly, toe first, for the receiver can feel a jarring heel on the pool bottom right up through the practitioner's body. The foot actually slides lightly in contact with the bottom. The challenge in taking steps

in the water is to maintain back and hip alignment while moving. Destabilizing factors are 1) the giving up and finding again of support, and 2) the water resistance offered by the the practitioner and receiver's bodies.

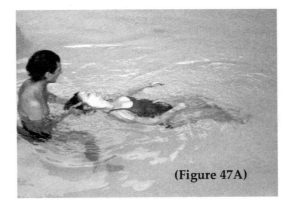

(Figure 47A)

The Head Wave of Healing Dance is created by rapidly walking backwards.

With every step, whether on land or in water, the nervous system is making adjustments without conscious involvement. However in water, these skills must first be learned and imprinted before they become automatic. 'Geisha' steps, backing up, are another way to create circle and figure eight shapes. Large diagonally backward 'Godzilla' steps are used to generate wave movements

for the receiver. When traveling backwards, a beneficial low-pressure area is generated immediately in front of the practitioner the receiver rides in a sort of 'water pocket', similar to the draft created by lead cars and bicyclists in races. The practitioner may visualize that he cuts a canyon through the water and pulls his receiver between its walls. By traveling quickly, he generates virtual currents in which the receiver rides. There is a sense of going forward, of leaving the old behind.

On land it is more efficient walking forwards than backwards. In water the reverse is true; walking backwards is clearly easier and faster. Why is this? First of all, our weight is already falling backwards without effort. Secondly, the back is more streamlined than the front of the torso, allowing water to slip around it more easily. When we walk to the front our thigh leads, but in walking backwards, the heel is the first part of the body to cut through the water, and it offers minimal resistance. In contrast to walking forward in water, when walking backwards the foot is in complete contact with the bottom for a longer time, resulting in more leverage and hence more push from the bottom to power the walk.

The step is a metaphor for transition and uncertainty. From a place of familiarity and support, a step reaches out into new territory, already reducing support by half. It then falls into the unknown, where it is necessary to re-establish balance and security. Steps present the greatest body mechanics challenge for students of aquatic bodywork to master, just as transitions are the most difficult of life phases.

5) *Creative Imbalance*

Walking on land entails a fall forward onto the foot receiving the body's weight. Moving in water also includes an off balance phase. Yet moving in water is not at all the same on land. It is much slower due to water's viscosity. In water a practitioner can lean and fall sideways or backwards and still have plenty of time to smoothly recover equilibrium. This enables a new logic of moving: conscious slow motion falling, or

what I term creative imbalance. It is the most effortless way to generate movement. The practitioner's own body weight transmits movement to the partner. The fall begins with the head. As it tilts in the desired direction, the vertebrae, one by one from the top down join in the movement like a stack of blocks tumbling. At the same time a body state activates in which the leg tenses in the direction of the head tilt in preparation for receiving the body's weight.

We don't always need to be in balance. Life is less a stable phenomenon than a constant process of course correction, of zig zagging, one movement arising opportunistically out of another. Equilibrium then is a process, not the static moments of weight centeredness. Natural movement is alternately losing and recovering balance. What shall we call it? Creative imbalance.

6) *Just Do Half*

Water buoys the receiver. Trusting the water to help and overcoming the fear of dunking the receiver form a stage in the development of practitioner technique. An experienced practitioner does not over-support, but allows the water to do half the work. He thinks of himself as an extension of the water, becoming like water, even identifying with the water. Similarly, he needs only to power half the movement; when given an impulse, the body will follow through. Our role in offering movement includes allowing the receiver the time and space to continue moving freely, lightly and weightlessly on her own. This entails observing and placing our mind in our partner's body, even becoming our partner. In summary, let the water do half the work, let the receiver do half the movement.

7) *Breath*

Relaxing the entire body is achieved by breathing into the belly. It is especially important that the upper body not get rigid with tension. Tension there crystallizes the physical structure, making it top heavy, less grounded and more liable to topple off balance. Exhaling and sinking is a way to release stress and stay in touch with surrender, the quality most important for a practitioner to model.

Breath cannot only relax and ground, it can be a source of movement. By entering an intuitive, non-thinking state, breathing synchronizes with movement and actually becomes a source of movement. Ueshiba Morihei, the founder of Aikido, taught that through the breath we could be in tune with other people and with our surroundings. The Master termed this 'kokyu,' or the Breath of Life, the fundamental rhythm of life that energizes and fills the universe. (Ueshiba, 1984) It is as attainable in aquatic bodywork as it is in Aikido.

8) Ideokinesis
The Greek roots of this word mean 'idea' and 'movement.' Ideokinesis is the concept developed by Lulu Schweigard (Schweigard, 1974) describing the process whereby an idea held in the mind is executed in movement without the doer consciously knowing the means. He need only have a mental picture of a movement, and the nervous system recruits all the right muscles to perform it in the most economical fashion. Another way to state this principle would be, "Visualize movement shapes."

9) Scanning
Years ago, I learned a way to check and improve body mechanics from Maxine Mahon, one of my ballet teachers. It consists of mentally roaming through the body and monitoring what is going on. The purpose of this continual head to toe scanning is to keep correct placement, timing and coordination. It is a way to refresh and restore muscular responses as they begin to fatigue. Over time, with enough practice, all these responses become second nature, like walking, and require little maintenance.

In aquatic bodywork the same technique of scanning can be used, but with one improvement: we ask a question. It is the nature of the universe to respond immediately to a question; several New Age healing modalities work on this principle. In the Trager Approach, for example, the practitioner wonders to himself as he works, "What could be lighter? What could be freer?" With such an inquiring attitude there arises a receptivity and attunement to a response from the receiver, thereby evoking one. The bodymind's answer is non-verbal — a letting go, a shift in body state. This works reflexively, too, when we ask ourselves questions such as, "Am I grounded in my breath?" "Is my body in comfort and flow?" "Am I effortlessly present?" Having a wondering attitude produces results without any conscious action.

10) Get the power from as low down as possible.
When moving in water the practitioner must counter the forces that destabilize by consciously creating a chain of leverage, beginning with the pool bottom and passing sequentially through the ankles, knees, hips, spine, shoulder joints, elbows and wrists to the hands.

The elbows are often braced against the sides of the ribcage, like dolphin flippers, to more efficiently translate power from the torso to the hands. Each part of the body has a role to fulfill. If strength and control are not present low in the body, the higher segments must work extra hard to compensate. Ballet dancers strengthen their feet and legs more than in any other movement discipline. This frees their torsos and especially their arms to relax and express. They thrust down into the ground to jump up, to move laterally or to maintain equilibrium. Practitioners of Tai Chi sink their weight downward. An aquatic practitioner will be nearer one of these two poles of thrusting and sinking, depending on how yang or yin a given movement is.

11) Dance!

The final word on body mechanics points beyond what I've discussed so far. In dance, technique is learned to be forgotten; in performance one gives oneself to the dance. "Just dance it," says the coach to the dancer

heading on-stage. He might add, "Don't think, don't worry, just do it."

We each have a very private mode of being that from the outside appears as movement and is called dancing. Perhaps it is a way of entering into the Greater Flow or the Universal Ecstasy. Whatever it is, this dance has a rightness and power to it. It expands us and attunes us to our environment. The imagery around dance is endless: "Dance with yourself, dance with your partner, dance with the water, dance in the Light, dance from the heart." In short, dance!

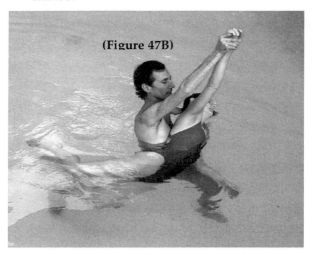

(Figure 47B)

Basic Support

The basic position of support in aquatic bodywork has the receiver floating supine out in front of the standing practitioner. The head will be supported in the hand or elbow crook of the practitioner's 'head arm' (the arm closest to the receiver's head); the practitioner's 'foot arm' will support under the pelvis or the knees, and the receiver's arm nearest the practitioner will either float in front of his chest or wrap around his back.

Most aquatic sessions begin in stillness in such a pose. Many processes are set in motion during these quiet moments. First, the horizontal fosters Being, as the vertical fosters Doing. The receiver is free to embark upon an inner journey.

Secondly, the horizontal body position is that of rest, ease in the musculature and balanced circulation.

Third, as the receiver feels the practitioner's touch and experiences his support and sensitivity, his credibility is established, paving the way for further relaxation. This is a step beyond the degree of trust a purely verbal exchange can foster.

Fourth, a transition takes place from self-responsibility and independence to dependence and receptivity. This is a retro-journey, a return, and takes time. By entrusting the practitioner to carry her and keep her nose out of the water, the receiver, on some level, is placing her very survival in the practitioner's hands.

Fifth, a state of self-healing arises, referred to as 'cellular breathing.' In moments of stillness and well being the body's wisdom asserts itself and the cells come into a state of dynamic attunement with their environment. They attend to housekeeping, metabolizing nutrients, excreting toxins and releasing shock (Sawyer, 1999).

There are no perfect positions; at some point they all must be abandoned for change. Like a sleeper who shifts her position at intervals during the night, the receiver needs slight variations to refresh her neck. She must not be held for too long in one position. By varying the head's support, the muscle fibers in the neck will be fired more randomly and fatigue from repetitive firings in a static position will be delayed.

The practitioner neither overstabilizes nor understabilizes the head. Instead, he supports like a wise parent: setting limits, but allowing a degree of freedom so that tiny adjusting movements are possible. This will also allow movement to sequence through the spine. An occipital-sacral counter-traction facilitates this, working with water's natural joint decompression effect.

The receiver's head will be over-supported unless at least one ear is submerged. Over-support of the head occurs as an expression of caring by beginners until they clarify their technique. When the head is too far out of the water and becomes weighted, the neck tends not to release completely. As James McMillan, the founder of the Halliwick Method formulated, tone is a function of weight. This means that so long as the proprioceptors sense weight, muscle tone is maintained. Therefore, when the head is held out of the water, tone in the neck muscles is generated. The head must ride low, with the water line covering the ears, but not too close to the corners of the eyes. The practitioner senses the weight of the head and the degree to which the water can support this weight. He works in "teamship" with the water, trusting its buoyancy and letting it do most of the work. Because the body's specific gravity averages less than that of water, (0.974), nearly 100% of body weight is supported by the water.

The waterline submerges the receiver's ears and crown; the chin and eyes stay dry. It traces the edge of a mask around the face; the head is more than half submerged. When the water laps at the corners of the eyes and mouth, a conscious or subliminal hypervigilance on the part of the receiver is the outcome; quite the opposite of the safe, peaceful space the practitioner wishes to establish.

Paradoxically, the properly supported head appears to float. All else being equal, the head should be supported only enough to maintain the waterline below the eyes, nose and mouth, and to afford enough weight for occipital traction.

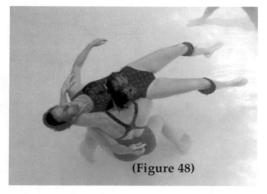

(Figure 48)

The crown and the ears are submerged.

To support the hips correctly, maintain the pelvis just below the surface and guard against lumbar hyperextension. Supported supine at the surface, the body is not truly horizontal. With the head at the surface and the hips maintained discreetly submerged in the water, the body angles slightly downward from head to foot, though the legs stay well away from the bottom of the pool.

The point of pelvic support is beneath the apex of the sacrum. The forearm provides broad, even support across the back of the hips. The back of the hand can also lever the sacrum well. Supporting with the palm on the sacrum may be too intimate for some receivers, especially at the outset of a session.

The vertebrae from the 12th thoracic down to the hip joints constitute a linked chain of articulation, in which compensation through the pelvis and lumbar spine facilitates leg movements at the hip socket in all directions (Kapandji, Vol. 3, 1974). The strong Y ligaments across the front of the pelvis require that support be under the sacrum, lest the weight of the legs tilt the pelvis forward and hyperextend the lower back. This can be alleviated by moving the supporting arm down to the apex of the sacrum or even onto the backs of the thighs. Use of the Third Arm, as employed in the Jahara Technique, accomplishes the same thing.

Leg flotation must allow some heft in the legs, otherwise hip support cannot gain purchase across the pelvis and there can be no traction. Moreover, over-flotation of the legs obstructs their natural movement and prevents the hips from rising and falling with the breath.

Supporting under the pelvis is not ideal. Many receivers exhibit some tendency to protect the lower back with contraction of the abdominal muscles. Counter-traction between the occiput and the sacrum serves to protect the low back, alleviating compression at L5-S1. Support under the knees, on the other hand, allows the lumbar curve to reverse, stretching the back muscles in a safe position for those with lower back problems.

More About the Head and Neck

Over 12% of Americans suffer from pain and dysfunction in the neck and head. Aquatic bodywork has the potential to alleviate these conditions, or, when practiced without awareness, it can aggravate them. The greater a joint's range of motion, the greater its susceptibility to injury. The cervicals, from the atlanto-occipital joint down to the C6-C7 intervertebral joint, form the most mobile segment of the spine. The upper segment of the neck is anatomically and functionally distinct. It consists of the atlanto-occipital and the atlanto-axial joints. Their range of motion in flexion-extension and rotation equal that of the remaining cervical joints. (Hoppenfeld, 1976) This is to say that the neck, already quite mobile, is even more so in its upper, suboccipital segment. It requires special attention in the form of precise support, stabilization and traction.

Not surprisingly, in aquatic bodywork the neck is more vulnerable to misapplied technique than any other area of the body. It is not designed to lie passively, face up in water. The neck is designed for action, primarily in the vertical, bipedal stance. The muscles crossing its suboccipital segment (suboccipitals, longus cervicis, rectus capitis anterior and rectus capitis lateralis) have the strength to stabilize and move the head in a balanced vertical alignment. They are not equipped for sustained periods suspended backwards without head support, as in the water. In this case, practitioner support takes over for the muscles.

Two infantile reflexes (Moro's reflex and the startle reflex) are activated by the sudden loss of head support. Although they are apparently no longer operative in an adult, the infant part of the mind is often reached and re-experienced in aquatic bodywork. It is conceivable that subliminal fear and consequent distrust could ensue from mishandling of the head, especially later in a session when a deeper level of vulnerability is attained. Moshe Feldenkreis, founder of the Feldenkreis Method, posits that the startle reflex is operative throughout life, generating misalignments of posture and disturbances in breathing, regardless of age (Feldenkrais, 1991).

The bony structures on which the head arm gains purchase to support and traction are the naturally round area of the back of the head, the external occipital protuberance and the superior and inferior nuchal lines. Support is with the forearm (palm turned downward) or in the crook of the elbow (palm facing up). If support is given slightly inferior to the occipital bone beneath the atlanto-occipital joint, there is the possibility that compression of the delicate soft tissue structures there will become painful. Also, in the absence of traction, the head will fall back, giving rise to hyperextension.

A certain amount of neck curvature, cervical lordosis, is natural. It promotes a level bite, the equilibrium of the head anterior to the fulcrum point of the occipital condyles, and the normal, level gaze of the eyes. Reid's base line, from the inferior margin of orbit through the center of the auditory canal and the center of occipital bone, will be horizontal when the neck has a slight, posterior concavity (Kapandji, *op.cit.*).

Some receivers are extremely sensitive to the slightest degree of neck hyperextension in the water. Others are quite comfortable with a bit of extension through the neck, even arching into the position. (This can be embarrassing for a teacher demonstrating to a class.)

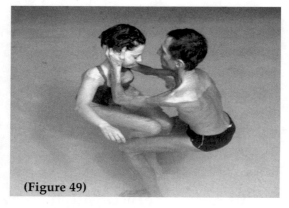

(Figure 49)

This head traction illustrates one of aquatic bodywork's many stretches for the neck.

how to keep the neck correctly aligned. Been there.) When cervical lordosis becomes accentuated through misapplied support in the middle of the neck, rather than tractioning at the juncture of the neck and skull, discomfort is immediate. In almost all cases of hyperextension, the practitioner's responsibility is to

resolve it by repositioning his arm and applying proper traction.

Effects and Applications

Aquatic bodywork is significant neither for a pleasing philosophy nor for how aesthetic it may appear to the onlooker, but for its practical results. Aquatic bodywork brings relief to stressful lives. It sets a new standard for relaxation and well-being. Receivers routinely declare at the end of their sessions, "That was the most nurtured, the most relaxed I have ever felt in my life." Aquatic bodywork is the treatment for some neurological and orthopedic conditions that nothing else can reach. It is direct, without interruption or interpretation; emotional processes are not spoken of, they are experienced and given the space to unwind piece by piece to their resolution. Aquatic bodywork demonstrates to the receiver how satisfying contact with one's own self can be. It shows a healthier way of living, more like water, in allowing energy and feelings to flow unfettered through our being. Watsu, WaterDance, Healing Dance and

Jahara Technique are modalities in which one can legitimately speak of healing taking place, not merely the cessation of symptoms.

For many people, Watsu is the initiation, the entrance into a closer relation with self and with water. Its safety and nurturing contact appeal precisely to those needing or fearing intimacy, including abuse victims. Watsu is the ideal setting to overcome fear of water. Watsu has shown itself to be the perfect prescription for everyday stress and insomnia. Physical therapists have adapted Watsu for successful treatments. (Peggy Schoedinger, PT, one of Watsu's most brilliant practitioners and teachers, developed a training precisely to address such special conditions.) Watsu has proven invaluable when integrated into therapeutic situations calling for bonding, such as couples and family therapy. The 'unconditional positive regard' bestowed upon the receiver raises the self-esteem of the elderly and of those fighting substance abuse. Its gentleness and comfort have found it a place in hospice work.

Not everyone needs to receive Watsu as his or her first experience of aquatic bodywork. Some fall in love with WaterDance from the moment they witness it and are ready to go underwater with complete comfort. These are very often swimmers, divers, surfers and those free souls who feel an affinity for water and dolphins. As receivers explore their relation to water, which for some is quite profound, even central to their being, they tend to gravitate to the advanced subaquatic techniques offering more movement, space, adventure and challenge. WaterDance and the underwater work in Healing Dance appeal to these aquanauts. WaterDance is not without its therapeutic applications; Erez Beatus, one of Israel's most gifted water professionals, has been successfully using it in Eilat to treat children and adults with special conditions. WaterDance, along with the Jahara Technique, is only slightly size graded; large receivers can be easily accommodated.

The first appeal of Healing Dance is to those who love water and stretching, who wish to experience beauty and grace, and surrender to the power of movement. More than any other technique, it is the Dance. It brings the experience of physical freedom, especially poignant for those who are unable to stand or walk. For the athlete, martial artist, dancer and would-be dancer, the movements of Healing Dance are a delight and an invitation to playfully participate by allowing their own movement impulses expression. Healing Dance's waves with the receiver lying on her side are beneficially disorienting and excellent for releasing holding patterns of a psychological origin. These waves, with the multiple joint mobilizations they offer, are good for spinal problems; receivers often report that their backs feel much better following a session. As receivers soon discover, there is much of stillness and nurture in the Healing Dance, too — moments to expand into oneself while being safely held.

The Jahara Technique is used in spas and private practice and is finding many applications in rehabilitative aquatics. This technique is providing relief for patients with limited range of motion during recovery from injuries, or suffering from herniated discs and chronic back pain. Physical therapists are turning to the Jahara Technique to treat disabilities such as cerebral palsy, and chronic conditions like rheumatoid arthritis. It is especially effective with larger individuals due to the assistance in support provided by a cylindrical closed-cell foam flotation device called the "noodle" or the "Third Arm." Its slow, gentle approach is well suited to working with the more fragile elderly.

The Jahara Technique is excellent for first time receivers as it entails less physical closeness than the other techniques and also allows time for the neck and head to release.

The Aquatic Bodyworker

Each of the four techniques has a particular appeal. According to his or her temperament the prospective student will be drawn to study one or several. One who wishes to nurture and share his heart might feel most at home in Watsu. The person who loves movement and the experience of freedom might focus on Healing Dance and WaterDance. The student for whom effortlessness, flow and meditative expansion are core values would be attracted to the Jahara Technique. The kind of population that a bodyworker already treats or contemplates working with will also influence his choice.

For some students the goal of becoming aquatic bodyworkers is most appealing. Just as a massage therapist often combines modalities, such as circulatory, deep tissue, joint mobilization and energy work, in one session, an aquatic bodyworker is one who trains in more than one technique and is able to draw from his toolbox the particular approach required in the moment. This

synthesis leads to greater creativity, a richness not present in any one massage modality. Even instructors of aquatic bodywork tend not to specialize in any single technique, but qualify to train students in two or more.

Watsu, WaterDance, Healing Dance and Jahara Technique have all borrowed moves and ideas from each other and have much in common. In their advanced levels, all lay emphasis on creatively adapting to the receiver, whether it is her size, flexibility, buoyancy, or her spontaneously arising movements and feelings. All are a mixture of movement and stillness, space and closeness, the dynamic and the serene. All are adept at accessing trance states with their accompanying memories, visions and insights. All have broad therapeutic applications. All point the receiver toward her Self while demanding the same commitment to awareness and growth of their practitioners.

With their potential to extend out from a few isolated hours to all his

waking moments, the sublime states attained offering aquatic bodywork beckon to the practitioner. He begins to realize how the serenity and attunement of the water experience serve as a model of being and relating. Then, just as the masters of the spiritualized arts of the Orient sought not merely to practice art, but to *become* it, he can transmute his craft into a way of life.

Over time, a personal philosophy evolves, not to talk about, but to live. It differs for each individual, as each is a unique creation embodying an unrepeatable frequency of love.

Those who feel the calling to share aquatic bodywork choose a path with heart, worthy of devoted commitment. Aquatic bodywork is a container broad enough and deep enough for the soul's expansion through a lifetime.

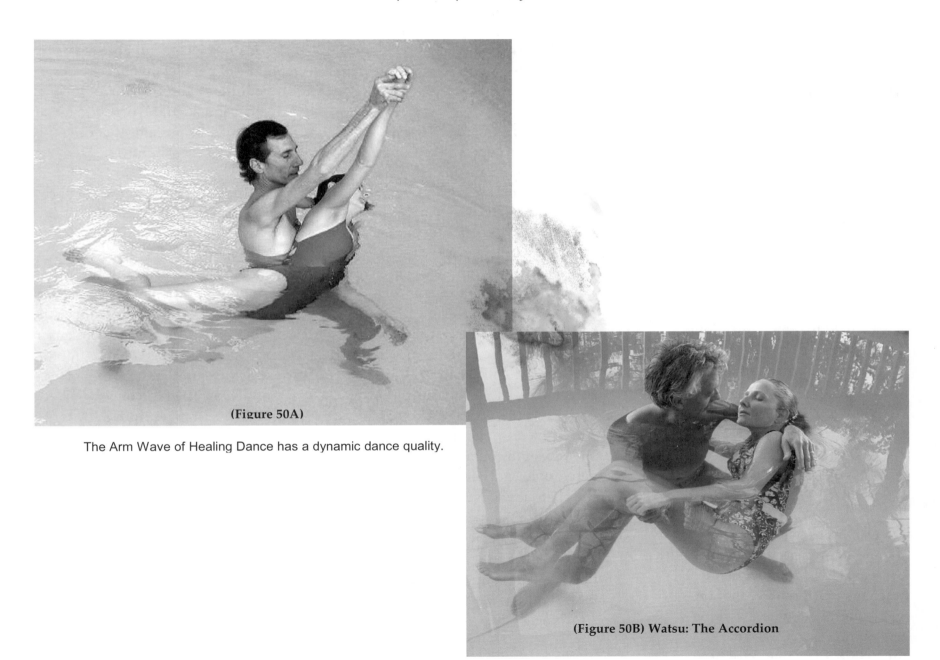

(Figure 50A)

The Arm Wave of Healing Dance has a dynamic dance quality.

(Figure 50B) Watsu: The Accordion

Chapter 3
Contractile Physiology in the Pool

Chapters 3-16 are by Douglas Bedgood

Muscle Tissues

To arrive at where we are as a species, developmental changes have required billions of years of selection and adaptation. The physiological efficiency of life represents an enormous duration of evolutionary events that only the human intellect can begin to discover or even have an interest in comprehending.

We will not neglect the adaptive efficiency of muscle physiology in this text. Our study of its biochemistry will be comprehensive to the molecular level.

The properties of muscles are excitability, contractility, extensibility, and elasticity. The purposeful functions are voluntary motion, maintenance of posture and tone, generation of heat, vascular circulation, digestive activities, respiratory assistance, function of reproductive ducts and the urinary system, reflexes and sensory functions that require movement.

"Myo" means muscle. "Fascia" means surrounding, beneath the skin. Fascia is both superficial and deep. Subcutaneous fascia is loose connective tissue. Deep myofascia is dense, irregular connective tissue containing collagen. Muscles are enveloped and supported within independent compartments for separate fibers with a mesh of fibrous connective tissue fascia called epimysium. The bundles of muscle fibers, or faciculi (Figure 52), are surrounded by perimysium. The individual fibers or muscle cells are surrounded by endomysium. The endomysium contains a rich capillary network for nutrient and oxygen supply to the muscles. Epimysium, perimysium, and endomysium are extensions of deep myofascia that extend beyond the contractile muscle fibers, merging into dense connective tissue tendons for periosteal bone attachment.

A skeletal muscle is a bundle of fibers, fasciculi. The fasciculi fiber is a bundle of parallel myofibrils. The myofibril is a thread of myofilaments, myocin and actin. Myocin and actin are contractile proteins that can be excited by nerve impulses.

A motor unit is one somatic motor nerve fiber and all the muscle fibers it innervates as a functional unit for neural control and motor activity. Neural contraction signals originate in the anterior portion of the spinal cord. Each spinal nerve may contain 6,000 motor nerve fibers and 12,000 sensory nerve fibers (Kardas, 2003). A motor nerve fiber stimulates myofilament contraction. The ratio of nerve fiber to muscle fiber ranges from 1:100 to 1:2,000. The neurons that innervate fewer muscle fibers are used first during contractions requiring a greater variance of response for fine, precise movements. When more force is required for brute control of large movement using large muscles, neurons are recruited that innervate a higher volume of over a thousand muscle fibers per neuron.

The outer membrane of a muscle cell is the sarcolemma. Within this membrane is the sarcoplasm or the muscle fiber cytoplasm. The sarcoplasm contains the fluid where most of the chemical reactions occur, the fluid that contains adenosine triphosphate (ATP, Figure 57), creatine phosphate (CP), myoglobin, myofibrils, glycogen, ribosomes, mitochondria (Figure.61), and more than one nucleus. The sarcoplasmic reticulum (Figure 53), is a communications network that spreads nerve impulses through transverse tubules that are open at the sarcolemma and penetrate into deeper parts of the cell. The terminal cisternae are lateral calcium ion storage sacs on the muscle cell.

Several peripherally located nuclei in each muscle cell provide DNA for protein synthesis. Mitochondria use oxygen and carbohydrates for cellular respiration and ATP production. Ribosomes are the layered and folded surface organelles in the cell used for protein synthesis. Glycogen (Figure 66B) is glucose (Figure 66A) stored as a branched chain of twelve glucose

molecules in the muscle cells and liver. Myoglobin, a red pigment, binds oxygen, releasing it when demand is heavy. ATP and CP contain high-energy phosphate bonds. When their bonds break, energy is released like a trillion mini-explosions within the muscle cells for use in contraction.

A muscle twitch is a response by muscle fibers to electrical stimulation from a nerve impulse in vivo or from external sources. A stronger impulse increases the quantity of muscle fibers that are stimulated with higher amplitude, and vice-versa. Rapid successions of impulses produce overlapping twitches called summation. If the frequency of stimulation is fused and constant, not pulsing, the result is tetanus, a sustained contraction of fibers. When a muscle fiber contracts it contracts to the fullest extent or not at all (Kardas, 2003). A neuron will either fire at the same intensity every time or it will not fire at all. A depolarizing refractory period determines the maximum firing rate, the rate determined by information

conveyance rather than the nature of one impulse. A pre-synaptic neuron can inhibit a post-synaptic neuron from firing. This excitation and inhibition greatly increase the neuronal conveyance of information. Excitation can strengthen from temporal summation or from spatial summation (Kardas, 2003). The former is more likely to fire a post-synaptic neuron due to repeated pre-synaptic excitatory firing. This can be conversely inhibited. Spatial summation occurs when three pre-synaptic neurons each deliver excitation at the same time to one post-synaptic neuron. These simple variables can create enormously complex neural circuits with as few as twenty neurons. Muscle fibers, depending on their type, twitch at different times, sometimes many fibers at one time and sometimes only a few fibers at a time for a long duration. They are able to repeat a response after relaxation, referred to above as the refractory period. There are three phases of a muscle twitch: latent period, contraction period, and the refractory period.

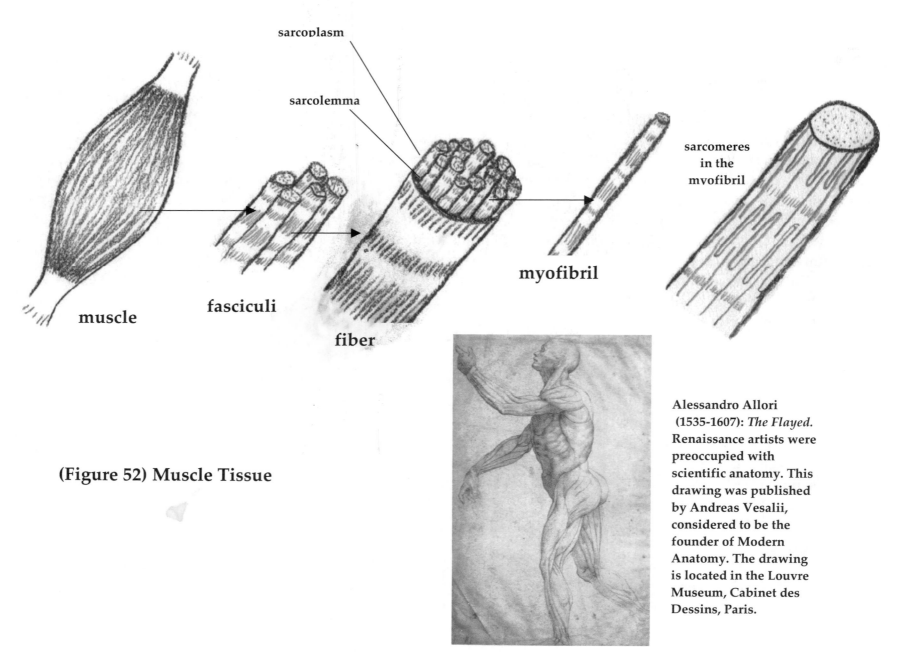

sarcoplasm

sarcolemma

sarcomeres
in the
myofibril

myofibril

muscle

fasciculi

fiber

(Figure 52) Muscle Tissue

Alessandro Allori
(1535-1607): *The Flayed*.
Renaissance artists were
preoccupied with
scientific anatomy. This
drawing was published
by Andreas Vesalii,
considered to be the
founder of Modern
Anatomy. The drawing
is located in the Louvre
Museum, Cabinet des
Dessins, Paris.

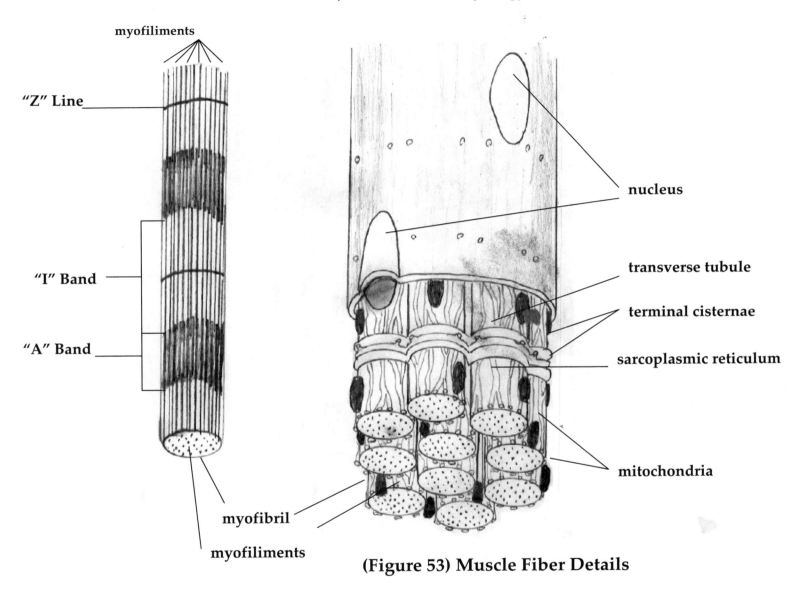

myofiliments

"Z" Line

"I" Band

"A" Band

myofibril

myofiliments

nucleus

transverse tubule

terminal cisternae

sarcoplasmic reticulum

mitochondria

(Figure 53) Muscle Fiber Details

The myofilaments in Figure 53 are individual protein strands. Hundreds of geometrically oriented filaments are in a sarcomere (Figure 52 and 53). The thick filament is myosin. Each myosin filament contains around 500 myosin heads. The thin filament is actin. The dark striation in Figure 53 is both myosin and actin. The light striation is actin alone. In Figure 54 the "A" band is anisotropic. The "H" zone through the middle is myosin alone. The lateral band is where the actin filaments overlap. The length of the "A" band remains unchanged during contraction and relaxation. The "I" band is actin alone, anchored to the "Z" line. The sarcomere is the section between the "Z" lines that shortens during contraction. As the "I" and "H" zones compress, the "A" band remains constant. On the right (Fig. 54) is a simple illustration representing sarcomere contraction.

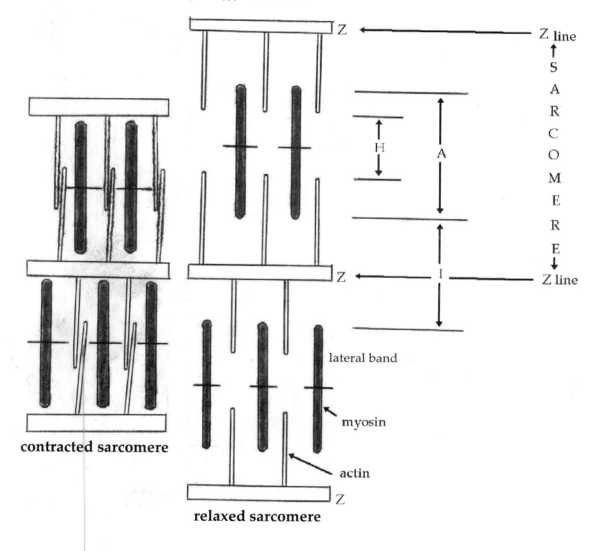

(Figure 54) Sarcomere Contraction

(Figure 55A)
Actual photo of a sarcomere
showing myosin, actin ,
"Z" lines and the "A" Band

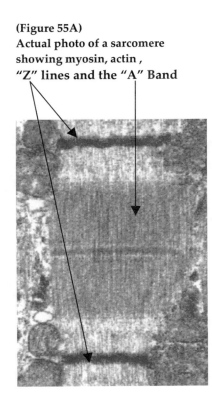

Many biology and human physiology textbooks illustrate myosin with two heads that leverage together or separate, looking away from each other. It is far from realistic and should resemble the myosin filament in Figure 55B.

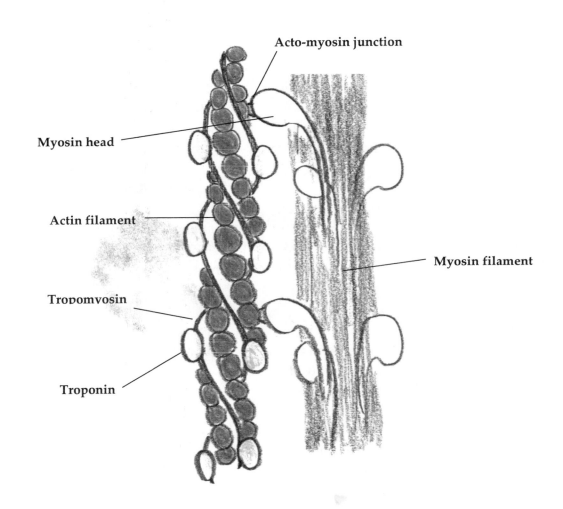

(Figure 55B) Actin-Myosin Filaments

If you look at the electron crystallography image of myosin (Fig. 58A-B) you will see that the binding site in the giant molecule is like a mouth that opens and closes on the actin receptor site (Rayment, 1993). Myosin has the hooks and actin has the loops.

G-actin is globular actin, a monomer. As a dynamic polymer, F-actin is a long filament of two strands twisted into a helix, each containing 300-400 G-actin molecules. Actin filament elongation is stabilized by the hydrolysis of ATP nucleotide. The mechanical properties of G-actin and F-actin are influenced by the bound nucleotide and the divalent cations Mg and Ca. Mg-actin has a more closed nucleotide binding cleft relative to Ca-actin. Currently there are investigations into the role of water molecule diffusion into the nucleotide-binding site and it's influence on ATP hydrolysis. There are also ongoing studies of G-actin monomer interactions within the F-actin polymer filament.

Basically, the regulatory proteins that prevent contraction are troponin and tropomyosin. Tropomyosin is a thin, rigid thread of 40-60 molecules per filament located in the longitudinal groove along the surface of the actin helix between the two strands of actin. It covers the receptor sites where myosin binds to the actin when the receptor sites are not covered. A tropomyosin molecule spans about seven G-actin molecules (Huxley, 1985). Scientifically, the G-actin molecules in the filament are called subunits of the actin polymer, but we will refer to them here as molecules. Troponin is a globular molecule on top of the tropomyosin. Immediatly prior to contraction, Ca++ concentration in the sarcoplasm is very high and it combines with troponin. This interaction removes tropomyosin from blocking the receptor site. The cross bridges of myosin are then able to bind to the actin and allow the power stroke of muscle contraction.

Cross bridges are oriented on opposite sides of the sarcomere allowing the actin filaments to be pulled towards its center. Prior to myosin cross bridges binding to actin, the mouth-like binding site of myosin functions as myosin ATPase enzymes to split ATP (Figure 57) into ADP(Figure 56) and P. ATP splits from a triphosphate into a diphosphate plus one phosphate.

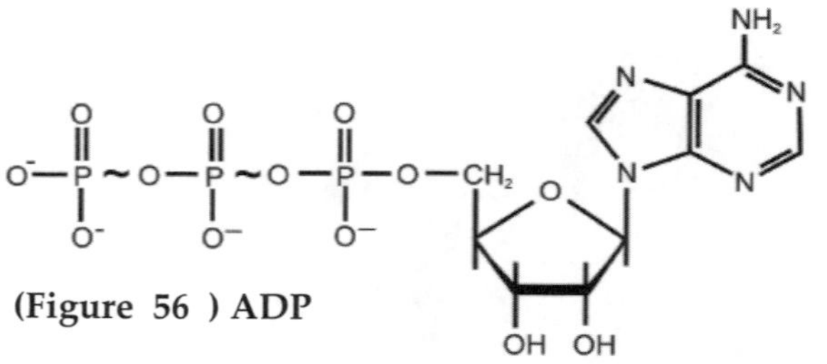

(Figure 56) ADP

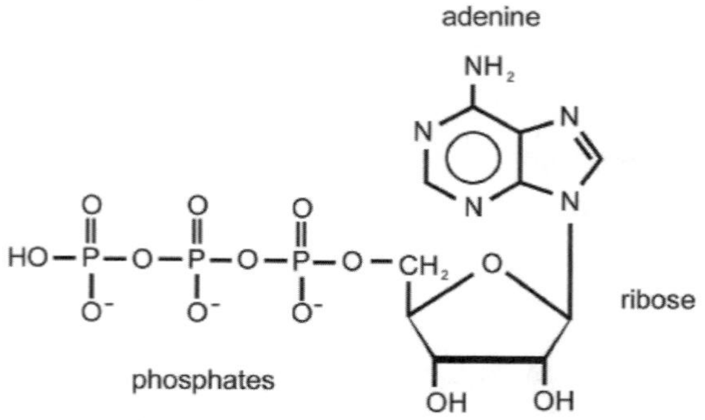

adenine

phosphates

ribose

(Figure 57) ATP

ADP+P are bonded to the site until the cross bridges connect to actin. ADT + P are then released and the actin filaments are moved by the myosin towards the "A" bands. When the power stroke is complete, new ATP molecules bond with the cross bridges on the myosin, the connection with actin is broken, and the filament is then at rest, ready for another contraction. The rigor complex occurs when a muscle contracts but there is no ATP available to release the actomyosin bond.

Muscle contraction is initiated when [Ca++] calcium ion concentration in the sarcoplasm is rapidly increased above a specific molar, 0.01M. Relaxation occurs below that concentration, when Ca++ is actively transported into the sarcoplasmic reticulum for storage in the terminal cisternae. Nerve stimulation releases Ca++ from the sarcoplasmic reticulum for attachment to troponin. The calcium pump is an active process in the sarcoplasmic reticulum membrane that requires ATP to rapidly move Ca++ back to the sarcoplasmic reticulum. Two proteins assist the

process, calsequestrin and calcium ATPase.

The transverse tubules between the terminal cisternae, seen in the details of the muscle fiber illustration (Fig.53), have pore openings through the sarcolemma and conduct electrical impulses from the cell membrane. The new electrical impulses from the motor neuron axon terminal stimulate the neurotransmitter acetylcholine at the synapse. This diffuses to a muscle fiber, changing sarcolemma permeability and opening the transverse tubule pores for sodium and potassium ions which then produce muscle fiber electrical impulses. The impulses enter through the pores and through the transverse tubules, causing the Ca++ to release from the sarcoplasmic reticulum, stimulating contraction as described above. This calcium concentration adjustment mechanism produces excitation-contraction coupling.

ATP is needed at two times in the contraction cycle. It is needed prior to ATP splitting and again to release the actomyosin cross bridge. Endurance

conditioning increases the ATP available in the muscle fiber for contraction.

In most certification manuals for personal trainers, muscle physiology is generally explained, at best, as follows: Contractile tissue contains actomyosin, a complex of the two contractile protein filaments that interact with each other— actin and myosin. When stimulated in the presence of adenosine triphosphate (ATP), the thicker myosin molecular filaments and the thinner actin molecular filaments slide into an overlapping position, shortening the sarcomere. Hydrolysis of the ATP provides the needed energy. After hydrolysis, the link is broken and the contraction is relaxed, and the muscle is prepared to repeat the contractile cycle. This is a very simplistic explanation of muscle contraction, usually with an equally simplistic diagram of the contractile proteins. Introductory certification programs for beginners in personal fitness training would benefit the profession by supplementing simplified explanations of muscle physiology with references to more comprehensive texts (e.g.Wilmore, 1999).

The computer graphics (Figures 58A-E) from the Molecular Biomechanics Laboratory at the University of Virginia, are molecular simulations, ribbon representations, and electron crystallography images of actin and myosin contractile proteins. These images are: myosin, G-actin, F-actin, the actomyosin complex, kinesin, and an acto-myosin model. Some of the other contractile proteins not included in these graphics are: Mg-actin, Ca-actin, calcyclin, myosin I, myosin II, myosinV, troponin C, calmodulin, calbindin, squidulin, tubulin, CDC31, caltractin, Ca-dependent protein kinase, ATP & ADP-bound kinesin, other forms of kinesin and many dyeins that are microtubule motor proteins. These are all extremely large and complex molecules. For instance, one of the smaller molecules in the group, G-actin, in the thin actin filament, contains over 5,000 atoms.

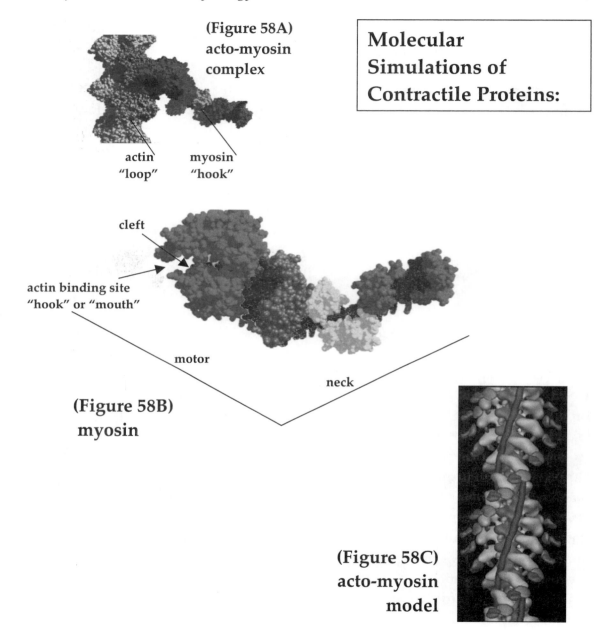

**(Figure 58A)
acto-myosin
complex**

actin
"loop"

myosin
"hook"

cleft

actin binding site
"hook" or "mouth"

motor

neck

**(Figure 58B)
myosin**

**Molecular
Simulations of
Contractile Proteins:**

**(Figure 58C)
acto-myosin
model**

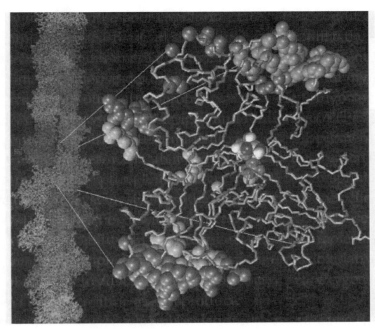

**(Figure 58D)
G-actin**

When viewing micotubules in a cell, tubulin protofilaments are seen as longitudinal striations. The filamentous dimeric subunits are chain-like associations of strong alternating alpha and beta tubulin monomers almost identical in structure at opposite ends of the molecule. The difference is in the amino acid sequence. Each monomer has a binding site for guanine nucleotide, for other proteins, and one for taxol that prevents cell division in cancer cells (www.lbl.gov/Science-Articles/Archive/taxol-site.html). The tubulin molecule has polarity. At the positive end more dimers are added than released and at the negative end more dimers are released than the re-association of new dimers. This function of polarity propels vesicle transport and direction-dependent cellular events.

Kinesin (Figure 58E), a motor protein, generates mechanical force by using energy from ATP hydrolysis. Kinesin performs organelle transport and chromosome segregation. It binds to and moves on or walks along

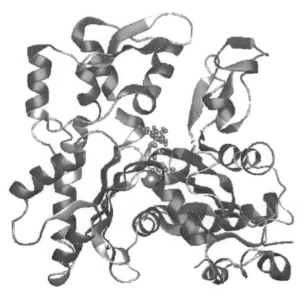

**(Figure 58E)
kinesin
ribbon representation**

microtubules. I have seen a close up digital video of this molecule walking along, end over end, on a microtubule. This walking action of changes in protein-microtubule interactions results in an eleven-degree rotation of the ATP-kinesine head relative to ADP-kinesine. Besides conventional kinesine, C-kinesine, kinesine I and II, and recent molecular discoveries, there are different forms of kinesin yet to be identified and their motor polarity determined. C-kinesine is most abundant as a retinal synapse photoreceptor. These kinesine motors transport mitochondrial and vesicular cargo along microtubules, accounting for orchestrated sliding between microtubules, and are involved in spindle motility. Kinesine II is concentrated in the axon and connecting cilium, inner segment, and synapse of photoreceptors. It assembles and maintains motile and sensory cilia.

Contraction is not exclusively proprietary to myosin and actin. Skeletal, smooth, and cardiac muscles are not the only cells in the body that incorporate contractile proteins. In fact, every cell in our body has them. Consider how life is able to duplicate itself. What force actually pulls the chromosomes in opposite directions (Figure 58F) during cellular division? What force moves cilia and flagella? How does a spermatazoa move its tail? What in the epithelial lining of the fallopian tube moves an ovum towards the uterus? What causes mucus to be transported out of the respiratory system? What force shortens the intercellular microfilaments and microtubules or rapidly reorganizes the cytoplasmic structure that is the inner lattice and tubulin cytoskeleton of a cell that supports enzymes and organelles, holding the hundreds to thousands of mitochondria in place within the cell? What causes the spindle apparatus in mitosis to function?

(Figure 58F) mitosis

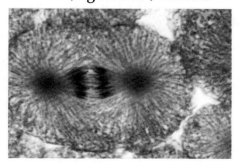

The answer is contractile proteins. Looking at it this way, all cells in our tissues contain proteins with contractile ability. All contraction requires energy.

Consider for a moment the amoeba entamoeba histolytica, a protozoan parasite and one of the simplest animals on Earth that use aquatic propulsion to move. What is the physiology of amoeboid movement? All systems are within one cell including the function of "muscle" contractility. What is the mechanism of contraction in an amoeba? Actin polymerization drives forward movement of the lamellipodium extension, which contains an extensive branched network of actin filaments. The positive end of these polar filaments is oriented toward the plasma membrane. Other proteins participating with actin at the leading edge of lamellipodium movement modify G-actin into it's ATP-bound form, bind to the sides of filaments to nucleate new growth, stabilize the network, bind to the plasma membrane pulling it forward along a growing actin filament, and depolarize and disassemble actin farther back from the leading edge. These other proteins with actin are: profilin, Arp2/3 complex (Actin-related proteins Arp2 and Arp3), cross-linking proteins, myosin I, cofilin and gelsolin.

In the regions being retracted at the rear of the amoeba are bipolar assemblies of myosin II that contract the tail end by sliding the actin filaments. Other binding proteins activate other proteins that in turn activate the proteins that nucleate actin polymerization at the leading edge.

Does the simple amoeba begin to sound complex? It is as complex as the human body on a single cell scale. To take this further, phospholipase C is signaled to activate and hydrolyse a protein that locally increases profilin, cofilin, gelsolin, and calcium ions. The cytosolic calcium accumulating at the tail end of the moving amoeba starts the actin-myosin II interaction. Actomyosin contracts the back as the actin filament assembly stretches out the front. ATP supplies the energy.

The amoeba moves forward through water. The next time you drink some bad water or eat contaminated food in a developing country and get amoebic colitis or dysentary, think of all those little aquatic exercisers developing endurance in your intestines in an aquatic class of their own.

Pathways to Energy

Anaerobic endurance is the efficient use of stored muscle-cell ATP to contract muscle fibers against resistance. It does not require external oxygen. Aerobic endurance is the duration and capacity of ATP production using external oxygen to contract slow twitch muscle fibers. Strength is a one-time event, an all-out full contraction of maximal fiber quantity; it does not require endurance, external oxygen, or duration under resistance. Power is the fast use of maximum strength, involving fast twitch fiber contraction through a range of motion.

Muscular endurance combines aerobic and anaerobic energy, utilizing contraction of the maximal muscle fibers of all types to deliver power over an extended time.

Proteins in general are polymers of amino acids in sequence. There are millions of different proteins unique to each species. These polymerized amino acid macromolecules are involved in the structure and function of every living organism.

Other examples of proteins, besides the contractile muscle proteins, are the hemoglobin that forms from an oxygen globular protein, collagen that forms from fibrous protein, and nucleic acids that are the linear polymers of nucleotides. For us, the nucleic acids carry all genetic information including traits like the quantity of muscle cells we have and the proportion of muscle fiber types.

We can develop efficiency of one muscle fiber type over another with training and conditioning programs designed for each type of muscle fiber. The growth in size of a muscle is an expansion of individual fibers, not an increase in the number of fibers.

Muscle fibers are classified as type I, IIA, and IIB. Oxydative ATP delivery is considered aerobic and glycolytic ATP delivery is considered anaerobic.

Type I are aerobic slow-twitch oxidative muscle fibers with high fat storage for fuel and a good capillary supply to deliver oxygen. Type I can repeat light activity, contraction and relaxation with low intensity for a considerable length of time. Type I muscle fibers utilize ATP delivered from the citric acid oxidative system for energy (Figure 68, page 143).

Type IIA muscle fibers are intermediate-oxidative and glycolytic, both aerobic and anaerobic fast-twitch fibers with moderate fat storage and a moderate supply of capillaries. Type IIA is a very healthy compromise producing high power that can be conditioned for a moderate duration of repeated use to a couple of minutes. Type IIA muscle fibers utilize energy from ATP that is delivered from the glycogen lactic acid system for energy—Embden-Meyerhof Pathway (Figure 67, page 142). Type IIB are pure fast-twitch

glycolytic anaerobic fibers with low fat storage and a poor capillary supply. Type IIB are all strength, delivering an immediate surge in muscle power, and super fast for up to a few seconds of anaerobic contraction with rapid fatigue and no repeatability. Type IIB muscle fibers use energy from ATP that is delivered from creatine phosphate in the glycolytic system (Figure 101, page 194) for a brief extension of their contractile ability. In the process, creatine phosphate gives up phosphate to ADP, rapidly producing ATP with creatine as a byproduct. During recovery, phosphorylation reverses the reaction by restoring creatine phosphate throuigh the addition of phosphate from ATP.

Hydrolysis breaks the polysacharide bonds of mega molecules stored in the liver into glucose molecules. When muscle glucose is depleted these mega molecules are hydrolyzed into glucose and added to the circulating blood to find their way to the muscles in need of energy.

When muscles are specialized and conditioned for aerobic respiration like the heart, they contain high concentrations of larger mitochondria and myoglobin in the cells, with low myocin adenosine triphosphatase (ATPase). Myoglobin is a protein pigment like hemoglobin and it stores oxygen in the muscle cells. Aerobic respiration is combustion within mitochondria during which one glucose molecule yields 38 ATP molecules. In the type I slow oxidative fatigue resistant fibers, oxygen is the final electron acceptor.

Type IIA fast oxidative glycolytic fibers have low myoglobin content, high myosin ATPase, large neurons, and have fatigue resistance. In this faster respiration, the combustion takes place in the cell cytoplasm, as pyruvic acid changes to lactic acid with one glucose molecule yielding 2 ATP molecules. Type IIB muscle fibers are rapidly fatiguing fast glycolytic fibers, innervated with large, high-threshold neurons. They have fast twitch response time, low mitichondrial enzyme content, low myoglobin, and have anaerobic metabolic pathway enzymes.

Muscle fiber types are determined genetically but each type is capable of increased efficiency through training. It is apparent that type IIA is a compromise between the slow oxidative and the powerfully fast glycolitic fibers. Cardiovascular aerobic endurance exercise is best achieved using type I, strength and power using type IIB, and muscle endurance using type IIA muscle fibers.

Muscle endurance training and conditioning increase innervation, fuel storage, contractile speed, tissue capillary quantity, the size of the fibers and the volume of cytoplasm, thus increasing capacity and efficiency for metabolic processes.

The recruitment of many smaller muscle groups during full-body aquatic resistance exercise results in the predominance of the anaerobic energy pathway when comparing aquatic exercise to land-based or deep-water treadmill running because many smaller muscle groups are recruited (Michaud, 1995). There is more muscle involvement caused by the need for more coordination and balance during complex movements under water's high resistance.

What is VO2max? It measures maximal oxygen consumption at the cellular level in liters per kilogram of body weight per minute and represents the capacity for aerobic resynthesis of ATP for cardiorespiratory endurance. Maximum oxygen consumption occurs when mitochondrial oxygen intake cannot increase despite an increase in exercise intensity. It is at a plateau. Exercise is anaerobic beyond that point, resulting in high levels of blood lactate. This point is the anaerobic threshold. Lactic acid (Figure 59) begins to accumulate quickly in most people before they reach their VO2max.

(Figure 59) Lactic Acid

Knowing the percentage of VO2max that is the anaerobic threshold and maintaining that percentage for a prolonged duration can improve aerobic potential. An untrained person has an anaerobic threshold of 55-60% of VO2max while endurance athletes have 85-90% thresholds. The rate of blood lactate accumulation is the same but the onset is delayed until higher exercise intensity and duration are reached. This threshold is the most important quantification of endurance because it determines how much aerobic potential is utilized. VO2max is primarily determined by genetics but is influenced to a large extent by training habits and the proportion of tissue that is metabolically active, i.e. by lean body mass.

VO2max is maintained among aerobically trained runners when deep water running is substituted for running on land. Maximal oxygen consumption, maximum heart rate, and ratings of perceived exertion were all lower for chest-deep aquatic exercise in a research study comparing it to land-based treadmill running (Hoeger, 1992).

Maximum heart rate is independent of fitness level and gender and is influenced by age (Tanaka, 2001). There is a new formula (Schnirring, 2001) that now replaces the inaccurate formula used since 1970. The old formula, 220 – age, has concerned cardiologists for a long time. Maximum heart rate was overestimated for young adults and underestimated for older adults, intersecting with the new formula at age 40 (Tanaka, 2001). The new formula for determining maximum heart rate is 208-(0.7 x age). It is the result of 351 cross-validated studies on 18,712 subjects. The research at the University of Colorado was published in 2001 in the *Journal of the American College of Cardiology* and noted as the first proposed new equation based on age and fitness-level ranges of healthy subjects. This change has repercussions with other calculations that use the old maximum heart rate formula. One is the land-based Karvonen Formula:

(220-age) minus (Resting heart rate) x (maximum target of 85%) + Resting heart rate = Maximum training

threshold. The range from the minimum to maximum target is 50% to 85%. From the beginning of the formula there is a widening error as the age becomes younger and older than 40 years old compared to using the new Maximum heart rate formula in the calculation (Fig.60).

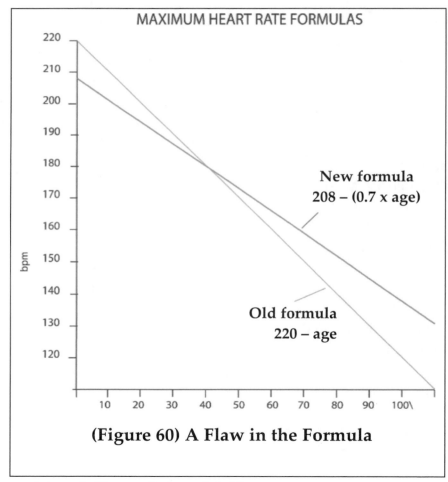

(Figure 60) A Flaw in the Formula

Sophisticated heart rate monitors that automatically display maximum heart rate, training thresholds, or any other displayed results using the commonly used old formula are only accurate at age 40. All the simple 220-age charts on gym walls are also inaccurate. For a fifteen-year-old it is overestimated by 7.5 bpm. For an 80 year old it is underestimated by 12 bpm.

Aquatic exercise instructors learn in their Aquatic Exercise Association training to deduct 17 bpm from the Karvonen Formula for calculating the aquatic training heart range. Why? When an individual exercises in colder water the heart rate is lower compared to exercising on land with comparable oxygen consumption (Avellini, 1983). The reason is due to a shift in blood volume from the periphery, as much as 700ml, to the body core's central circulation when exercising in chest deep water (Arborelius, 1972). Heart stroke volume increases with higher cardiac output and higher venous pressure (Haffor, 1991). The water pressure on leg veins just under the skin and

water pressure compressing the abdomen and rib cage increases transport of blood toward the heart. There are approximately 10 liters of blood plasma stored as peripheral interstitial (i.e. lymphatic) fluid. When a person is in cool water, some of the reserves are partially directed into the blood circulation (Lieb, 2003). This reduces the blood viscosity. The immediate adaptive physiological response to this peripheral decrease in fluid is for the heart to stretch its muscle fibers to increase in volume and contractile strength so as to pump more blood with each stroke (Lieb, 2003). This adaptation is called the Frank Starling Mechanism. The stroke volume becomes 35% larger (Arborelius, 1972). More blood is pumped per stroke so the frequency of pumping is less. Heart rate is decreased by up to 20 beats per minute (Mougios, 1993). Other similar studies yield from 10 to 17bpm lower (Sova, www.aeawave.com). However, in very warm water heart rate increases due to a rise in peripheral circulation. Therefore individuals with hypertension should avoid full

immersion in hot water for more than a few minutes.

Strength and power evolved for effectiveness in daily living situations: to build shelter, to carry fuel, to dig, fight, climb, protect and mate. Cardiovascular aerobic endurance meets a variety of challenges such as a lengthy hunt; a long journey of relocation like natives of Tahiti following bird migrations to the north and paddling canoes for thousands of miles to be the first human inhabitants of the Hawaiian Islands; the pursuit of a more promising homeland or more natural resources; seasonal migration, a lengthy harvest, food gathering, traveling trade routes, gathering and harvesting over vast distances, and evading an enemy.

It is a reasonable hypothesis that the production of ATP for anaerobic endurance began in evolution with a prokaryotic amoeboid. Using this assumption aerobic endurance began with bacteria. Then along came the eukaryotic amoeba that surrounded an aerobic non-photosynthetic bacterium and instead of enzymatically ingesting it, the bacterium was put to use in a symbiotic relationship. The bacterium survived as a mitochondrion within the amoeboid. The organism then had aerobic and anaerobic ATP production. This is the amoeba whose motility we described above. On and on it went through evolutionary time with many failures and very few successes. Natural selection ruled life's development. We have mitochondria in every cell of our body with the exception of mature red blood cells. Similarly, the ingestion and endosymbiotic establishment of these spirochetes, the bacterium, gave the ameboid organism aerobic energy for use by its contractile proteins, providing mobility and one of the basic foundations of the animal kingdom.

Mitochondria (Figure 61) are like factories containing biochemical laboratories within the folded inner walls of their membranes. Substances in a cell's cytoplasm enter the mitochondria and are broken down into constituentn parts for

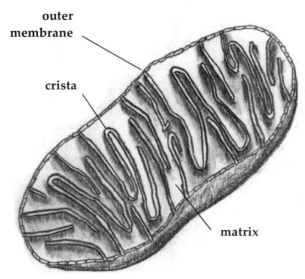

outer membrane

crista

matrix

(Figure 61)
Mitochondrion

reformulation into new suibstances and then released. Mitochondria increase in quantity and individual size from endurance training (Van De Graaff, 1995).

Mitochondria are genetically different from our cell nuclei. DNA and RNA are nucleic acids. The DNA (dioxyribonucleic acid) in mitochondria are double-stranded closed circles. DNA in cell nuclei are stranded helical spirals (Figure 62). RNA (ribonucleic acid) is a single

strand formed from one of the two spiraled DNA strands for the purpose of carrying out DNA directed activity in the cell cytoplasm. Purines and pyrimidines are nitrogen containing compounds. There are purines (Figure 65A) and pyrimidines (Figure 65B) that covalently bond the two DNA chains of pentose sugar-phosphate nucleoside polymers with phosphate linkages (Figure 63) together like a ladder (Figure 64). The pentose in DNA is deoxyribose and the pentose in RNA is ribose. The two purines, adenine and guanine, with the two pyrimidines cytosine and thymine, make up the four base components that are arranged and bonded in pairs on either side of the DNA "ladder" at a constant distance of 20 Å (angstrom) between the strands. 20 Å = 2 billionths of a meter in length. The pyrimidine, uracil, replaces thymine when the one-sided sequence is translated to RNA during its formation.

Mitochondrion ribosomes that function at sites of translation during protein synthesis resemble the ribosomes of bacteria and are different from the cells own cytoplasmic ribosomes in the cell. Mitochondria are similar in size and morphology to bacteria. They are independently self-reproducing and live within eukaryotic cells with their membrane-bounded nuclei. We could not live without mitochondria. We are at the tip of an evolutionary mountain that incorporated mitochondria to be the site of Krebs cycle reactions: aerobic respiration, oxidative phosphorylation of ADP to ATP, and the electron transport system of the mitochondrial cristae.

The chemical schematic of Energy Pathways is in two parts. On the left (Figure 67) is the glycogen-lactic acid system referred to as the Embden-Meyerhof pathway. It is anaerobic, without oxygen, and takes place in the cell cytoplasm. By glycogenolysis, glycogen stored in muscles is broken down into glucose-6-phosphate forming ATP, transforming glucose to lactic acid by hydrolysis. The lactic acid diffuses into the interstitial fluid and blood. Fatigue occurs from depletion of muscle glycogen and accumulation of lactic acid faster than

it can be carried to the liver to be recycled. Figure 68 represents aerobic energy production for muscular activity using the Krebs Citric Acid Cycle that takes place within the mitochondrion. The fuel is pyruvic acid, manufactured during glycolysis (Figure 67)

For aerobic endurance, ATP is produced by the mitochondria in the Krebs cycle using oxygen supplied by the blood. For anaerobic endurance, ATP is produced in the cell cytoplasm using stored fuel within the cell, the primal source of energy in what is called the Emden-Myerhof pathway (E-M) pathway (Figure 67). Anaerobic respiration in skeletal muscle cell cytoplasm involves the use of stored glycogen from dehydration synthesis of carbohydrates in muscle cells and in the liver. Glycogen (Figure 66) is animal starch. Similar to glycogen, starch is used for energy storage by plants. Glycogen is a polysacharide of joined glucose molecules in a highly branched configuration.

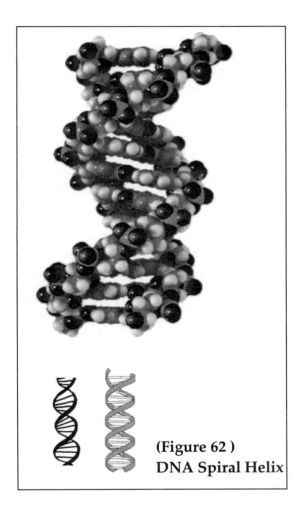

(Figure 62)
DNA Spiral Helix

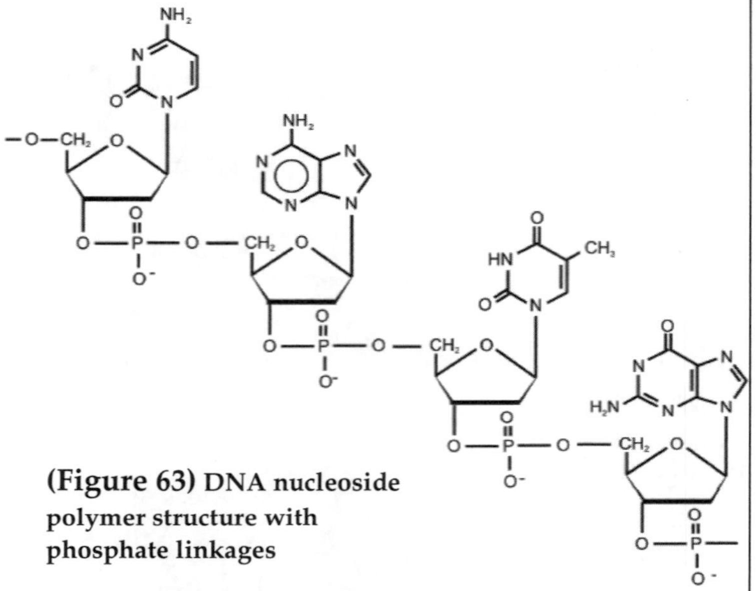

(Figure 63) DNA nucleoside polymer structure with phosphate linkages

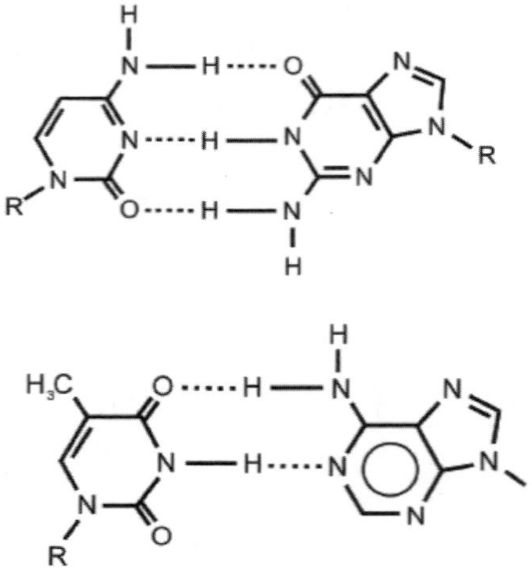

(Figure 64) Hydrogen bonded component bases between nucleoside polymer spirals (R)

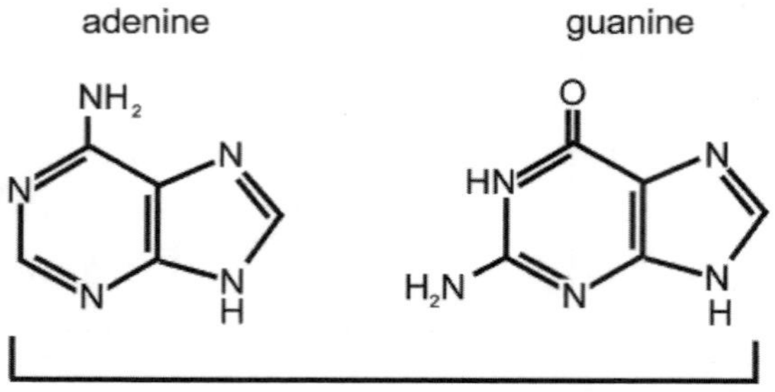

cytosine/guanine pair

thymine/adenine pair

adenine

guanine

cytosine

thymine

uracil

(Figure 65A) Purines in nucleic acids

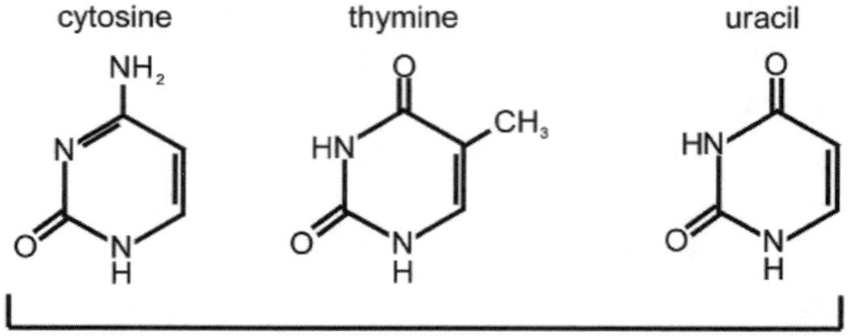

(Figure 65B) Pyrimidines in nucleic acids

Purines and Pyrimidines in DNA

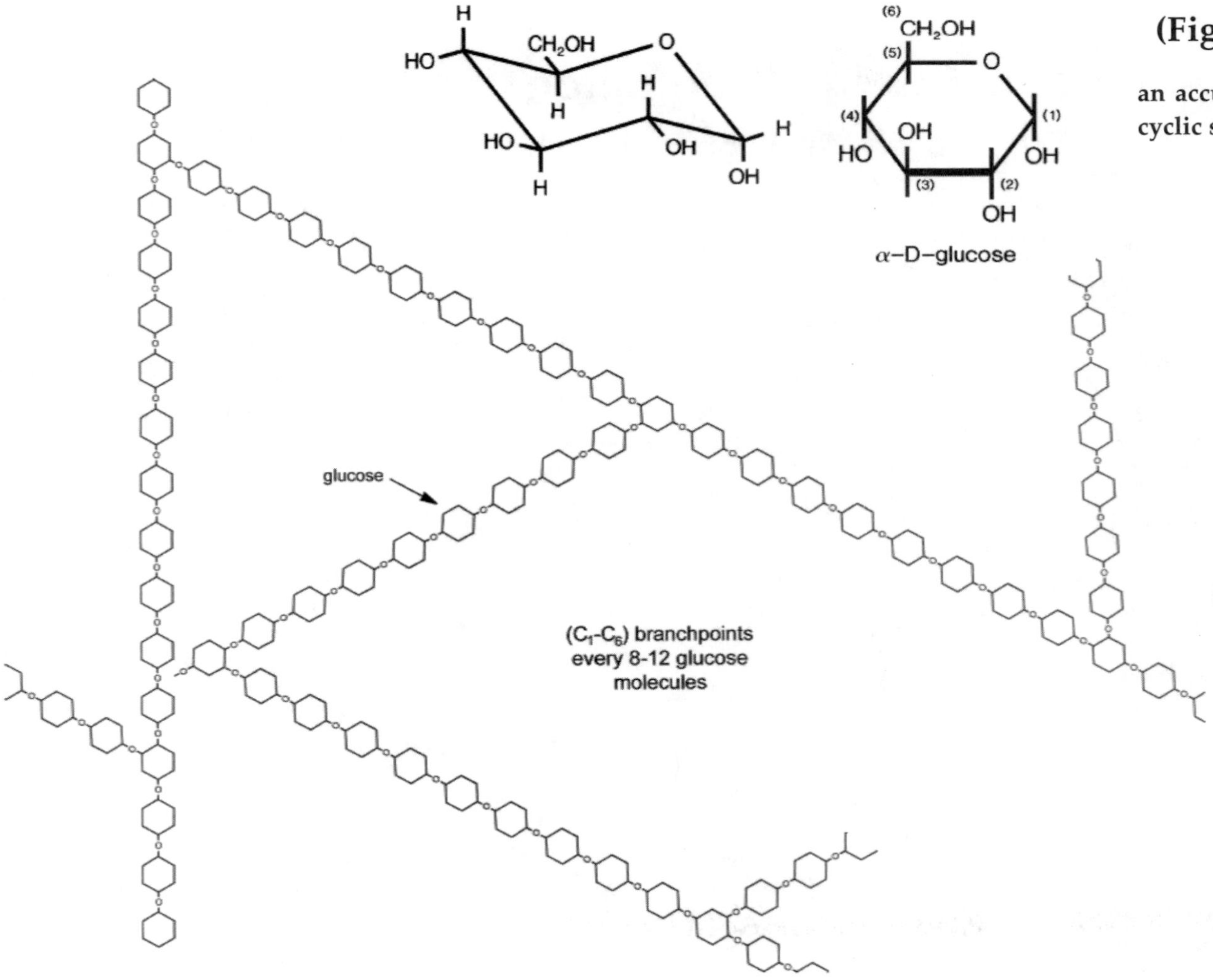
CH₂OH
HO
OH
(1)
(2)
(3)
(4)
(5)
(6)
α–D–glucose
glucose
(C_1-C_6) branchpoints every 8-12 glucose molecules

(Figure 66A)

an accurate representation of the cyclic structure of α-D-glucose

(Figure 66B) Glycogen, a Glucose Polymer

(Figure 67)

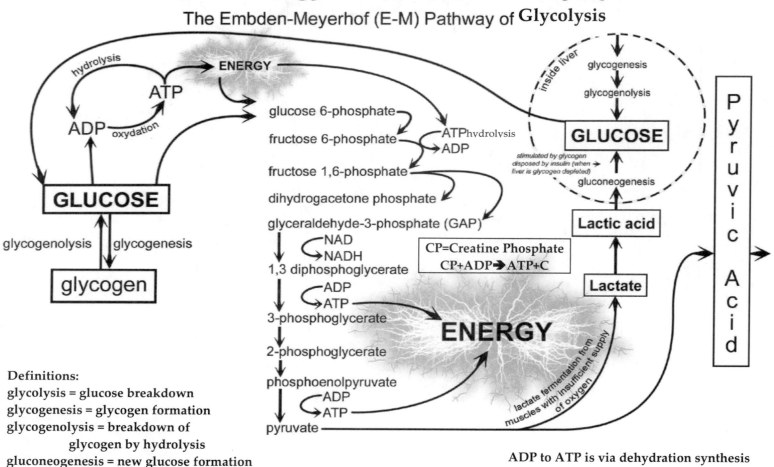

Anaerobic Energy Production in cell cytoplasm

The Embden-Meyerhof (E-M) Pathway of Glycolysis

Definitions:
glycolysis = glucose breakdown
glycogenesis = glycogen formation
glycogenolysis = breakdown of
    glycogen by hydrolysis
gluconeogenesis = new glucose formation

ADP to ATP is via dehydration synthesis

The anaerobic energy pathway is older than aerobic respiration from an evolutionary perspective due to the lack of oxygen in the early atmosphere.

(Figure 68)

Aerobic Energy Production inside mitochondria

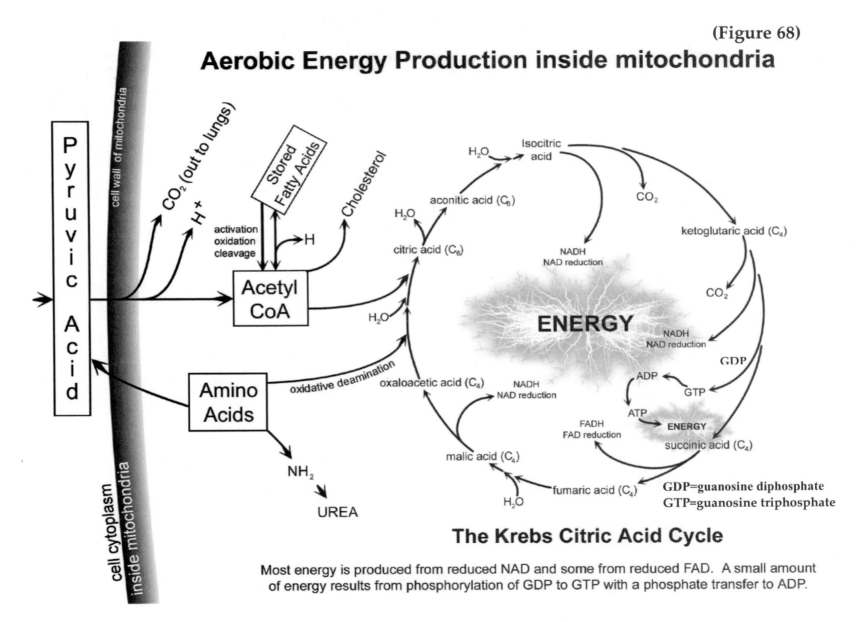

The Krebs Citric Acid Cycle

Most energy is produced from reduced NAD and some from reduced FAD. A small amount of energy results from phosphorylation of GDP to GTP with a phosphate transfer to ADP.

Nalu: The Art and Science of Aquatic Fitness, Bodywork & Therapy

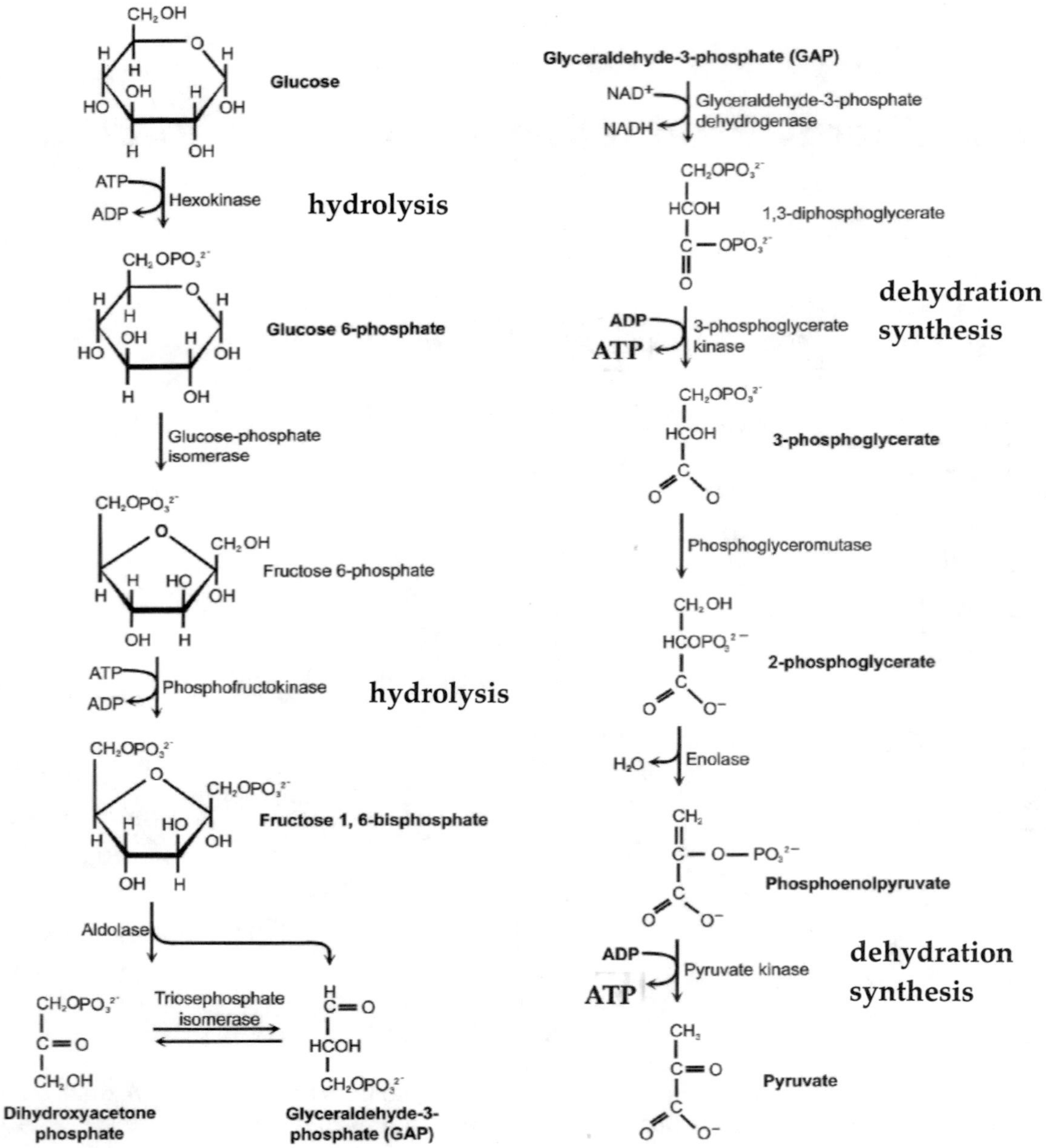

(Figure 69)
Anaerobic Energy Production, Up Close;
Glucose to Pyruvate

(Figure 70)

The Krebs Cycle up close

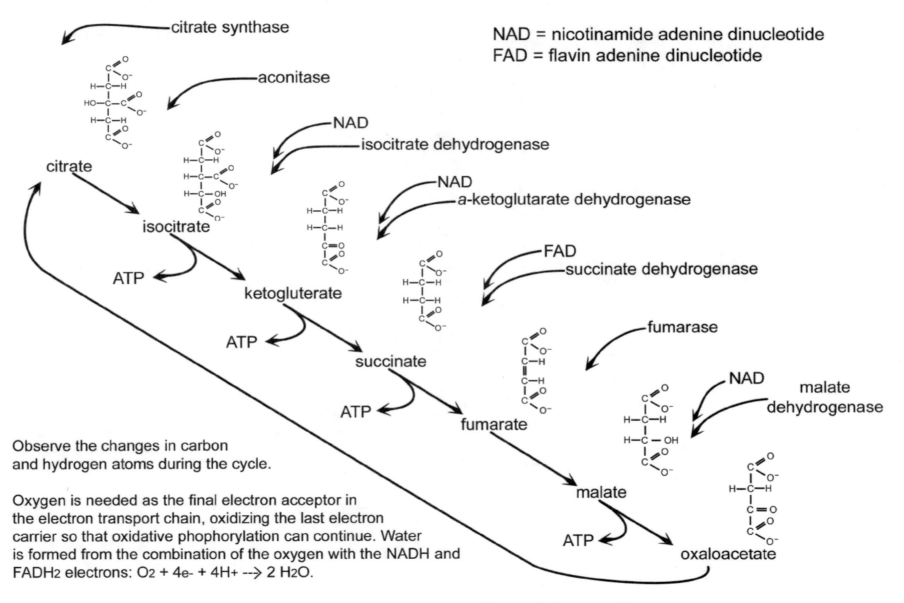

NAD = nicotinamide adenine dinucleotide
FAD = flavin adenine dinucleotide

Observe the changes in carbon
and hydrogen atoms during the cycle.

Oxygen is needed as the final electron acceptor in
the electron transport chain, oxidizing the last electron
carrier so that oxidative phophorylation can continue. Water
is formed from the combination of the oxygen with the NADH and
$FADH_2$ electrons: $O_2 + 4e^- + 4H^+ \rightarrow 2 H_2O$.

Nalu: The Art and Science of Aquatic Fitness, Bodywork & Therapy

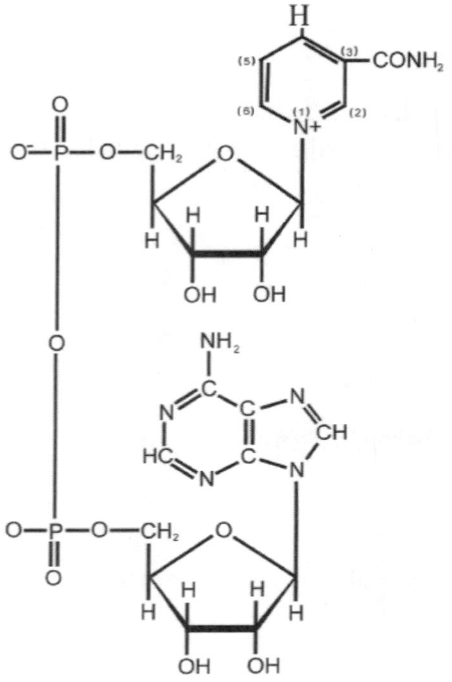

(Figure 71) NAD

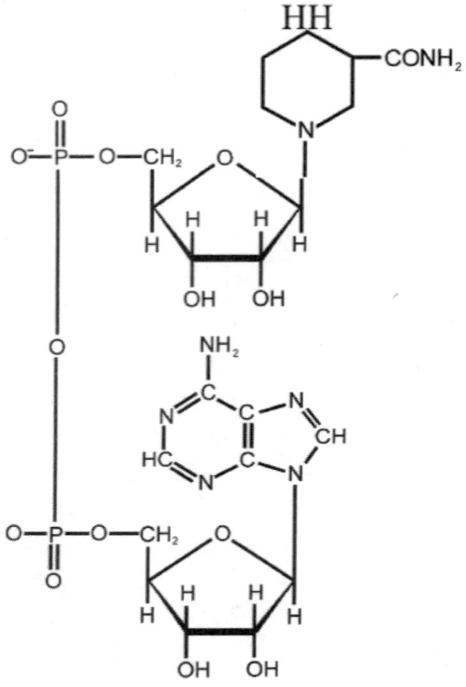

(Figure 72) NADH

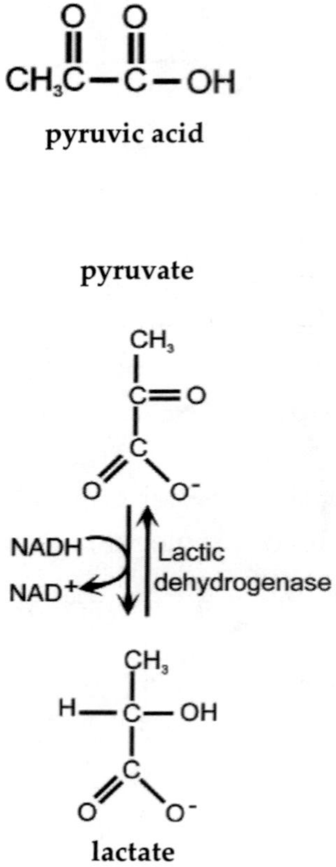

pyruvic acid

pyruvate

NADH / NAD+   Lactic dehydrogenase

lactate

**(Figure 73)
Lactate from Pyruvate**

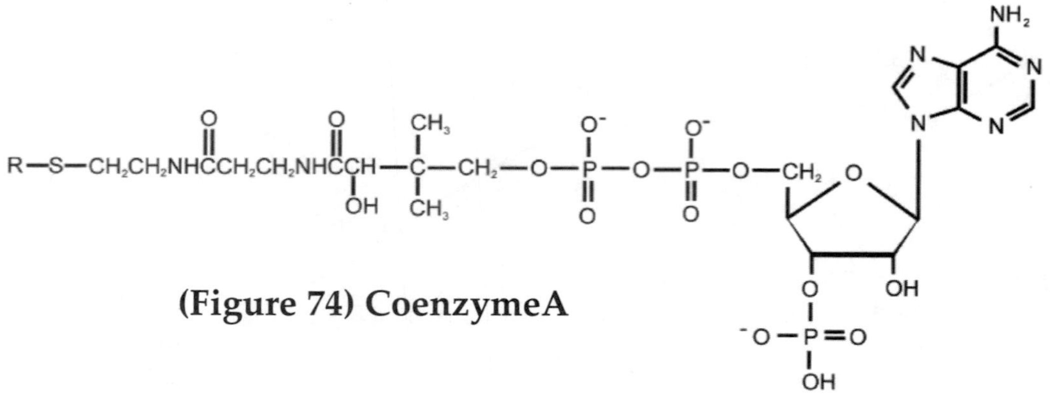

(Figure 74) CoenzymeA

Detailing anaerobic respiration, glycolysis metabolically and enzymatically breaks down glucose in the cell cytoplasm into pyruvic acid releasing hydrogen in the process. This released hydrogen reduces a coenzyme that transfers pairs of hydrogen atoms between adenine dinucleotide molecules, NAD (Fig.71). The hydrogen reduces the number of electrons as opposed to oxydizing or adding electrons. The result is two free hydrogen ions and two NAD molecules per glycolysis of one glucose molecule or 2x NADH (Fig.72).

The oxidative pathway to ATP production called the Krebs cycle is highly efficient and productive. During aerobic endurance training the Krebs cycle by itself does not become more efficient. Hemoglobin oxygen transport does become more efficient with an increase in capillaries and blood volume. There is an increase in the number of mitochondria. That is where this cyclic metabolic process takes place, oxydizing the acetic acid portion of acetalCoA, providing substrates coupled to the formation of

ATP. More mitochondria in a type I muscle cell increase the amount of energy that can be produced.

The Krebs cycle is slow. Anaerobic cell respiration is almost three times faster than aerobic respiration. Being fast has the advantage of quick action under high resistance. Being slow has the advantage of much energy production over time. Aerobic respiration is slow due to the complexity of the Krebs cycle. Pyruvic acid (Fig.73) enters mitochondria and is changed to carbon molecules that bind to coenzyme A (Fig.74) yielding acetyl CoA. CoenzymeA combines acetic acid with oxalic acid to form citric acid. Carbon dioxide is released. Three NAD convert to NADH+H. One FAD reduces to $FADH_2$. Oxidized iron ions gain one of the electrons and pass it on in the electron transport chain. Through the reduction and oxidation (redox) chain in the electron transport system occurring in the mitochondrial membranes, ATP is formed by oxidative phosphorylation, providing energy. Finally the electrons are given

to oxygen, which is reduced with two hydrogen atoms to form water. In the electron transport system within mitochondria during aerobic cell respiration, electrons are passed as pairs on electron carriers in the chain. This is demonstrated with the most common form of coenzyme-Q (ubiquinone) found in mammalian mitochondria (Johnson, 1983). During the Krebs cycle FAD is reduced, passing electrons to ubiquinone (Fig.75). Ubiquinone is reduced to ubiquinol, passing electrons in pairs.

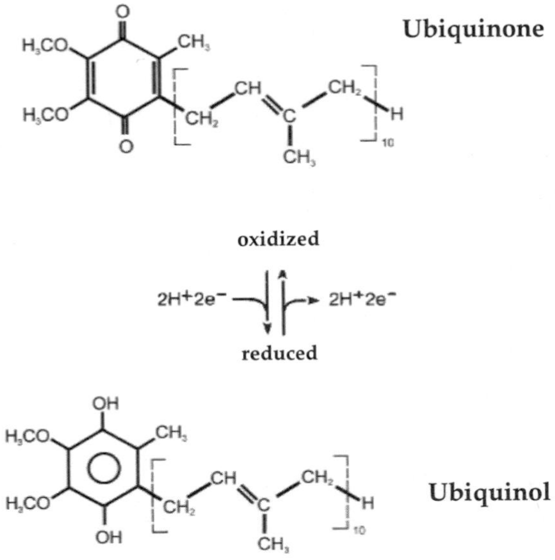

(Figure 75)

Water is the source of the oxygen we breathe. Oxygen comes from plant photosynthesis in a cell organelle called a chloroplast that functions as an energy producing "laboratory" equivalent to mitochondria in animal cells. The electron transport system functions in chloroplasts too. Phosphorylation of ADP to ATP occurs in chloroplasts and in mitochondria. Interestingly, like mitochondria, chloroplasts also have their own DNA and propagate independently from the cell; both synthesize proteins at translation sites called ribosomes that resemble the ribosomes of bacteria. The chemical process in a chloroplast is to absorb a quantum of red/blue spectrum sunlight providing the energy required for driving the chain of redox reactions that manufacture carbohydrates with oxygen as a byproduct. The resulting product is carbohydrate stored as starch. The carbohydrates we eat come from water and carbon dioxide during plant photosynthesis. Carbohydrates become "our fuel" and oxygen is "our fire".

The evolution of endurance began with and in water, a polar molecule with a negative charge at the oxygen end and a positive charge at the two hydrogen ends that are separated by an angle of sixty degrees. Other polar molecules can be attracted to these polar charges in a water molecule.

Going far, far back in time, how did the water molecule hold together and how were organic compounds formed? Atoms share electrons through covalent bonds. Ionic bonding is a transfer of electrons. In time, molecules and organic compounds form from water, carbon and nitrogen. Carbon is from carbon dioxide, and the nitrogen is ionized by lightening from the air. Organic compounds form into monomers which then form from macro-molecular polymers. Water molecules are removed by condensation reactions and are added by hydrolysis reactions. Monomers separate from one another.

Water insoluble membranes form from lipids. These boundaries become plasma membrane for cells. In plants the cellular membrane is cellulose. A cell's cytoplasmic matrix is 90% water, the environment for the organelles. Prokaryotic bacteria, blue-green algae, and eukaryotic nucleated cells emerge. Membranes compartmentalize cells to contain the organelles like the chloroplasts and mitochondria that are truly aquatic. The polymers become proteins, nucleic acids, sugars and carbohydrates, structural polysaccharides and membranes in an orderly sequence. Membranes are the basis for cell formation. Adaptation to the need for more endurance of any kind takes place within cell membranes.

*A*t the end of aerobic endurance

I was in a six man outrigger canoe in a long distance practice race up and down the Kona coast of the Big Island, from Keauhou Bay to Kawaihai and back, a long way to paddle at a competitive pace for miles and miles in a strong cross wind with rough water. "Hitting the wall" during the last ten miles happened to all six of us. For me it was not only being out of energy with the added burden of an oxygen debt, it was truly a wall. I traversed into a quiet world beyond numbness. The paddling motions were still there, the canoe kept going, but there was no sensation of touch. The other senses were distorted too, almost to the point of hallucinations. All I could feel was my breathing muscles. It was like a vehicle out of gas that kept going entirely on it's own momentum.

*A*t the end of anaerobic endurance

I was rock climbing at the southern edge of the Mojave Desert with a carpenter partner, Mingo. Our mission was to document new climbs for the Sierra Club, be the first to rock climb up difficult boulders, cliffs and outcroppings of majestic proportions. I was leading on one particular climb, placing the protection into crevasses and cracks. Mingo followed, keeping the rope tight, collecting the hardware, and being an anchor should anything go wrong at my end. It did go wrong. We had been

ascending difficult climbs all day. This would be the last one. Near the top I came to a ceiling I couldn't get past — it was hanging out 7' from the cliff wall and extended horizontally some thirty or forty feet. A narrow, irregular two-inch wide ledge became the tip toeing walkway and across I went to get to one end of it to perhaps go around the obstacle. I wedged the last protection in a crack and yelled for some slack in the rope to do a horizontal maneuver. The soft rubber tips on my tight climbing shoes clung to the smallest protrusions - now less than one inch wide. It was like tip toeing sideways in small steps. At the same time I could only grip the smooth white granite rock surface with my curled-over fingertips like stiff vices hooked onto the smallest of cracks and bumps. My elbows were already bloody from jamming them into larger cracks on the way up to insert metal wedges with carabiners for the rope to go through, so I was not exactly in a comfort zone.

I was very tense. All my muscles were contracted. There was fear and the

fear is what caused so much tension and unnecessary muscle contraction. It was constant. I slowly made my way across part of the ledge under the overhang. Mingo was a long ways down the cliff standing firm on a rock outcropping, holding the rope around his waist but still letting me have some slack to make progress. He could see me. I suddenly began to hurt all over. There was total muscle pain throughout my body. I was out of energy but the need for it was still maximal. I froze. Further progress was impossible. Lactic acid saturated every muscle. I yelled down to Mingo to brace himself and before I could finish the request, everything released and I went flying into a backward flip, end over end. It was a giant pendulum fall, like Tarzan, only I went careening into the side of a solid rock cliff on the other side of our climbing route. When I stopped swinging I was amazed that I was hanging there in the air with Mingo anchoring me from below and all the vertical wedges that I placed on the way up holding in place. I was anxious for Mingo to give me lots and lots of rope, to let me down to a wide ledge in case the top-most protection failed, the carabiner that held the pendulum swing. Yes, I was enveloped in abrasions from bouncing off the cliff. I was thankful to be wearing a helmet, a strong climbing harness and to have an experienced climbing partner. That was the limit of anaerobic endurance.

Metabolically, this is what was happening. The rigorous ascent to the overhang depleted muscle glycogen. Being the lead climber with protection only being placed below me and being in a very precarious position with all my body weight placed on the tips of my toes and fingers, I was tense. There was simultaneous, maximal neuronal firing of nearly every major muscle group and no glycogen for fuel. As a result, extracellular potassium accumulated at the axons, temporarily interfering with impulse production. The fatigue became severe. I felt frozen in one place as I clung to the granite. It was painful. I couldn't move.

In my liver the Cori Cycle was started—this is gluconeogenesis or reverse glycolysis, a life-saving attempt at recovery. The need for energy was critical. The lactic acid that was delivered from muscles to the liver was quickly being converted into pyruvic acid. Liver enzymes converted pyruvic acid into glucose 6-phosphate for glycogen synthesis or the secretion of glucose back into the blood for energy. Fast-twitch muscle fibers were then recruited and utilized, converting glucose back to lactic acid. There was a subsequent increase in hydrogen ion concentration from the lactic acid that temporarily lowered the pH in my muscle cells. The acidity reduced ATP production by inhibiting specific glycolytic enzymes. The need for overall major muscle contraction was greater than the production of energy.

Then came failure. Suddenly there was no pain and no muscle contraction. I could feel my body depart from the cliff wall. Without ATP, calcium ions could not accumulate by active transport in the sarcoplasmic reticulum. ATP is the source of the energy needed to pump the calcium ions into the terminal cisternae of the sarcoplasmic reticulum during the relaxation phase of muscle contraction. The relaxation phase is a prerequisite to calcium release for attachment to troponin for stimulating muscle contraction. This compromised the excitation-contraction coupling so the muscles could not respond to electrical stimulation. They instantly gave up.

Life needs glycogen and ATP. The totality of the muscle failure was a last resort to prevent brain death. The central nervous system is always the priority when it comes to survival so the muscles shut down and I went tumbling into space.

⤜«((((O⪢   ⤜«((((O⪢   ⤜«((((O⪢

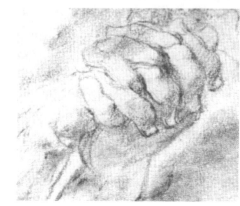

Chapter 4
Mobility

The Contractile Element

It's time to close your chemistry and physics books for a moment and turn to your most detailed anatomy books. Search for each muscle, look at their attachments to bones, and visualize how their contractile force creates each action listed below. Movements at joints are: flexion, extension, abduction, adduction, rotation, circumduction, inversion, eversion, protraction, retraction, elevation, and depression.

Muscle Actions Chart

(Excluding Phalanges and Face)
* =prime movers

Rotation of head
Sternocleidomastoid (unilateral) *
Splenius capitis (unilateral)*
Splenius cervicis (unilateral)*

Flexion of the head
Splenius capitis (unilateral)*
Slenius cervicis (unilateral)

Flexion of neck
Sternocleidomastoid *
Scalenes (unilateral & bilateral)

Extension of the neck
Splenius capitis (bilateral)*
Splenius cervicis (bilateral)*

Abductors of the wrist
Flexor carpi radialis*
Extensor carpi radialis longus*

Adductors of the wrist
Extensor carpi ulnaris*
Flexor carpi ulnaris*

Flexors of the wrist
Flexor carpi radialis*
Flexor carpi ulnaris*
Palmaris longus

Extensors of the wrist
Extensor carpi radialis longus*
Extensor carpi radialis brevis*
Extensor carpi ulnaris*

Pronators of the forearm
Pronator teres*
Pronator quadratus*

Supinators of the forearm
Bicept*
Supinator*

Extensors of the elbow
Triceps*
Anconeus*

Flexors of the elbow
Biceps(short head)*
Brachialis*
Brachioradialis*
Pronator teres

Medial rotators of the humerus
Anterior deltoid*
Pectoralis major*
Subscapularis*
Teres major*
Latissimus dorsi*

Lateral rotators of the humerus
Infraspinatus*
Teres minor*
Posterior deltoid*

Adductors of the humerus
*Pectoralis major**
*Coracobrachialis**
*Latissimus dorsi**
*Teres major**

Abductors of the humerus
*Supraspinatus**
*Middle deltoid**

Flexors of the humerus
*Anterior deltoid**
*Pectoralis Major (clavicular head)**
*Coracobrachialis**
Bicept (short head)

Extensors of the humerus
*Latissimus dorsi**
*Teres major**
*Posterior deltoid**
*Infraspinatus**
*Teres minor**
*Triceps (long head)**
*Pectoralis major (sternal head)**

Horizontal abductor of the humerus
*Posterior deltoid**

Horizontal adductors of the humerus
*Anterior deltoid**
*Pectoralis major**

Upward rotators of the scapula
*Upper trapezius**
*Lower trapezius**
*Serratus anterior**

Downward rotators of the scapula
*Levator scapula**
*Rhomboids**
*Pectoralis minor**

Protractors of the scapula
*Pectoralis minor**
*Serratus minor**

Retractors of the scapula
*Middle trapezius**
*Rhomboid**

Elevators of the scapula
*Upper trapezius**
*Levator scapula**

Depressors of the scapula
*Pectoralis minor**
*Lower trapezius**

Flexors of the spine
*Interenal oblique (bilateral)**
*Iliocostalis (unilateral)**
*Longissimus (unilateral)**
*Spinalis (unilateral)**
*Intertransversarii**

Extensors of the spine
*Iliocostalis (bilateral)**
*Longissimus (bilateral)**
*Spinalis(bilateral)**
*Semispinalis(bilateral)**
*Multifidus (bilateral)**
*Rotatores**
*Interspinalis**

Rotators of the spine
*Semispinalis (unilateral)**
*Multifidus (unilateral)**
*Rotatores**

Rotators of the trunk
*Internal oblique (unilateral)**
*External oblique (unilateral)**

Flexors of the trunk
*Rectus abdominus**
*External oblique (bilateral)**
*Quadratus lumborum**

Compressors of the abdomen
*Rectus abdominus**
*External oblique (bilateral)**
*Internal oblique (bilateral)**
*Transverse abdominus**

Inspirators and expirators
*Intercostals**
*Diaphragm**
*Serratus posterior superior**
*Serratus posterior inferior**

Lateral rotators of the hip
*Piriformis**
*Gemellus**
*Obturator internus**
*Gemellus inferior**
*Obturator externus**
*Quadratus femoris**
*Bluteus maximus**
*Iliopsoas**
*Sartorius**

Medial rotators of the hip
*Gluteus medius**
*Gluteus minimus**
Tensor fasciae latae
Pectineus
Adductor longus
Adductor brevis
Adductor magnus (horizontal fibers)

Flexors of the hip
*Iliopsoas**
*Pectineus**
Tensor fasciae latae
Adductor brevis
Adductor magnus (anterior portion)
Rectus femoris
Sartorius

Extensors of the hip
*Gluteus maximus**
*Biceps femoris (long head)**
*Semitendinosus**
*Semimembranosus**
Adductor magnus (posterior portion)

Abductors of the hip
*Gluteus medius**
*Gluteus minimus**
Tensor fasciae latae
Sartorius

Adductors of the hip
*Adductor brevis**
*Adductor longus**
Adductor magnus8
*Gracilis**
Pectineus

Lateral rotator of the knee
*Biceps femoris**

Medial rotator of the knee
*Semitendinosus**
*Semimembranosus**
*Popliteus**
Gracilis
Sartorius

Extensors of the knee
*Vastus lateralis**
*Vastus intermedius**
*Vastus medialis**
*Rectus femoris**
Tensor fasciae latae

Flexors of the knee
*Biceps femoris**
*Semitendinosis**
*Semimembranosus**
Sartorius
Bracilis
Gastrocnemius
Plantaris
Popliteus

Dorsiflexors of the ankle
*Tibealis anterior**
Extensor digitorum longus
Peroneus tertius
Extensor hallucis longus

Plantar flexors of the ankle
Gastrocnemius*
Soleus*
Plantaris
Peroneus longus
Peroneus brevis
Tibialis posterior
Flexor hallucis longus
Flexor digitorum longus

Invertors of the foot
Tibialis anterior*
Tibialis posterior*

Evertors of the foot
Peroneus tertius*
Peroneus longus*
Peroneus brevis*

Slowly study the muscle origins and insertions at attachments to bones using more than one anatomy book. They will show different anatomical views for a better perspective. A muscle origin is usually medial or proximal, and is closer to the spine. Muscle insertions are usually lateral or distal, and farther from the spine. Look at each bone landmark, groove,

projection, and prominence carefully to see exactly where the attachment is located on the periosteum of the bone. Visualize the contraction of the muscle and the direction of force on the bone. Learn the actions, muscles, tendons, ligaments, bones, landmarks on the bones, and muscle attachment points. This will take considerable effort to permanently input the data and images into your memory until you can speak confidently without hesitation using this knowledge. There is a study method described in the section on *Articular Surroundings*. This takes time.

The muscle we will analyze is the powerful psoas major with the iliacus (Figure 76). The psoas major crosses several joints at the central core of the body: L-5/sacrum, sacroiliac, and the iliofemoral joint. The psoas muscle originates on the bodies and transverse processes of lumbar vertebrae T12 - L5, passes the sacrovertebral joint, and merges with the iliacus that originates on the iliac fossa. Together they pass between the inguinal ligament and the iliopubic eminence and over the iliofemoral

joint to their common insertion on the lesser trochanter of the proximal femur. We will consider the iliopsoas as one muscle. The action of the iliopsoas is femur flexion and rotation, and vertebral column flexion when the femur is in a fixed position. The iliopsoas is the strongest hip flexor.

The one skeletal muscle that remains the strongest in the body for the longest time, well into the geriatric years, is the iliopsoas. It is important to keep it strong as long as possible because the iliopsoas is the walking muscle. It is the first initiator of hip flexion. The beginning of taking a step is from contraction of the iliopsoas. It takes the first step and the last step in a person's lifetime. When it is weakened by pregnancy, the other hip flexors do the initiating. This causes a "duck walk." When it is weakened from atrophy by doing too much sitting, older people have difficulty beginning to walk. Taking that first step becomes an immense challenge.

*T*heo walks barefoot in the sand.

For a couple of years I took Miss Theo Vickery for a thirty to sixty minute walk in Old Town Key West late every afternoon. Some call her Miss Vickery or Vicky. I call her Theo. She was a Bell Telephone Operator during WWII when there were a lot of sailors in Key West. She is a near-centenarian at 97 years old, was living independently in her own home, doing her own grocery shopping, pushing her own shopping basket, taking care of herself. In her worn down Birkenstock sandals, she would take a small pail of grain to feed the wild chickens that live around the Key West library and in its Palm Garden. Theo is so interested in watching the chicks grow, in smelling flowers along the way, looking at airplanes descending to the island, saying hello to her neighbors, watching her wild Jasmine bloom after a storm, admiring the growth of her productive tropical fruit trees (papaya, banana, avocado) and talking about Key West history, visiting the large graveyard where most everyone she ever knew is located now, petting friendly sidewalk cats and dogs behind fences, and she is fascinated by unusual architecture.

(Figure 75)

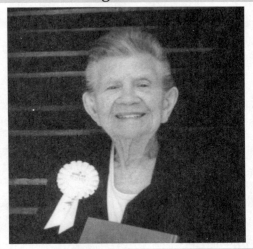

Miss Theo Vickery (2003)
Key West, Florida

One special enjoyment for Theo has been walking barefoot in the dry, fluid-like, fine Bahama sand at Higgs Beach, stepping high, gazing out across the Caribbean blue towards Havana. There and elsewhere she talks about horse and buggy days in North Georgia where she was born in Hart County, now under Lake Hartwell, about her father's first "Tin Lizzy" in Sanford, Florida, and her nephew John Schneider who was the blonde kid in " The Dukes of Hazard." Theo has witnessed the change of horses to automobiles, trains to airplanes, out-houses to indoor plumbing and oil lamps to rural electrification. She has a lot to say. In the last hundred yards of our walks back to her house on Love Lane, she wanted to walk fast, more or less like a sprint to the finish. Suddenly she will say "gettyup, gettyup, gettyup", propelling all of her nearly ninety-seven years and seventy-six pounds down the lane at her full walking speed with me keeping up at her side for safety. I was just a grab bar and a friend.

It was the development of her iliacus and psoas muscles (Figure 76) which enabled her to do what she could without ambulation equipment (wheelchair, walker, cane). Two years previously Theo had been living in a convalescent center using a wheelchair and a walker to go from her room to the cafeteria and back three times a day. She was recovering from two recent surgeries and two past strokes. She hated the place and wanted to live by herself at home again on Love Lane, originally called Johnny Cake Alley. In the convalescent center she could see that the patients never do go home again. They live out their weakening lives and die in those institutions.

At the convalescent center I began to take Theo on walks to get her out into the fresh air every day. At first I pushed her in the wheelchair. After a while, out in the parking lot, I would face her from a short distance away and ask her to stand up. Carefully, with great focus, she would rise to a standing position. In a short time she was taking three or four tiny wobbling steps forward, then having to sit down again in the wheelchair. In a matter of a week she was using a walker, one difficult step at a time for several minutes. After two months she was walking slowly for up to fifteen minutes while holding my hand. Then we found some steps to climb across the street at the college campus. That was a pivotal moment because it was hard work and her iliopsoas muscles responded by

gaining strength and muscle endurance. The iliopsoas is the strongest muscle in her body and is the reason why this near-centenarian was able to walk so well again. Without the endurance of the iliopsoas muscle, humans would not have migrated out of Africa and would not have crossed the Bearing land bridge to inhabit the American Continent. We may have become paddlers instead of both paddlers and walkers.

The walks became more than a desire for outdoor fresh air and nature. They became regular exercise and a way to get away from the convalescent center indefinitely. And that she did, not by asking her doctor but by telling him what she was going to do and when she was going to go home. Theo became stronger and let go of my hand on a long walk through the quiet Truman Annex development over two years ago. She only held my hand when crossing the street or is approaching a curb. She expressed a desire to find a pool for rehabilitating from immobility and pain in her left thigh and for physically conditioning

her whole body with water resistance. Theo wanted to improve her balance to complete her remarkable recovery, a testament to willpower. So to the pool we went one afternoon concentrating on treating her left adductor magnus that had been the source of her complaint. The slow stretching and warm water were a perfect preparation for the exercises that followed and the rehabilitation was successful. Now Theo wants to return to the pool again.

><((((○>   ><((((○>   ><((((○>

When assisting elderly individuals in an aquatic program or in any other situation, the most rewarding and successful outcomes result when the caregiver fosters an environment of self-motivation, socialization, as much independence as is safely possible, and daily regularity for both physical and mental exercise. Mental exercise involves lively and interesting conversations that include dates, times, years, history, travel, experiences that have stimulated the senses, very recent activities and short-term plans.

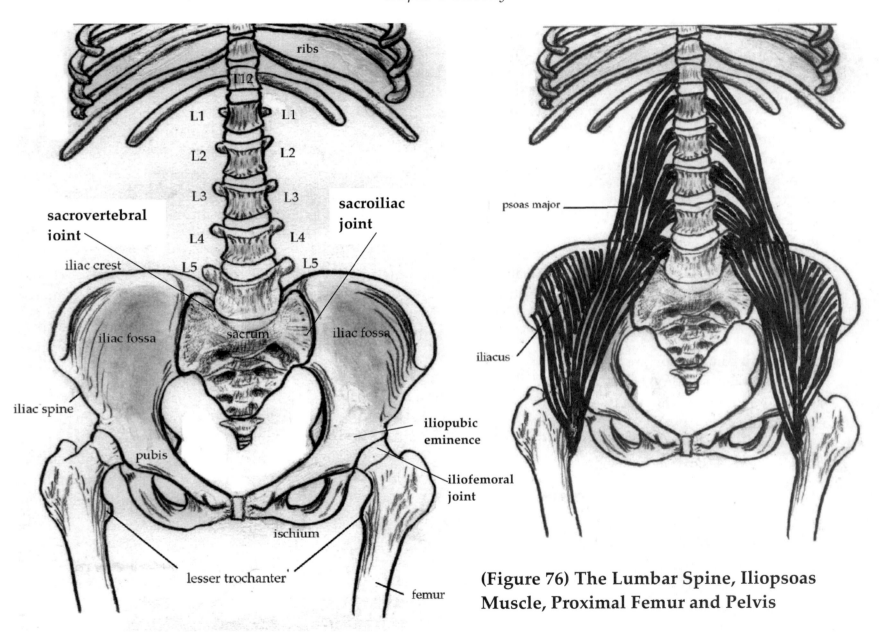

ribs

T12

L1   L1

L2   L2

L3   L3

sacrovertebral joint

sacroiliac joint

iliac crest   L4   L4

L5   L5

iliac fossa   sacrum   iliac fossa

iliac spine

iliopubic eminence

pubis

iliofemoral joint

ischium

lesser trochanter

femur

psoas major

iliacus

(Figure 76) The Lumbar Spine, Iliopsoas Muscle, Proximal Femur and Pelvis

Tendons stretch and recoil, storing potential energy during the stretch and returning elastic strain energy during the recoil. Tendons contain just enough elastin for optimal elasticity while still maintaining tissue strength. Recoil velocity is faster in tendons than contraction velocity in muscles (McNeill, 2002). Tendon elasticity affects control of muscle, not control of limb position. This will be an exploration into the series elastic element and its relationship to exercise performance.

Tendon and ligament composition are similar. They are both dense fibrous connective tissue but their functions are different. Ligaments, not always well defined, connect bones to bones while tendons link muscles to bones. They both adapt to specialized functions with variations in their properties throughout the body.

The tendons, as well as ligaments, have a low vascular supply. The blood comes from the peremysium that covers the tendon, from surrounding tissue, and from the blood supply at the periosteal insertion. They don't need metabolic energy because they don't contract. Tendons respond to load application structurally and mechanically.

Tendons have a hierarchical structure (Figure 77). The sheath-covered tendon structure surrounded by the layers of the peritenon splits into tertiary, secondary, and primary bundles of fascicles containing fibrils and parallel rows of fibroblasts, the tendon-forming cells. A fibril has a waviness or crimped pattern that can be stretched out until the collagen fibril is stiff. The wavy crimped pattern and its ability to recoil back from straightened stiffness to its original shape are the key to efficient tendon behavior. The fibril pattern contributes to the stress strain relationship where the recoil force is greatest at maximum extension. The collagen fibrils are composed of subfibrils which contain microfibrils.

Tendons have a major role in proprioception. Golgi tendon organs and mechanoreceptors sense tension and resistance to muscle contraction.

Another function of tendons as well as ligaments is energy storage. In a study measuring elastic energy storage in runners, the energy stored in the Achilles tendon, quadriceps tendon, and in foot ligaments was as much as 50% of the requirement for running (Alexander and Bennet-Clark, 1977). During recoil after flexion, most of the stored energy is released by the tendon.

The dry weights of both tendon and ligament have percentages of mostly type I collagen, the primary ingredient, that are not far apart, ranging from 70-85%. Type I collagen is a protein blend of glycine, proline, and hydroxyproline. Tendons and ligaments have a similar small percentage of proteoglycans to reduce friction when compressed by adjacent bones. The major difference in the dry weight percentages between tendon and ligament is the amount of elastin. Tendon has 3% or less elastin and ligament has up to 15% (Martin, Burr, Sharkey, 1998).

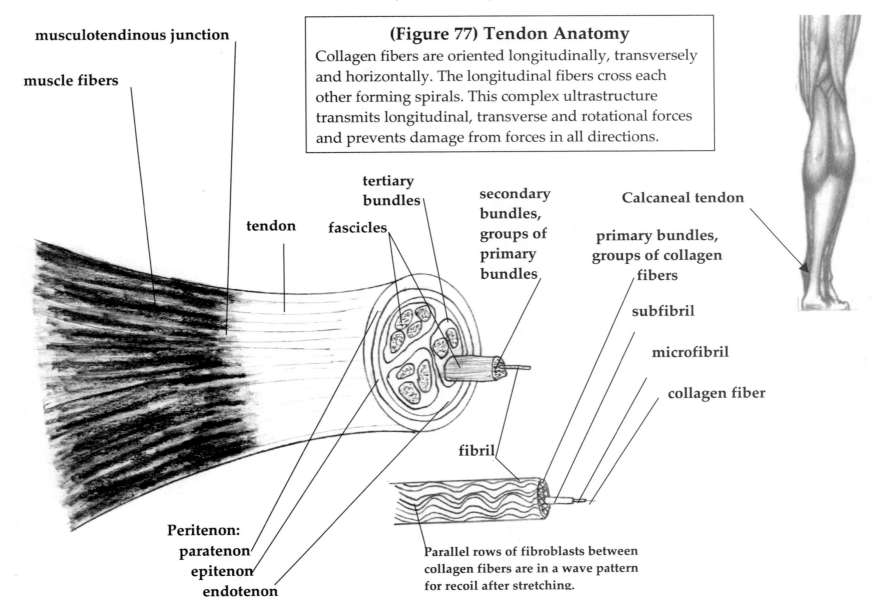

musculotendinous junction

muscle fibers

(Figure 77) Tendon Anatomy
Collagen fibers are oriented longitudinally, transversely and horizontally. The longitudinal fibers cross each other forming spirals. This complex ultrastructure transmits longitudinal, transverse and rotational forces and prevents damage from forces in all directions.

tertiary bundles

secondary bundles, groups of primary bundles

Calcaneal tendon

tendon   **fascicles**

primary bundles, groups of collagen fibers

subfibril

microfibril

collagen fiber

fibril

Peritenon:
paratenon
epitenon
endotenon

Parallel rows of fibroblasts between collagen fibers are in a wave pattern for recoil after stretching.

In the absence of research data and with studies on aquatic exercise limited primarily to cardiac improvements, we will proceed with the reasonable hypothesis that aquatic exercise increases tendon and muscle length because of greater opportunities to stretch and move isokinetically through a full range of motion. Longer muscles and greater elasticity of tendons increase the efficiency of exercise performance in the muscle-tendon unit that includes the contractile and series elastic elements. The entire unit comprises the muscle, musculotendinous junction, tendon sheath, tendon, and the osteotendinous junction. Within the unit are sensory organs monitoring the characteristics and changes that occur during activity.

Tendon mechanics is both nonlinear and viscoelastic. The viscoelastic property of tendons indicates time-dependent mechanical behavior. In addition to extension, the stress-strain relationship depends on the duration of load application and is not constant. Stress is reduced during constant deformation and deformation increases under a constant load.

The long flexor tendons show high strength compared to extensor tendons and they are stiffer to conserve more energy, though they are the same at birth before functional adaptation (Shadwick, 1990). Compared to extensor tendons, flexor tendons are like biological springs. During deceleration, extensor tendons are not elongated so they do not need higher strength.

The amount of force developed in a movement is dependent to a large extent on the tendon condition and the timing of stimulation in relation to the successive changes in length, the length-change cycle (Johnston, 1991). The range of velocity is narrow for optimum efficiency of the muscle contraction itself. Peak power velocities have a broader range. A very wide range of velocities of power and absorption is needed for locomotion. The generation of power by a muscle is quite limited without the series elastic element. Tendon elasticity is crucially important to exercise performance because it increases cycle velocity and conserves muscle energy. The amount of series elastic compliance can strongly affect the efficiency of a muscle contraction without dramatically changing the generated muscle force (Ettema, 1996). Both stiff and compliant muscles have equal series elastic efficiency demonstrating that muscle efficiency is not better or worse due to storage and re-utilization of series elastic energy (Ettema, 2001). The improvement is in the utilization of energy (Biewener, 2000).

Tendon elasticity decelerates a mass, and accelerates a mass with the recoil effect from stored energy. Body mass has an influence by being in balance with the amount of tendon elasticity in the mass/spring system. During optimal exercise performance tremendous elastic energy is stored and released by the tendon, as the muscle only needs to work nearly isometrically to keep the cycle going. The tendon stores energy as potential energy, not kinetic energy. Kinetic energy is similar to pedaling an old-fashioned treadle sewing machine after it gets going, or the large wheel of a seated treadle sharpening stone used for sharpening a farmer's mule-powered discs and plows, or the energy contained in a moving wagon. Kinetic energy only takes the slightest little push to maintain an optimal velocity. Stored elastic energy is potential energy. It is available when it is released during the recoil phase as a component of the entire series elastic element.

Getting back to Theo's walks in the sand at Higgs Beach, tendon elasticity doesn't have a chance to show off its characteristics there. This has a profound effect on mechanics and energetics. Using a force platform and testing oxygen consumption, walking and running in sand were compared to the same activities on a hard surface. There is a big difference between walking on sand and on a hard surface. It takes more energy to walk on sand because there is more mechanical work and muscle/tendon efficiency is decreased. Walking on sand doubles or triples the work that would be needed at the same speed on a hard surface. Running on sand is

only slightly more mechanical work, needing 1.6 times the energy compared to running at the same speed on a hard surface. Depending on the running technique, an initial heel strike would be inefficient because the heel touchdown is in front of the vertical line of body's center of gravity. In a constantly efficient running technique like the Pose method (Romanov, 2002), developed by Dr. Nicholas Romanov, there is no heel strike and the forefoot touch-down right under the center of gravity allows for full use of Achilles tendon length to recoil for most of the energy needs. The effect is gravity and momentum tending to stretch the series elastic element, then recoil of the tendon in a repeating cycle. Muscle effort is minimal and energy is conserved.

Walking on sand is relatively more work than running on it because running at least has the advantage of momentum. Like running inefficiently with an initial heel strike, walking on soft sand is all muscle contraction with no chance to incorporate the recoil qualities of the Achilles tendon.

Elastic energy storage and utilization enhance jumping efficiency much more than jumping performance (Anderson, 1993). There is no difference in jumping height but there is a large difference in energy expenditure. Equal elastic strain energy is stored in both types of jumps but more of the stored energy is lost as heat during counter-movement jumping (Anderson, 1993). The source of the strain energy in counter-movement jumping comes from gravitation and momentum during downward movement and stretching of proximal extensors, while the stored energy from squat jumps comes from the contractile element.

Stored strain-energy required for increased load-bearing ability in tendon tissue is increased molecularly by the prevention of flexible regions from further stretching, regions where mineralization is initiated within collagen fibrils (Silver, 2001). The amount of stored energy and the elastic spring constant are proportional to the mineral content in the collagen. Charged amino acid residues are thought to initiate the mineralization.

Static stretching reduces tendon stiffness by lowering structural viscosity and increases elasticity with no effect on maximal voluntary contraction (Keitaro, 2001). Tendon elasticity decreases with age. A regular stretching program can slow the loss of elasticity. During aging, tendon fibrils increase in diameter with a corresponding increase in ultimate tensile strength and stiffness.

Strength training with weight resistance in old age increases human tendon stiffness (Reeves et al, 2003) and thus reduces the risk of tendon injury. It also increases production of contractile force and velocity in motor activities. However, less strain energy is stored in stiff tendons so cyclical tasks require more energy. Aquatic resistance exercise oriented towards isokinetic muscle endurance is not expected to stiffen tendons among the elderly population, but research is needed. High load-bearing flexor tendons become stiffer, stronger, and

less extensible with age. Due to material properties, mature flexors are designed more for elastic energy storage than extensors are (Shadwick, 1990). Tests on a general population concluded that with endurance exercise, repeated contractions for longer duration increased tendon compliance with more elasticity (Keitaro, 2001). Isometric training increased stiffness of tendon structures (Keitaro, Kanehisa, et al, 2001), shortening electromechanical delay but reducing tendon elasticity and efficiency of the entire unit. There may be an advantage to overall quality of articular and muscle-tendon unit health using water for isokinetic muscle endurance training instead of isometric or isotonic weight workouts.

- Isokinetic exercise enhances tendon efficiency for potential energy storage in the series-elastic element more than isotonic or isometric exercise.

- Water is better suited to isokinetic exercise than land.

- Therefore, water is logically best suited for tendon enhancement and therapy.

Immobilization harms both tendons and ligaments. The effects of several weeks of immobilization on tendon structure and function can be severe due to a loss of fibers. Wolff's Law, detailed in Chapter 7, *Bone Density and Aquatic Exercise,* applies to all connective tissue. The effects of immobilization are significantly more rapid than structural and functional increases from exercise. Like money, you can spend it in a hurry but it takes a long time to save it.

During immobilization, adhesions can form between the tendon and the tendon sheath. Passive exercise during tendon repair after an injury helps to prevent these adhesions and promotes tendon function during the healing process. Because there are more complex movement possibilities in water than on land, passive aquatic bodywork methods during healing are an excellent choice for physical therapists.

Fascial fibers and ligamentous attachments become shortened with the possibility of compressing nerves and causing pain when they are suddenly chilled or if they experience excessive strain tears. Ligaments also loose elasticity and shorten with age. Joint mobility in old age is largely dependant on ligament elasticity. Minimizing this loss of ligament elasticity involves a constant awareness of good balance, good posture and development of the kinesthetic or proprioceptive sense. Poor balance punishes the ligaments more than any other structure in the body (Billig & Loewendahl, 1949). Poor balance causes shortening of ligaments that bind and adjust to poor posture, compressing nerves and causing chronic pain in the process.

Posture correction should focus on mobility rather than on alignment. Aquatic bodywork is commendable for this purpose. See Chapter 2, *Aquatic Bodywork,* for details on useful techniques. Fascial and ligamentous shortening caused by chronic poor posture is effectively corrected with precise and frequent passive and active mobilization to restore ligament elasticity.

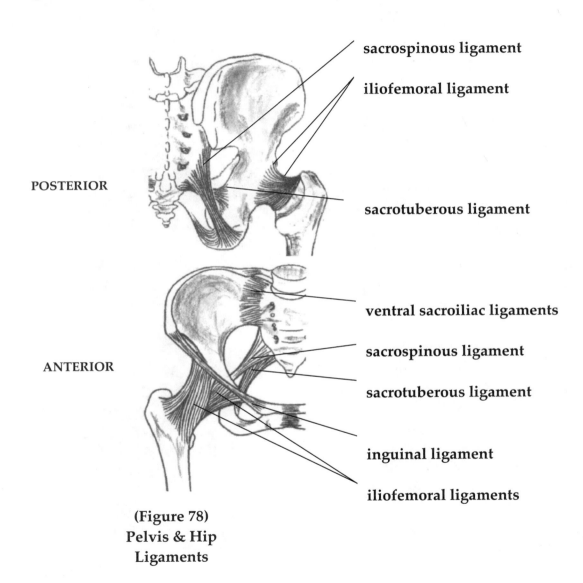

sacrospinous ligament

iliofemoral ligament

POSTERIOR

sacrotuberous ligament

ANTERIOR

ventral sacroiliac ligaments

sacrospinous ligament

sacrotuberous ligament

inguinal ligament

iliofemoral ligaments

**(Figure 78)
Pelvis & Hip
Ligaments**

Chapter 5
Articular Surroundings

Joints

You will want to become anatomically familiar with the synovial joints prior to investigating tendon pain.

While earning a degree in Health Science I developed a successful study method to learn musculoskeletal anatomy. It was a guaranteed 'A' in any level anatomy class. Luckily there were two large empty walls to fill up with my drawings.

Borrow or purchase several of the most detailed human anatomy books you can find. One can be a book of photographs of the real thing. Another book can be fine illustrations and another book can be simplified drawings. They should include everything. Work with joints, one at a time. Select a joint and start with its bones. Have a pencil, eraser, and lots of paper. Draw the bones that are involved until the proportions

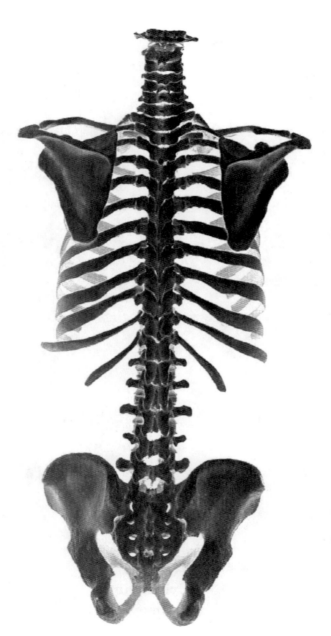

(Figure 79) Spine & Core Articulations

are accurate. Include every groove, projection, bump, and rough spot. Write their names pointing to each landmark on the bone. Now add the other articulating bone joined to the first one. Make over a dozen copies of your bone drawing. On one page, draw the connecting ligaments that connect the bones to each other at that joint. Confine your study to the specific, local area of the joint and the ligaments that cross it. Write their names. Then go to the involved muscles and their tendon attachments. On separate pages of your bone copies, draw out each individual named muscle, one per page. List the points of attachment on the bone somewhere on each muscle page. To go deeper, study the nerves and vessels that pass through the region and the muscles that they feed and innervate. Do this for each joint. The spine (Fig. 79) will take the most drawings when you include all paraspinal muscles. It takes time to sink into your memory. It is helpful for you to draw freehand, slowly, concentrating on the tissue and it's nomenclature.

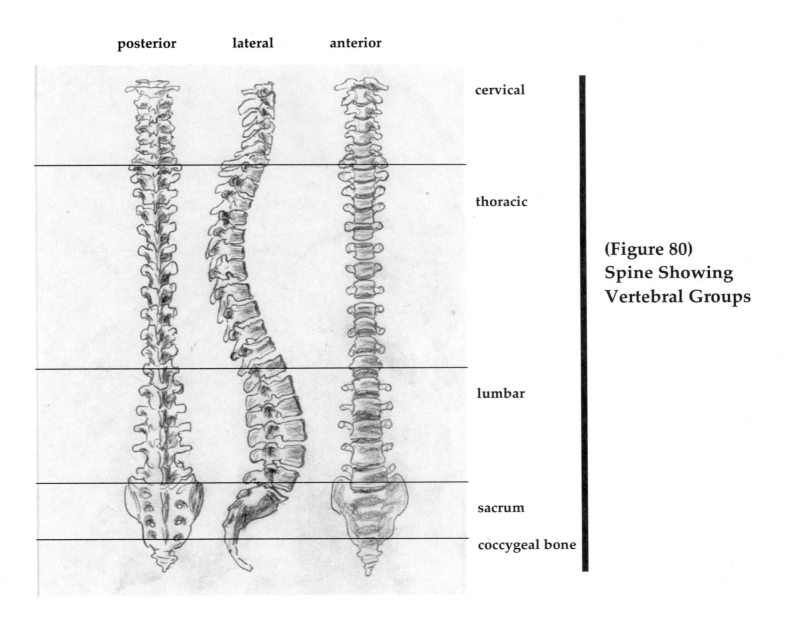

posterior   lateral   anterior

cervical

thoracic

lumbar

sacrum

coccygeal bone

(Figure 80)
Spine Showing
Vertebral Groups

Nalu: The Art and Science of Aquatic Fitness, Bodywork & Therapy

(Figure 81) Articulations of Rib with Thoracic Vertebrae

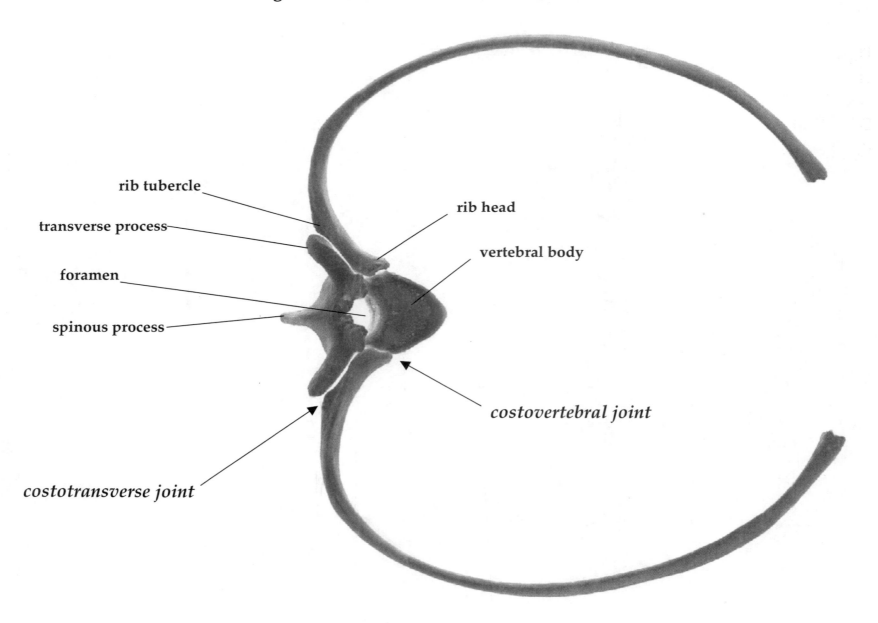

(Figure 82)

Thoracic, Lumbar Sacral & Coccygeal Vertebrae

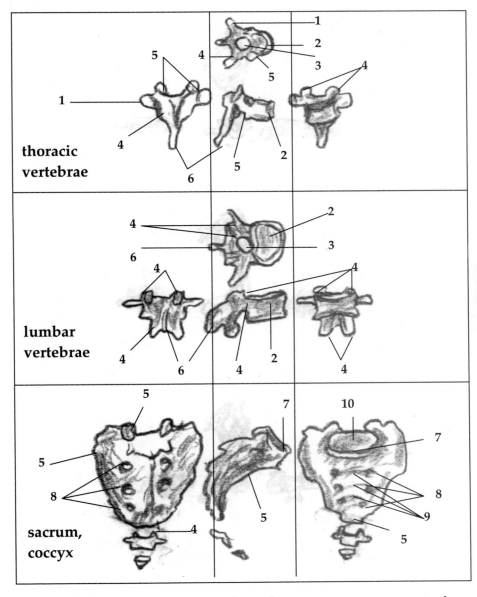

thoracic vertebrae

lumbar vertebrae

sacrum, coccyx

posterior   lateral   anterior

1. transverse process
2. body
3. foramen
4. articular process
5. articular surface
6. spinous process
7. promontory
8. foramina
9. fusion lines
10. base

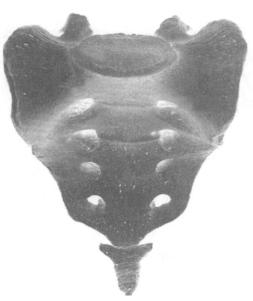

anterior sacrum & coccyx

Nalu: The Art and Science of Aquatic Fitness, Bodywork & Therapy

Diarthroses joints are freely movable. Amphiarthroses joints are slightly movable. Synarthroses joints are immovable. These are functional classifications. Structurally, fibrous connective tissue connects bones in a fibrous joint without an articulating cavity just as cartilage joins the bones of a cartilaginous articulation. Synovial joints are held together with ligaments that maintain support of bones in a joint cavity. We will describe synovial diarthroses joints.

Synovial joints allow free movement while maintaining posture. Limiting factors are: muscle actions, connective tissue strength, and bone shape at the articulation. Synovium, with a high concentration of lubricating hyaluronic acid, is a fluid secreted by the synovial membrane, filling the fibroelastic capsule. An avascular cartilage covers the bones at the articulation. It depends on joint compression and decompression for nutrient/waste exchange with the synovial fluid. Menisci are directional guides for articulating bones. They are also cushioning pads for fibrous cartilage in some joint capsules.

Bursae are flattened cushioning sacs of synovial fluid near articulations, between muscles or tendons and the bone (Figure 91). When they surround wrist and ankle tendons, they are tendon sheaths.

There are hinge, pivot, gliding, ball and socket, saddle, and condyloid synovial joints. Hinge joints (elbow & knee) permit flexion and extension. Ball and socket joints (hip & shoulder) permit the greatest range of motion in all directions. Two joints with an incongruity in dimensions are the hip and elbow. There are others. There are reasons for the way bones articulate. At the hip for example, there is a short ligament keeping the femoral head in the acetabulum. The acetabulum diameter is smaller than the diameter of the femoral head so that at low loads the pressure is on the perimeter of the articulation and at high loads the acetabulum stretches to conform tightly to the femoral head. The joint alternates from congruence to separation. This rhythm during walking facilitates lubrication in the joint for smooth ball-and-socket movement. There is much diversity in joint architecture, each with a different lubricating system.

The Rotator Cuff

As an example of joint articulations we will consider the anatomy of the rotator cuff and the shoulder here (Figures 83-92) because rotator cuff discomfort (most often the supraspinatus tendon) is one of the main reasons, along with the low back and knee, why people switch from heavy weight room workouts and free weights to aquatic resistance for muscle endurance conditioning.

The four muscles of the rotator cuff are: supraspinatus, infraspinatus, subscapularis, and teres minor. Following this anatomical review of the shoulder joint we will investigate some of the joint pain syndromes.

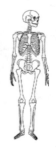
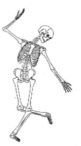

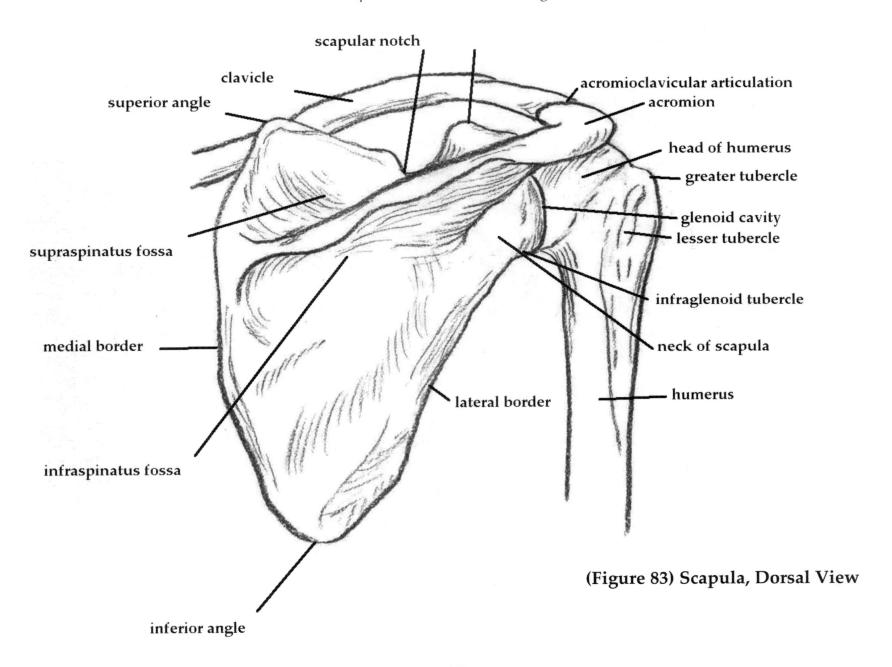

scapular notch

clavicle

superior angle

acromioclavicular articulation

acromion

head of humerus

greater tubercle

supraspinatus fossa

glenoid cavity

lesser tubercle

infraglenoid tubercle

medial border

neck of scapula

humerus

lateral border

infraspinatus fossa

inferior angle

(Figure 83) Scapula, Dorsal View

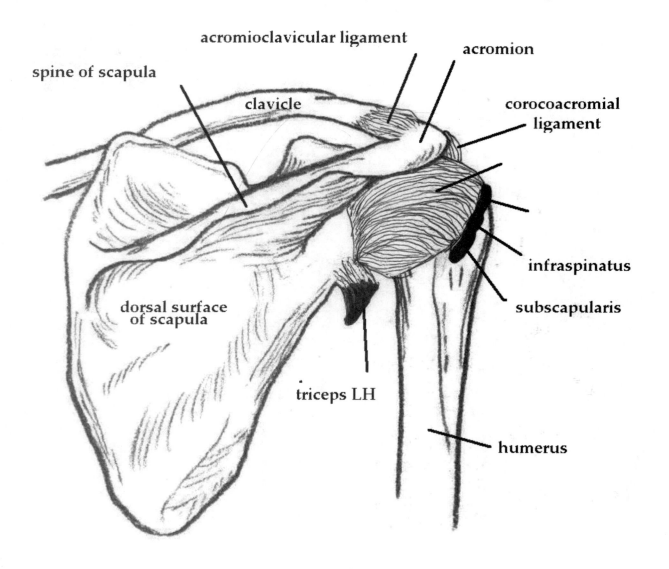

spine of scapula

acromioclavicular ligament

clavicle

acromion

corocoacromial
ligament

dorsal surface
of scapula

infraspinatus

subscapularis

triceps LH

humerus

**(Figure 84)
Shoulder Capsule,
Dorsal View**

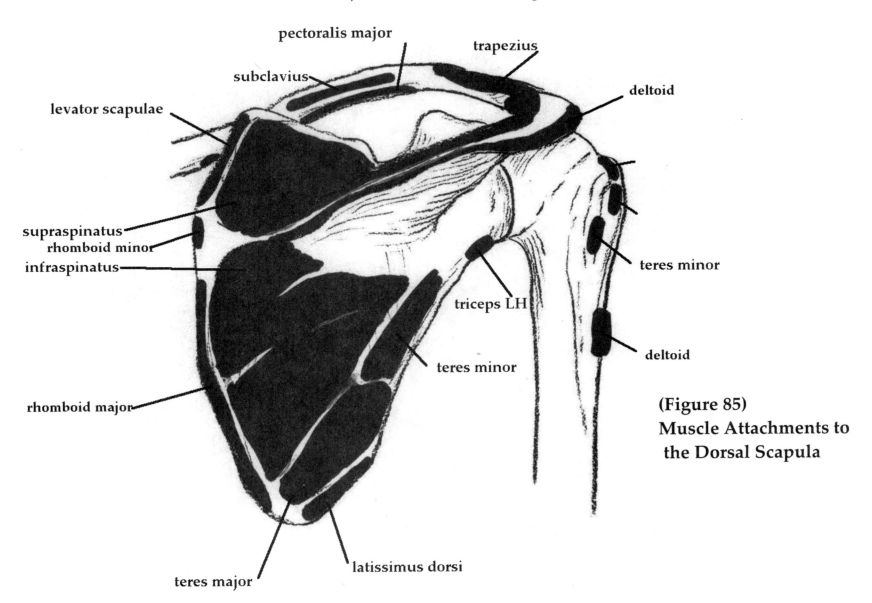

(Figure 85)
Muscle Attachments to the Dorsal Scapula

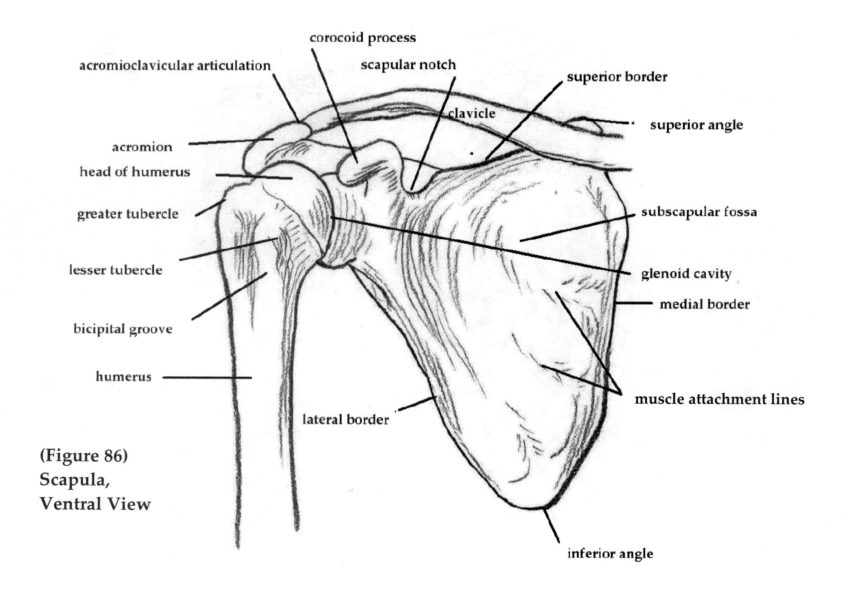

corocoid process

acromioclavicular articulation

scapular notch

superior border

clavicle

superior angle

acromion

head of humerus

greater tubercle

subscapular fossa

lesser tubercle

glenoid cavity

bicipital groove

medial border

humerus

muscle attachment lines

lateral border

**(Figure 86)
Scapula,
Ventral View**

inferior angle

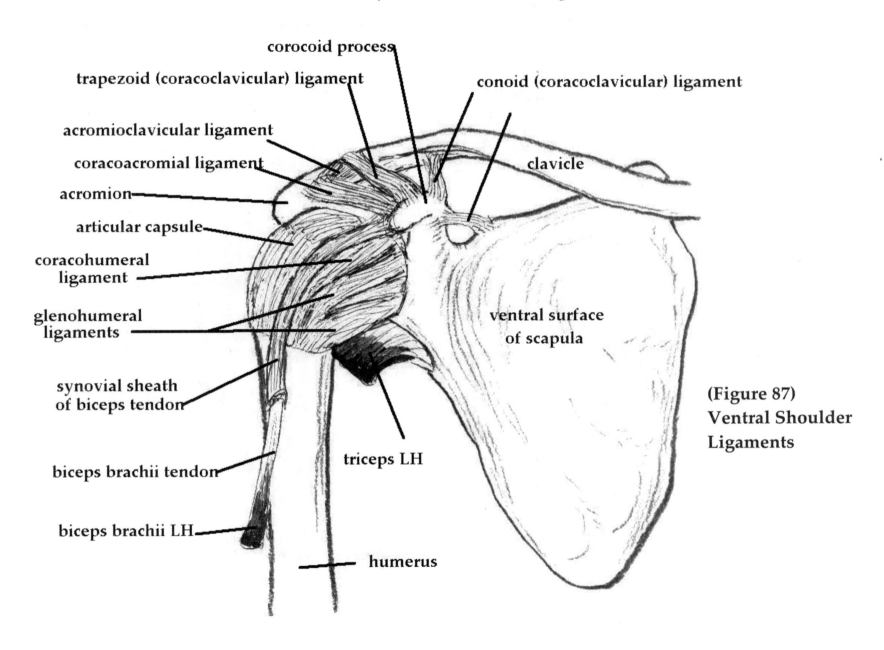

corocoid process

trapezoid (coracoclavicular) ligament

conoid (coracoclavicular) ligament

acromioclavicular ligament

coracoacromial ligament

acromion

clavicle

articular capsule

coracohumeral ligament

glenohumeral ligaments

ventral surface of scapula

synovial sheath of biceps tendon

biceps brachii tendon

triceps LH

biceps brachii LH

humerus

(Figure 87)
Ventral Shoulder Ligaments

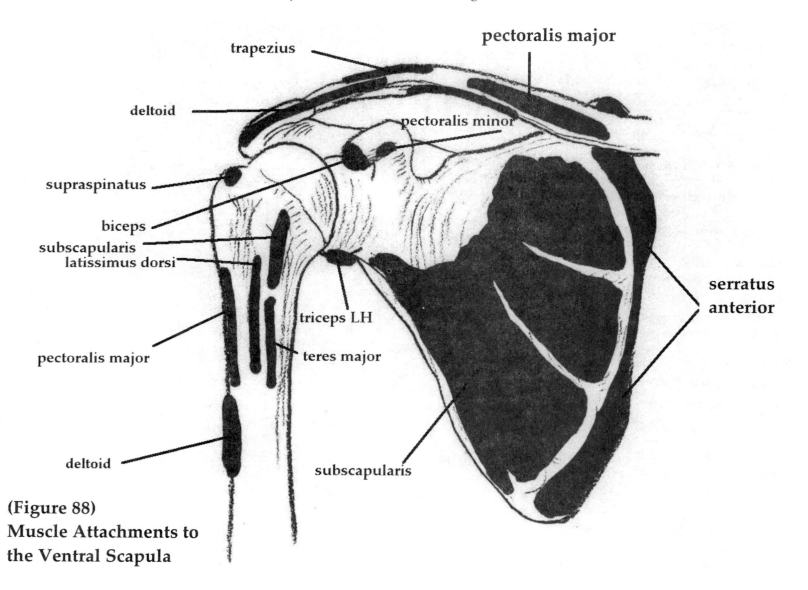

trapezius

pectoralis major

deltoid

pectoralis minor

supraspinatus

biceps

subscapularis
latissimus dorsi

triceps LH

pectoralis major

teres major

**serratus
anterior**

deltoid

subscapularis

**(Figure 88)
Muscle Attachments to
the Ventral Scapula**

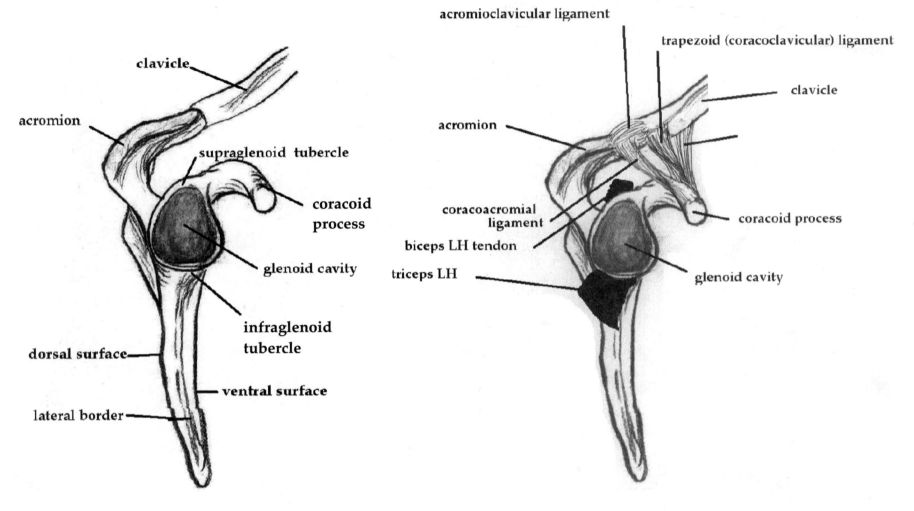

(Figure 89A)
Scapula, Lateral View

(Figure 89B)
Ligaments Between Scapula
and Clavicle, Lateral View

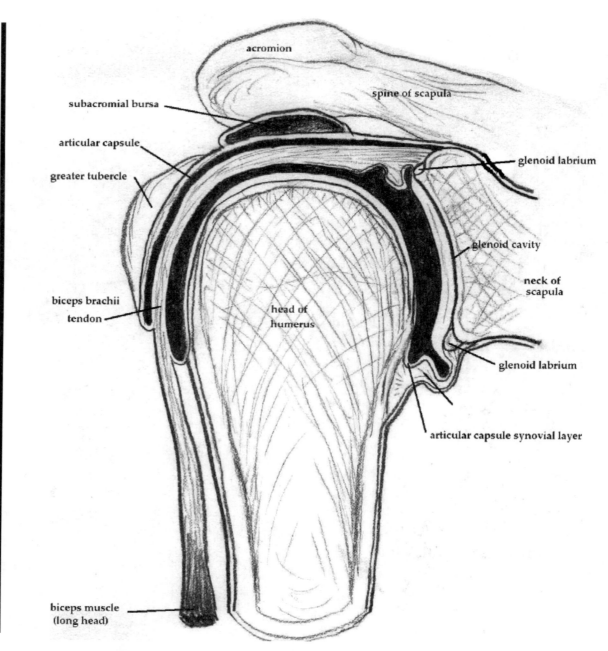

**(Figure 90)
Glenohumeral Joint
with Articular Capsule
and Subacromial Bursa**

acromion

spine of scapula

subacromial bursa

articular capsule

greater tubercle

glenoid labrium

glenoid cavity

neck of scapula

biceps brachii tendon

head of humerus

glenoid labrium

articular capsule synovial layer

biceps muscle (long head)

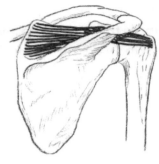

supraspinatus

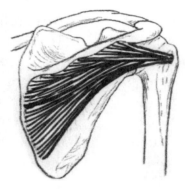

infraspinatus

(Figure 91)
Rotator Cuff Muscles,
Right Shoulder

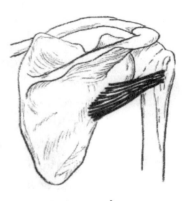

teres minor

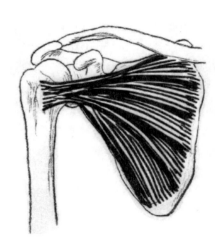

subscapularis

Tendon Pain

Overuse and repetitive stress without enough time for tissue recovery rather than direct, immediate trauma account for most of the painful conditions in sports, recreational activities, and certain laborious occupations. Overuse causes repetitive strain injury and is the same as cumulative trauma disorder. Aquatic therapy and water fitness cross training are key ingredients in an overuse recovery plan.

Aquatic exercise reduces pain in rheumatic disease and improves active joint motion (Templeton, 1996). Aquatic exercise as a rehabilitation technique increases overall joint flexibility and functional ability (Hoeger, 1992). Water exercise also minimizes age-related losses in function (Sanders, 1997). Tendinosis, among many other chronic causes, results in these losses.

Repetitive strain injuries are common with long distance runners. In one study (van Mechelen, 1992) runners report rates of annual injuries of up to 68%. These include painful trochanteric bursitis, avulsions, muscle strains, stress fractures, compression fractures, iliotibial band syndrome (snapping across the hip), groin pain from iliopsoas tendon irritation, and other tendinosis and tendonitis conditions.

The overuse "line" for tendons is genetically determined when all other variables are equal among athletes. There are differences in collagen ratios and differences in speed of tendon healing between individuals.

Tendons are made up of 65-80% collagen (mostly Type I), only 1-2% elastin, proteoglycans that trap water for absorbing external forces, and fibroblasts that synthesize this matrix. Like osteoblasts becoming osteocytes in bone matrix, fibroblasts in actively forming tendon become fibrocytes in mature tendon tissue. More specifically they are tenocytes: chondrocytes in cartilage, tenocytes in tendons, and osteocytes in bone are all fibrocytes.

Tendon collagen molecules are amino acid tripeptides of mostly glycene, proline, and lysine that assemble into fibrils. These fibrils then assemble into fibers. Collagen fibers are in bundles surrounded by a sheath.

Genetic defects cause abnormally weak collagen that is slow to repair. Tendinosis is a breakdown of collagen during repetitive motion. Chronic tendinosis, more common with age, is the result of a faulty repair process where the collagen produced by the fibroblasts is abnormal in quality. (Ledbetter, 1992; Liu, 1995). In the defective collagen: there is an imbalance of collagen types, breakdown exceeds repair, the bundle structure is disorganized, mitochondria in tenocyte nuclei are structurally abnormal, microtears in the weak collagen are visible, and vascularity is increased, among other conditions.

Enzymes that help break down proteins are proteolytic. They are utilized for tissue repair and remodeling. A low level of proteolytic enzymes, stromelysin in particular, is associated with individuals prone to tendinosis because they have a low rate of pre-injury collagen turnover (Ireland, 2001). High levels of proteolytic enzymes are also a problem because normal tissue remodeling cannot keep up with enzymatic protein brea-down. Normally there is a balance between the enzyme concentration and inhibitors to achieve optimal breakdown and repair. In tendinosis, injury rate exceeds repair rate so without a proper balance between the proteolytic enzymes and their inhibitors, tendinosis keeps getting worse (Erickson, L., 2002).

Tendinosis is characterized by a loss of collagen continuity with an increase in ground substance, vascularity, and cellularity from the presence of fibroblasts and myofibroblasts. There are no inflammatory cells present.

Tendinosis pain comes from irritating biochemicals at the injury and from inflammation of surrounding tissue, not from tendon inflammation (Khan, 2000). Tendonitis is tendon inflammation. It's as simple as four letters; "…itis" is inflammation and "…osis" is degeneration without direct inflammation.

Tendinosis is common. Tendinitis, tendon inflammation, is a rare condition (Kahn, 2000). Early tendinosis recovery takes 6-8 weeks. Early tendinitis recovery takes a few days followed by re-conditioning exercises. Eighty percent of full recovery from chronic tendinosis takes 3-6 months. Ninety-nine percent of full recovery from chronic tendinitis is achieved in 4-6 weeks (Cook, 1997).

The following tendon overuse syndromes are chronic.

- Achilles tendinosis (Maffulli, 2000)
- Rotator cuff tendinosis (Riley, 1994)
- Patellar tendinosis
- Posterior tibial tendinosis
- Digital tendinosis
- Tennis elbow
- Golfers elbow
- Carpal tunnel syndrome
- TMJD/ temporo-mandibular joint dysfunction (Westling, 1992; Gage, 1995)

Patellar tendinitis is a misdiagnosis and is unfounded (Maffulli, 1998). The patellar tendinopathy of localized, gradual-onset anterior knee pain associated with activity is tendinosis. Anti-inflammatory therapies are ineffective since there is no inflammation. Corticosteroids can cause necrosis of collagen tissue in tendons (Kraushaar, 1999). Complete rest is contraindicated. The most effective conservative treatment is tensile load strengthening to increase collagen production and alignment. However, loads should be reduced with less duration of activity.

The pool is the most appropriate venue for tendinosis therapy and an ideal environment for biomechanical re-education. It is worth mentioning here that a hot or warm water pool would prolong healing due to neovascularization and increased metabolism. Except when tendon pain is associated with inflammatory arthritis, there is an absence of inflammatory cells. Cold decreases tendon metabolic rate and promotes tendinosis healing (Rivenburgh, 1992). Inflexibility of the hamstrings (Cook et al, 2000), quadriceps, IT band and calf can increase patellar tendon load and cause patellar tendinopathy by restricting knee and ankle range of motion. Water enables greater and more diverse opportunities for stretching. Once the injury cycle starts, the pre-injury condition has little hope of returning. Weakness escalates injuries and the cycle continues. Activity levels have to change in frequency and modality. De-conditioning increases vulnerability. This is where aquatic rehabilitation is most effective.

Injury to the outer tendon layer of epitenon tissue that supplies nourishment, nerves, and lymph vessels to the tendon is paratenoitis, not the old term, tenosynovitis. This can occur separately or at the same time as tendinosis. The epitenon is surrounded with more connective tissue, the protective paratenon. Both together are the peritenon (Kahn, 2000)

There is a solid biomechanical rationale that aquatic therapy can rehabilitate tendinosis. Water spreads the load, attenuating it through the tendons at both ends of a muscle, reducing mechanical overload and correcting muscle imbalances that caused the collagen degeneration. Collagen production determines recovery from tendinosis. Tendon exercise without overload safely increases tensile strength by improving collagen alignment and stimulating collagen formation (Vilarta, 1989). Tendon strengthening is proven to successfully treat tendinosis (Woo, 1982). Therapeutic aquatic methods like the overall program offered at the Burdenko Institute (see Chapter 12) effectively correct motor patterns that lead to patellar tendinopathy. These methods concentrate on maintaining pelvic stability in deep water where resistance can stay within a functionally required range.

Bicipital tendinitis is a painful condition at the anterior humerus during shoulder flexion and occasionally during elbow flexion.

The pain is sometimes vague in locale but more specifically at the bicipital groove of the humerus (Figure 86, page 172) where the biceps long-head tendon crosses the humeral head and passes to the superior edge of the glenoid fossa (Sethi, 1999). The bicipital groove is between the lesser and greater tuberosities of the humerus. The pain of bicipital tendinitis is from the inflammation when friction against the tuberosities causes micro tearing of the tendon. Soft tissue palpation at the site usually elicits tenderness.

The tendon can be easily dislocated out of the groove if the transverse humeral ligament is injured (Murtagh, 1991). Bicipital tendinitis is associated with rotator cuff impingement syndrome because the long head tendon in its fibrous sheath within the bicipital groove passes between the tendons of the suprascapularis and subscapularis rotator cuff muscles. There can be inflammation and tearing of the entire group of tendons from compression into the anterior acromion during full humeral head abduction (Safran,

1998). Bicipital tendinitis is also associated with pathology of the glenoid fossa such as painful tears in the glenoid labrum, a band of fibro-cartilage that deepens the glenoid cavity (Fig.89).

A clinical assessment test for bicipital tendinitis is Speed's test. Supinating the palm in a 90° shoulder flexion with pressure applied downward on the distal arm produces pain at the anterior shoulder. Another test in a similar posture is eccentric contraction of the biceps with applied downward pressure.

Pain results from inflammation so the first intervention in bicipital tendinitis is edema reduction and overhead movement restriction without complete immobilization (Ellenbecker, 1995). After the elimination of swelling and pain, strength and endurance can be conditioned with careful and gradual progress. Stretching should be passive. The isokinetic properties of aquatic resistance allow for safer physical therapy than the use of gravity weights and machines. Too

much, too soon can cause tendon rupture or degenerative changes in the tissue (Safran, 1998).

Tendon Injuries: Tendons have greater tensile strength than bones. Long tendons have greater tensile strength than short tendons. The weakest zone in the muscle-tendon unit and the one most vulnerable to injury is at the myotendinous junction (Laszio, 1997). The risk of tendon injury is more likely to increase with: high-volume training rather than high-intensity training; long-term anabolic steroid use because it decreases tendon elasticity, energy absorbing capacity, and tensile strength; plyometrics and ballistic exercises; too rapid training progression; long workouts; prior injuries; musculotendinous units that have poor endurance; workout practices that ignore or diminish stretching routines; lifting techniques that are uncontrolled or not in balance; eccentric movement under load as a tendon is stretching; rapid muscle contraction; and with exercising too frequently (Moore, 1992).

Adhesive Capsulitis

Fibrosis of the shoulder joint capsule reduces active and passive range of motion and causes disabling pain. The primary condition, frozen shoulder, is distinct from arthritis or tendinopathy while the secondary condition is associated with trauma, disease, tendinopathy and arthritis. In fact, a significant pain source in capsulitis is rotator cuff dysfunction.

Capsulitis is more prevalent among diabetics. In a study published by the British Journal of Rheumatology, 19% of the subjects with diabetes mellitus had shoulder capsulitis while only 5% of the control group without diabetes had capsulitis. There was no difference with regard to age, sex, or type of diabetes (Pal, et al, 1986). The study also concluded that there is a 30% higher incidence of impaired joint mobility among subjects with diabetes mellitus.

The cause of the primary glenoid fibrosis in the shoulder is unknown. Most of the thickening is anterior at the coracohumeral ligament and superior glenohumeral ligament (Figure 87, page 173) with a decrease in synovial cells (Ozaki, 1989). There is a common treatment to reduce pain and increase range of motion with low incidence of complications, like cartilage or bone injury, which involves manually rupturing the fibrosis under anesthesia (Placzek, 1998). Ice or anti-inflamatories can help to control the pain but not solve the problem. Avoiding movements that cause pain will shorten its course.

Treatment with oral prednisone or intra-articular corticosteroid injection decreases pain but there is not much change in range of motion (Bulgen, 1984). Subacromial injections yield results similar to intra-articular injections (Rizk, 1991). Injecting air into the joint causes capsular rupture, decreasing the pain, still with only a moderate improvement in range of motion (Sandor, 2000). Surgically, manipulation or manual rupture under anesthesia shows a 50-80% improvement in range of motion (Plazek, 1998). Arthroscopic release of the contracted capsular structures

significantly improves range of motion with a 90% pain free and near normal condition within 3 months (Warner, 1996).

Physical therapy for adhesive capsulitis includes specific exercises that begin as subtle motions of gentle humerus pendulum swinging(Figure 92B), horizontal circular sliding (Figure 92A), rotating, and shoulder flexion with relaxed musculature, keeping the movement under the pain threshold (Figure 92B). Over-aggressive mobilization can worsen the condition (Sandor, 2000). Physical therapy can slowly advance to daily passive and actively assisted extensions and abductions kept under the pain threshold. The therapy pool is commonly utilized to treat adhesive capsulitis with exercise. With physical therapy the prognosis is nearly 100% successful in time (Sandor, 2000).

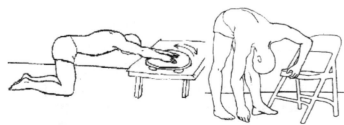

(Figure 92A)   **(Figure 92B)**

Complaints from the Sacroiliac

Dropping our focus to the pelvis, we see impact forces transmitted from two directions, the ground and the spine. The forces move all the pelvic joints like a kinetic chain. The very minimal nutational movements of the synovial sacroiliac joint in this multi-joint coordination are rotation and translation (Sturesson, 2000) but the axis of motion is dependent on the topography of the articular surfaces (Harrison, 1997). Mechanical adaptations to forces as subtle as leg length differences can cause damage to the sacroiliac joint and its articular surroundings. Athletes exposed to unpredictable forces are prone to sacroiliac joint pain syndrome. Decreasing the effect of gravity in aquatic therapy relieves stress on injured ligamentous support for the sacrum. One of the supporting ligaments, the sacrotuberous ligament, has attachments from the large biceps femoris and gluteus maximus muscles as well as the piriformis. No muscles act directly on the sacroiliac joint (Yung, 2002). The muscles, instead, attach to associated ligaments.

Pain is easily and quickly sensed in the sacroiliac joint because of the large concentration of unmyelinated nerve endings – proprioceptors and nociceptors (Bernard, 1991) and their association with adjacent neural structures (Fortin, 1999). This highly innervated region can refer pain to distant areas throughout the middle and lower body (Fortin, 1994). Classic SIJ pain is always present inferior and medial to the posterior superior iliac spine (Fortin, 1994) but never above L-5 (Dreyfuss, 1996).

*L*ava rocks from Hualalai,

an extinct volcano on the Big Island of Hawaii, were delivered to the job. I was building a rock wall along the pathways of a beautiful Kona estate and needed help so I recruited Timatea from the outrigger canoe club. He was a strong young fellow from Tahiti but spoke little English and I spoke no Tahitian. So we used sign language to get the big job done.

It was a repetitive act of bending down, lifting, bending down again and working, over and over for three weeks. One morning I filled the wheelbarrow with large lava rocks, grabbed the handles, and before the wheel even moved I collapsed on the ground with severe low-back pain. I was in good physical condition from practicing daily for the canoe races but my muscle endurance and strength were all upper body. I had neglected lower body conditioning. Hip abductors were weak and hamstrings were tight from not stretching.

><((((O> ><((((O> ><((((O>

Absent other low-back and hip pathologies, there is normal range of motion in the spine with sacroiliac joint pain syndrome. The causative weakness is in the abductors of the hip, mainly the gluteus medius. This causes tightness and overactivity in compensating muscles such as the quadratus lumborum which in turn can refer pain to the SIJ and the

piriformis with it's tendon attachments on the sacrotuberous ligament (Liebenson, 1996).

Provoking pain during movement identifies SIJ pain syndrome. There are other painful conditions that could be the cause of discomfort including myofascial pain from local trigger points, osteitis condensans from joint stress and laxity during pregnancy, spondylitis, ulcerative colitis, stress fractures to the sacrum among women with low bone density, degenerative joint disease among the elderly, metabolic conditions, trauma and pelvic fracture. The thoracolumbar fascia can also be involved in the syndrome because of the stabilizing erector spinae muscles that attach to it (Dreyfus, 1997).

Aquatic stabilization therapy includes coordinating and conditioning the muscles of the pelvis, hip, and low back. Exercises, land or aquatic, that increase pelvic stabilization increase the muscle endurance and strength of the hamstrings, abdominals, gluteus maximus, gluteus medius, latissimus dorsi and extensors of the back (Dreyfus, 1997) with a variety of loading conditions (Aitken, 1986).

Herzog's study (1999) on spinal manipulation has been referenced by many chiropractors as a clinically observed benefit that reduces the pain and muscle hypertonicity of the pelvis and surrounding area. Aquatic exercises under professional supervision, spinal manipulation, and massage therapy, in that order are an excellent sequence of conservative modalities that help reduce pain and correct the dysfunctions that produce sacroiliac joint pain syndrome.

"It's All in the Wrist"

We will conclude this chapter with the most distinctively primate and important joint in the development of human civilization, the only saddle joint in the body. It is the articulation in the wrist (Figure 92C) of the 1st metacarpal bone (thumb) with one of the smallest bones, the **trapezium** (Figure 92D). Both processes of this unique joint have a concave surface in

one direction and a convex surface in the opposing direction like the seats of two saddles that fit perpendicularly into each other. This allows for a wide variety of movements. Bipedalism allowed the potentials of this tiny articulation to become a giant among all life forms, past and present. The thumb is moved in opposition to the hand as it closes the thumb into the palm towards the fingers by the opponens pollicis muscle (Figure 92E) located deep to the abductor pollicis. It's all in the wrist.

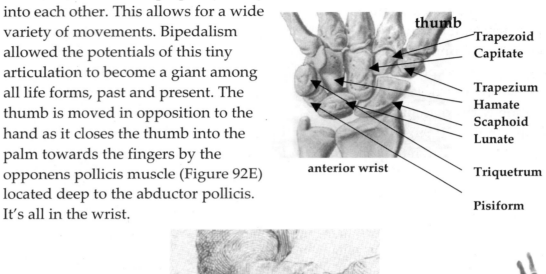

(Figure 92C) Wrist Bones

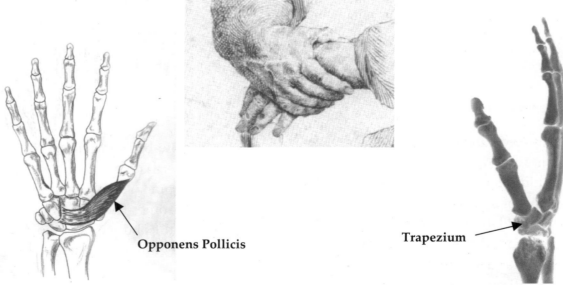

(Figure 92E) Opponens Pollicis of the Right Hand, Anterior View

(Figure 92D) Trapezium, Lateral View

Chapter 6
Aquatic Endurance Exercise

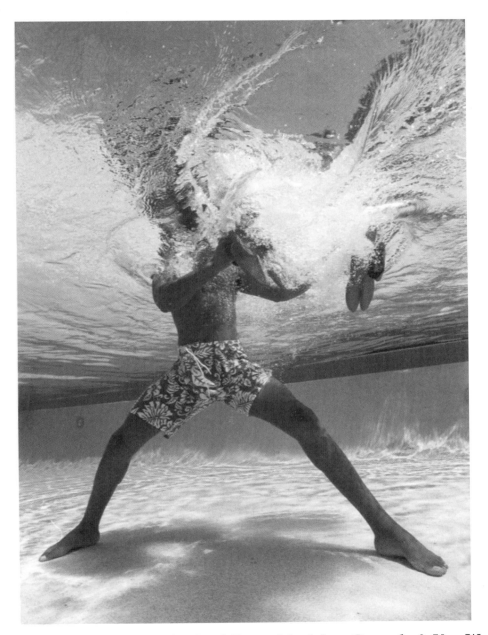

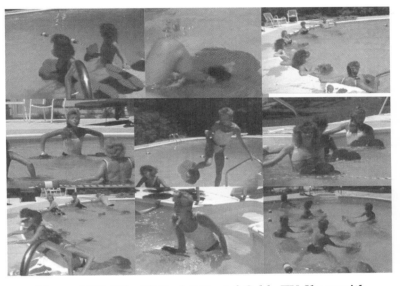

(Figure 93B) "The Fit Body" Centel Cable TV Show with Gabriella Detrich, using the Aquatoner

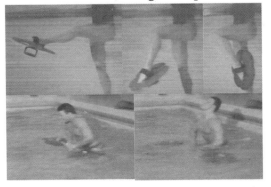

(Figure 93C) Scenes using the Aquatoner in National TV Ad.

(Figure 93A) Toko Irie: Steel Drum Musician, Grenada & Key West

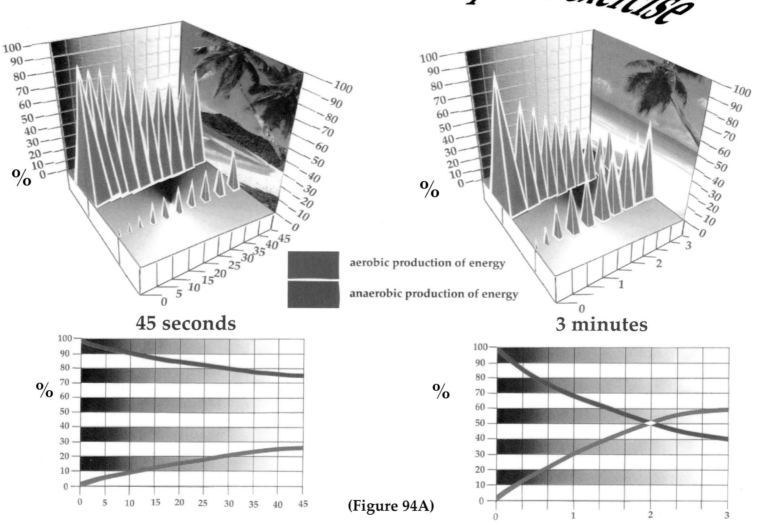

Aerobic & Anaerobic Energy Yield
during maximal-effort aquatic exercise

45 seconds

3 minutes

aerobic production of energy

anaerobic production of energy

(Figure 94A)

Nalu: The Art and Science of Aquatic Fitness, Bodywork & Therapy

The charted values in Figures 94A & 94B represent the respiratory contributions relative to the total energy output for conditioned performance of any exercise with sustained maximal effort, interpolated from Van de Graaff (1995) 271f, *Concepts of Human Anatomy& Physiology.*

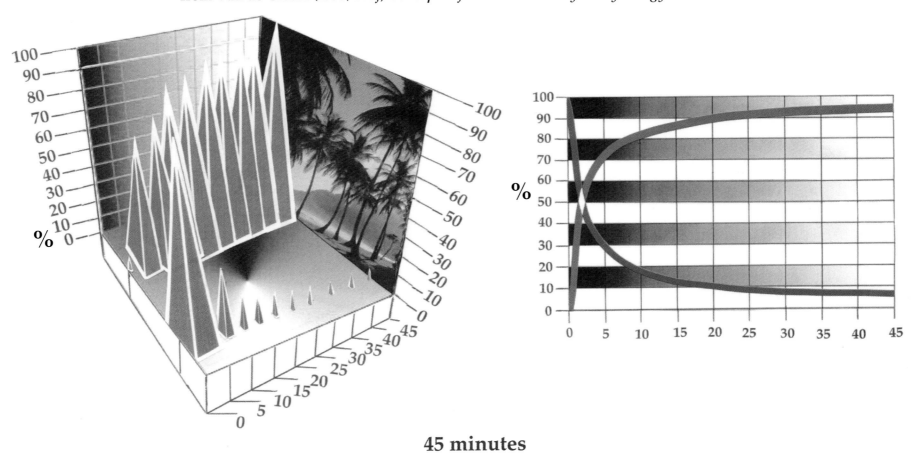

45 minutes

(Figure 94B)

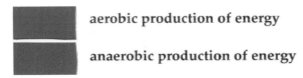

aerobic production of energy

anaerobic production of energy

Nalu: The Art and Science of Aquatic Fitness, Bodywork & Therapy

(Figure 95) Toko Irie using the Aquatoner

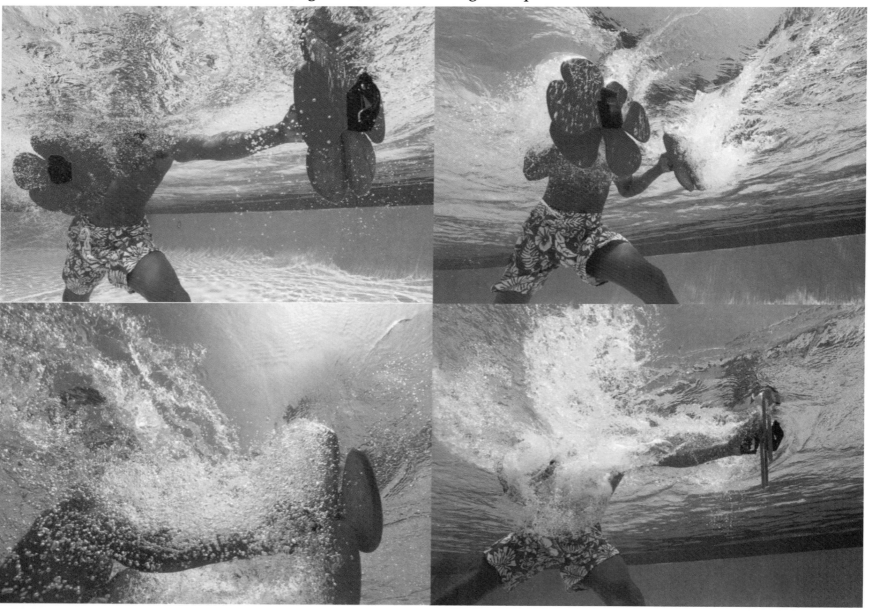

(Figure 96) Toko Irie , working out with the Aquatoning Bar

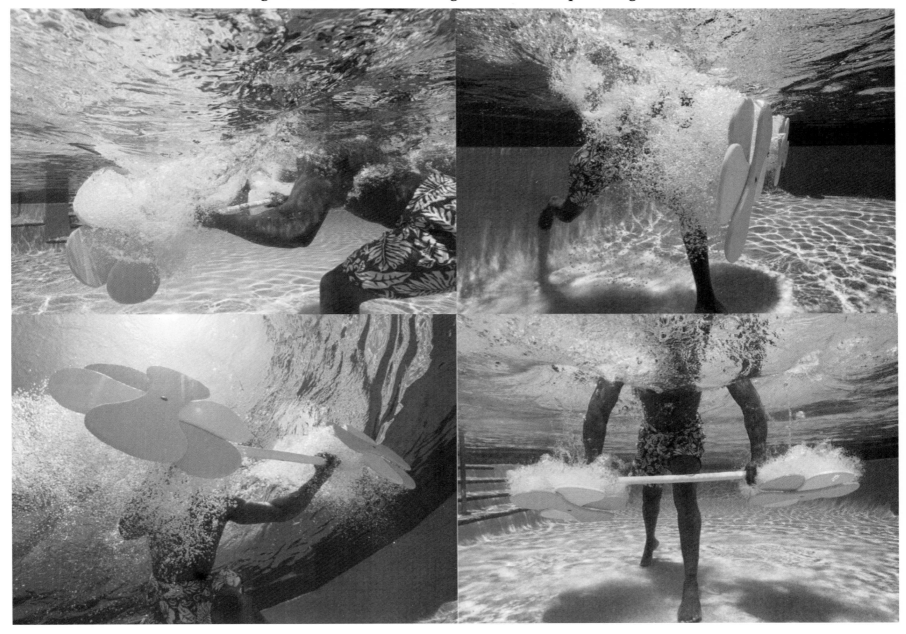

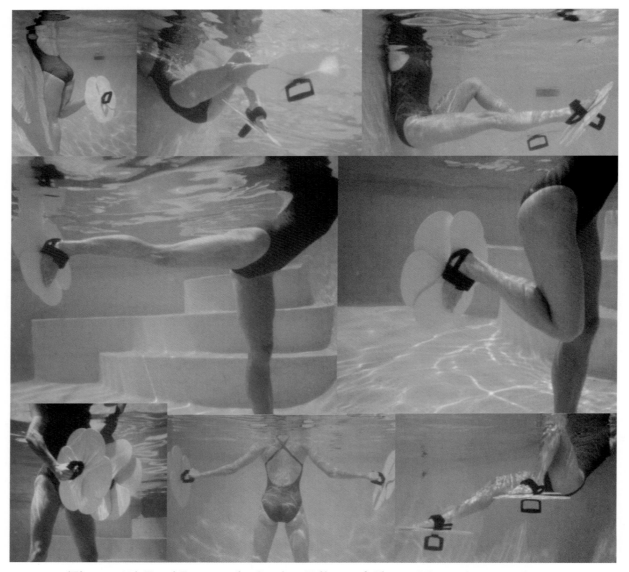

(Figure 97) Patti Loverock, Senior Editor of *Shape Magazine*, 1980's, performing comprehensive exercise with water resistance equipment

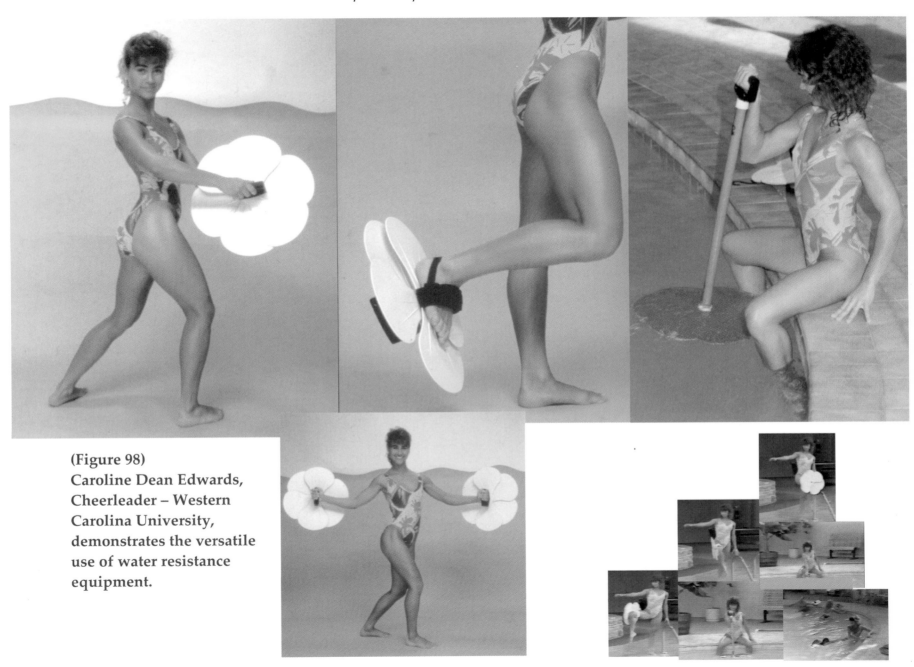

(Figure 98)
Caroline Dean Edwards,
Cheerleader – Western
Carolina University,
demonstrates the versatile
use of water resistance
equipment.

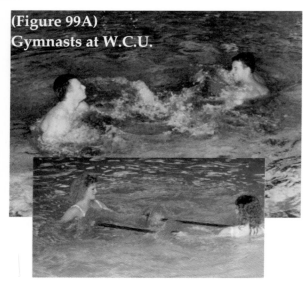

(Figure 99A)
Gymnasts at W.C.U.

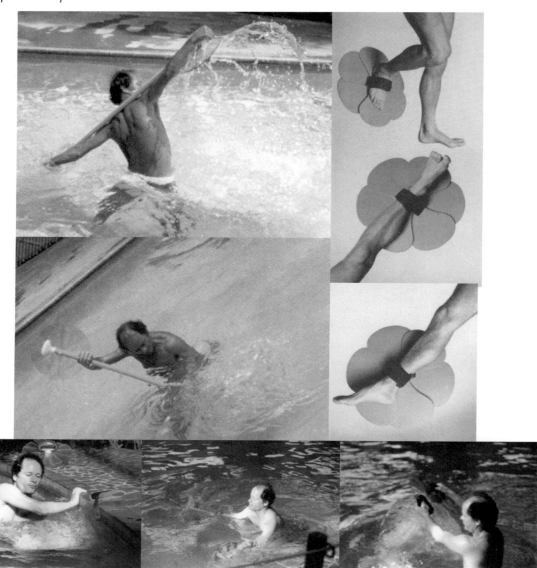

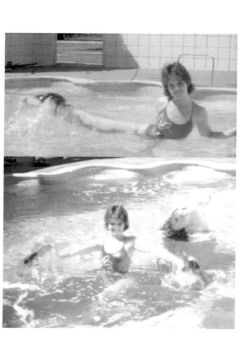

(Figure 99B) Marcia Lane, Jazz Dancer, using water exercise equipment at Palm Desert, California

(Figure 100)
Douglas Bedgood during early product development of aquatic muscle endurance equipment

Muscle Endurance

The healthiest people are not obsessed with one form of exercise over another. Extremes are unhealthy. Workouts that focus entirely on power or strength training and delete somatic qualities of movement are without a foundation. Exercise programs that exclude aerobic cardiovascular conditioning are detrimental to cardiovascular health. At the other extreme, an aerobics-only triathlon type obsession is abusive to the body, damages connective tissues, and leads to weak muscles and weak bones.

There is an upgraded compromise. I call it the aquatic two-minute series. Twelve to fifteen 2-minute sets are connected in a continuous series of high resistance full-body movements in deep and shallow water with the only break being to change or adjust resistance equipment. Together, they exercise all muscles in a thirty-minute continuity with variations of unplanned, multi-dimensional movements linked together in creatively spontaneous sequences.

Each un-patterned, unstructured series involves the eventual movement of all muscle groups. Keeping in mind the revelation that exercise geometry is infinite in water, each set repeats the concept but is not an exact duplication of the previous movements.

At approximately two minutes into intense exercise there is a point where aerobic and anaerobic energy yields are equal (Figures 94A and 94B). The aerobic energy rises from zero to 30% in the first minute while anaerobic energy drops from 90% to 70% in that time. At two minutes they are both at 50%, an ideal combination, then as the exercise continues to ten minutes, aerobic energy is up to 85% and anaerobic energy is down to 15%. In thirty minutes of continuous intense exercise, aerobic energy is way up to 95% of the total energy yield while anaerobic energy yield has dropped all the way down to 5% of the total. The exclusive extremes are unhealthy.

Using this data to evaluate energy pathways in one exercise session is interesting. For example: You exercise with high intensity continuously for thirty minutes. Assuming that the approximate time needed to elevate your heart rate to its target in this session is two minutes, the first two minutes increase aerobic energy yield from 5% to 50%. Using the energy yield graph at the beginning of this Chapter, I broke each minute into its anaerobic and aerobic components, added them up, and concluded the 30 minutes would be divided into 7 minutes anaerobic and 23 minutes aerobic. In Figures 94A & 93B, observe the rapid changes in the types of energy yield during the 20 second intervals of the first three minutes of maximal exercise as aerobic demands on the heart increase. Aerobic endurance training improves the conditioning of internal heart muscles.

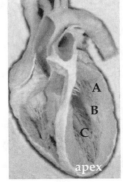

A) anterior papillary muscle tendons

B) anterior papillary muscle

C) posterior papillary muscle

(Figure 101A) Internal Heart Muscles, *The heart is more than one muscle.*

(Figure 101B) Exercise Duration and Energy Pathways Chart

Duration	Type of Workout	Fuel	Dominant Energy Pathway
More than 4 minutes	aerobic, low intensity, cardio endurance	more fats	Krebs cycle (page 143); O_2 needed; energy from fatty acids transferred to ATP through enzyme reactions; release of hydrogen; H_2 accepted by coenzymes; ATP formation; continual aerobic process in mitochondria; can metabolize fats & proteins.
2 – 4 minutes	anaerobic/aerobic	all sources	Transitional from glycolysis to mitochondrial energy production
20 seconds to 2 minutes	anaerobic, moderately high intensity, muscle endurance	more carbs	Glycolysis pathway (page 142); rapid production of ATP yielding lactic acid that is converted to glycogen for more energy; lactic acid eventually accumulates, lowering pH, causing fatigue from inefficient enzyme avtivity and create an oxygen debt; energy source is glucose and muscle glycogen with some glycogen contributed from the liver.
4 – 20 seconds	anaerobic, very high intensity, high velocity, power	only carbs	Creatine ATP – CP pathway (page 142); creatine kinase as the catalyst resynthesizes ATP from ADP and inorganic phosphate plus creatine; creatine supplies most of the energy; fast energy, eighteen times faster than aerobic energy; no need for oxygen; rapid fatigue.
1 – 4 seconds	maximum strength	only carbs	ATP only (page 142)

(Figure 102)
Recruiting Motor Units

motor unit #1
Innervation to white fast-twitch fibers; strength, speed & power; stored carbs for energy; anaerobic metabolism,

motor unit #2
Innervation to red fast-twitch fibers; high resistance up to two minutes; stored carbs for energy; beginning of fat utilization for energy; anaerobic and beginning of aerobic metabolism,

motor unit #3
Innervation to red slow-twitch fibers; cardio endurance; stored fat for energy; aerobic metabolism,

Preceeding complete exhaustion, motor units can be recruited in a #3-#2-#1 order or in a #1-#2-#3 order without complete exhaustion but with no remaining strength. To stay at #2 and delay exhaustion involves a sequence of changing muscle groups to recruit different motor units for continuous performance at high resistance.

In the aquatic two minute set method, all skeletal muscles are exercised through their full range of motion with high intensity in separate sets for two minutes each using anaerobic and aerobic energy. Both energy pathways, the Krebs citric acid cycle and the glycogen-lactic acid system, function simultaneously. Each separate muscle group set of exercises is equally aerobic and anaerobic at the two-minute point. Both fats and carbohydrates are used for fuel (Figure 101B, p. 194). With the initial warm up, stretching, warming up again with progressive resistance, the continuous sequence of aquatic two-minute sets, the cool down, and some finish stretches, the workout takes a good hour.

Aquatic muscle endurance involves is the ability to increase anaerobic power within a perfect isokinetic setting in water for compound, multi-angled, orbital motion. Aquatic resistance is the environment and the motion can continually change dimensions and forces simultaneously. This allows more

muscle tissue to be conditioned during each exercise excursion through the full ability of each range of motion.

Any movement of the body requires complex coordination of many parts. Movements are not truly isolated. To address individual needs in aquatic exercise, isolations can be a direction of focus but the primary benefits result from extensive coordination of many groups of muscles not ordinarily utilized in that way on land. The beauty of movement in water is that there are unlimited variations. The limitations on land relate to the unidirectional source of resistance. Against the resistive force of water, the speed of a motion can vary, and with it, the force required. Unstructured techniques are today's trend (Ogden, 2002). This creates the opportunity for massive stimulation of fast and slow twitch contractile fibers throughout the skeletal muscle architecture. Only in water's viscosity can this be experienced. Aquatic resistance equipment greatly enhances the stimulation.

Pure strength training is not possible in water. It is natural for the body to conserve energy for survival when energy is needed for fight or flight situations. During aquatic exercise, muscle tissue can develop endurance under the stress of repeated forces. An exercise of pure strength does not have leftover energy available to expend beyond one occurrence. It is isometric.

Power introduces isotonic speed into the equation. As an example of research on improvement of power from aquatic exercise, knee extensor power as final _mean_ peak force increased 13% with 8 weeks of shallow water running.The increase was at a contraction speed of 120°/sec. (Hamer & Morton, 1990).

In water, a protective instinct exists that balances all aspects of fitness so that the human organism conserves energy and is able to survive diverse challenges requiring a blend of power, anaerobic endurance, and aerobic endurance. As anaerobic muscle endurance conditioning allows the use of higher resistance

and velocity, there is an overlap with the efficiency of power at one end and cardiovascular endurance as a consequence at the other end. The assumption is that stopping, resting, and breaks in the sequence of exercises are kept minimal or non-existent. Without adequate resistance, only aerobic endurance would remain. The metabolic biochemistry of aerobic endurance is very different from anaerobic muscle endurance but they can be blended together as two parallel paths.

Resistance training increases lean body mass. Aquatic exercise without adequate resistance, such as in exclusive cardio workouts, is detrimental to the health of bones. They eventually lose density without adequate bone loading. (Martin, 1989).

Oxygen Transport

The physiological adaptation and efficiency of oxygen transport during aquatic exercise is a function of the frequency, intensity and type of training. The lungs and

cardiovascular system adjust to the demands, mainly by skeletal muscles, that require an increase in the delivery of oxygen to cellular mitochondria to maintain homeostasis.

In Chapter 3, _Contractile Physiology in the Pool: (Pathways to Energy),_ cellular physiology is described in detail. In this subchapter we will be concerned with the efficiency of delivering oxygen to the cell during exercise.

During aquatic endurance exercise, frequency of breathing increases. Along with the frequency is an increase in breathing volume (tidal volume) that benefits alveolar ventilation up to a point where the lungs become incapable of further expansion.

The ventilatory muscles are the diaphragm, the intercostals, the serratus posterior superior during inspiration and the serratus posterior inferior during expiration. Combined, this is a large, active muscle mass with an oxidative metabolism that requires more energy as exercise intensity and duration increase. The energy needed for ventilation during heavy exercise for a healthy, fit adult is high and can be as great as 15% of the total body needs including metabolism of massive skeletal muscles (Shephard, 1966). The ventilatory muscles are about 6% of total body weight.

The alveolar diffusion rate for oxygen is dependant on the gas exchange membrane area and proportional to the pressure difference of oxygen between the alveolus and capillary. There is a dramatic increase in cross-sectional membrane area and pressure difference triggered at the onset of exercise, increasing O_2 diffusion (Johnson, 1973). There is also an improved exchange of CO_2 that results from the increased pressure difference. Unused capillaries in the lung open so there is a larger gas exchange membrane area. The ventilation differences between resting and maximal exercise for a healthy adult are as follows (Pardy, 1984):

variable	resting	maximal exercise
total ventilation	6.0 L/min.	≈125 L/min.
tidal volume	0.5 L/min.	2.5 L/min.
breaths	12/min.	40/min.

Sympathetic nervous activity increases with exercise, vasodilating active muscles in a balance with vasoconstriction, redistributing blood flow, and increasing venous return with higher cardiac output (Christensen, 1983). During the type of exercise that involves simultaneous activity of many major muscles, like many aquatic fitness exercises, maximal vasodilation is limited by the sympathic nerves to protect against excess vasodilation in peripheal areas that would decrease cardiac output by decreasing venous return (Secher, 1977). Also, nutrient exchange is facilitated with the expansion of the vascular area caused by an increase in capillaries.

All of these adaptations affect oxygen delivery and utilization. Delivery, from lungs to yhe muscle cells, may be represented as D(O^2)=cardiac output x arterial O^2. Utilization between oxygen brought to muscle cells minus the oxygen carried away, or **U(O^2)=D(O^2)-Returned (O^2).** (Law & Birkwira, 1999).

Oxygen has arrived now at the muscle cell mitochondria where a continuous supply of is needed to produce ATP for the electron transport and oxidative phosphorylation system detailed in Chapter 3. It's time to take a stretch.

Stretching Aquatically

Range of motion can be limited by tight and tense skeletal muscles and by dysfunctional connective tissues. These limitations can affect core balance and coordination and can be reduced by stretching, which also helps eliminate soreness. Improved flexibility with pre- and post-event stretching is an asset in any physical activity. Stretching helps warm up muscle tissue to prevent injury and increase power through a wider range of motion. Stretching also increases muscle length and range of motion.

Loss of flexibility changes the muscle length/tension relationship so that muscle produces less peak tension, thus decreasing muscle strength. A gain in flexibility will produce more peak tension in a more lengthened state, increasing the strength of the muscle.

Participants in aquatic endurance exercise classes stretch on land first by pulling on grab bars, using body weight effectively, pushing on a bench or stretching on a ballet bar. Then they enter the water, warm up without resistance equipment through full body motions, and stretch again in the water.

Using aquatic exercise equipment in its highest resistance configuration will enable the water to assist in opposing your stretch. Move deliberately and slowly to feel the effects on all of your muscles and tendons. Use your entire body and reach as far as you can. You will not fall over in the water, so be daring. Have fun stretching. Look forward with anticipation to this important part of your aquatic workout.

Avoid stretching or straining to the point of any sharp pain. Exhale when slowly moving deeper into a stretch, and hold it between 30 and 60 seconds. Using the viscous properties of the water, it is possible to perform unusual stretches that are very helpful to joints. Stretches in water can be methodical or artistic and creative experiences that involve changing the angle of stretch in consecutive positions until all tendon connections near a joint are stretched. Return from a stretch gracefully as slowly as you went into it.

Follow the dynamic stretches with PNF stretching after a full warm-up. What is PNF stretching? Proprioceptive neuromuscular facilitation stretches are isometrically assisted. After dynamic stretches and a warm-up, PNF stretches are in order if there is an assistant, a training partner, or selection of grab bars and ledges in the pool adequate to oppose movement at the point of stretch. A foot can be anchored against a ledge and the body turned to accomplish a stretch without assistance. A hand on

a bar or ladder rail can work the same way. PNF stretching can use flotation products fastened to or held on the distal end of an appendage, but there are limitations that restrict the force to only an upward direction.

The best method of PNF stretching includes a training partner or assistant. Stretch passively to near the maximum point of stretch, hold, isometrically contract against the assisting force that produced the stretch, hold, relax in that position, then repeat the assisted passive stretch farther, hold, contract isometrically again against the assisting force, hold, relax and repeat until the increase in stretch is minimal.

Working Out in the Pool

As mentioned in Chapters 1, 2 and 16, the mind needs water fitness too. Free form aquatic exercise can be combined with emotion to initiate unstructured, unplanned movement in water as a way to release the emotions and express spontaneous feelings.

The time for the mind to take control of the body in a more structured way is when a person wants primarily to improve physical performance. The most effective physical fitness workouts for the body require basic discipline. There are three prerequisites to a safe diciplined workout: hydration, stability, somatic awareness, stretching, and progressive stimulation (ACSM, 1998). Gradually escalate activity level through a full range of motion to increase blood flow in muscles and elevate body temperature. Slowly stretch the myofascial and connective tissues, muscles and tendons. It can be done hurriedly but the healthiest time period from that hydrating drink of water to the beginning of the actual exercise session is about fifteen minitus or more. Do not stop exercising abruptly. Cool down slowly with a gradual lowering of intensity. Stretch again. A post-exercise massage can facilitate relaxation of the neuromuscular system and help heal dysfunctional tissues.

Before looking at some of the aquatic workout methods, we should learn about the effects of exercise on pregnancy, diabetes, cancer, and blood pressure.

A pregnant client benefits greatly from aquatic exercise. The water pressure alone facilitates lymphatic flow and it is a relief to take weight off of the feet. After the first trimester it would not be wise to relax in a prone position without support because the round ligament and broad ligament holding the uterus in place need to be kept strong without being over-stretched.

Sixteen million people have diabetes mellitus in the United States. Most, 90-95%, have type 2 non-insulin-dependent diabetes. Without exercise, sedentary lifestyles can precipitate diabetes (Kirk, 2003). Excess body fat increases the severity of the syndrome (Weyer, 1999).

The American Diabetes Association recommends exercise with high repetitions for diabetics. The American College of Sports Medicine recommends vigorous aerobic levels for diabetes and advocates prolonged, large muscle group exercises that are continuous (ADA, 2000). Exercise is the cornerstone in managing the disease (Colberg, 2000). Aquatic exercise makes it possible to meet the largest variety of individual requirements for type 1 and type 2 diabetes. Exercising vigorously as infrequently as once a week lowers the risk of developing the disease (Manson, 1991).

Aerobic exercise for type 2 diabetics is less likely to increase insulin sensitivity than anaerobic interval training due to an increase in glycogen storage (Eriksson, 1998). Training aerobically metabolizes more fats, sparing muscle glycogen and blood glucose for more effective blood sugar maintenance. The American College of Sports Medicine advises aerobic activity @ 55-85% maximum heart rate 3-5 days/wk for 20-60 minutes or longer to reduce fat for diabetics (Pollack, 1998).

Diabetics who also incorporate aerobics into the "off-days," can use resistance training in water fitness programs with up to 10 different multi-muscle group exercises 2-3 days/wk. Keep the number of repetitions at the high end, 12-15 per set. Unless insulin can be reduced before starting to exercise, avoid hypoglycemia during and after the workout by having carbohydrates readily available at the poolside. Hypoglycemia can actually result from exercise and is a serious risk. The risk is lessened during early morning exercise compared to workouts in the late afternoon (Ruegemer, 1990). Exercising under hyperglycemic conditions can be detrimental to metabolic control and cause dehydration (Colberg, 2000).

A conclusion in many research studies is that exercise lowers the risk for a variety of diseases such as hypertension and obesity (Engstrom, 1999), coronary heart disease (Haapanen, 1997), colon cancer (Thune, 1996), and breast cancer in a 15 year study of 4,000 athletes and non-athletes (Cromie, 2000; Thune, 1997). Exercise also reduces hormonally related cancers including breast, endometrial, prostate, and testicular (Schmitz, 2000), as well as mortality from all causes (Kampert, 1996). Exercise correlates with reductions ion prostate cancer growth of up to 30% (Aronson, 2001). Colon cancer, the third leading cause of cancer incidence and mortality in the United States, was significantly reduced with regular physical activity.

Systolic and diastolic blood pressure can be reduced with moderate, submaximal exercise by lowering cardiac output, peripheral resistance after training, and central fat deposition (Arrol, 1992). A study by the National Institutes of Health reports that moderate exercise among

70% of those tested reduced their blood pressure by over 10mm Hg (Hagberg, 1995). Maximal resistance exercise raises blood pressure during exercise but the myocardial oxygen demand is lower (Pollack, M., 2000). A conservative 30-60% maximal effort is recommended by the American Heart Association for modifying coronary risk factors like hypertension.

There are at least six basic aquatic workout methods for anaerobic muscle endurance and two or more methods for aerobic conditioning. In an aerobic pool workout, maintain your target heart rate for twenty minutes or more. Conventionally there are the repeated patterns of old style aerobic routines. Overall there is a healthy method that incorporates the series of the unstructured two-minute sets, described above, extended continuously through the duration of the aerobic session. This not only maintains heart rate, it also is motivating and stimulates an alert interest in what you are doing. In the process, balance, coordination, agility and reaction time improve. Lengthen the time as conditioning adapts to increased efficiency of the cardiovascular system. Go nonstop from one exercise to another, using exercises that require multiple muscle groups. The more muscle tissue that is engaged, the better the results. Exercise daily. During forced inhalation, the large diaphragm pushes up on the vena cava, giving much assistance to return blood flow through the largest vein in the body. Breathe deeply.

The six methods of pool workouts are:
- comprehensive workouts
- split routines
- free form movements (above)
- periodization within a workout
- periodization within a month
- isolations in one session

A comprehensive workout exercises all muscles in one session with one or two recovery days between sessions. A split routine divides each session into muscle groups such as chest/arms one day and back/legs the next day followed by one day off. Free form is not a routine. It is a powerful, comprehensive free-form movement

workout that includes all muscles through full ranges of motion. Progression involves increased intensity and duration.
A periodized workout within the same session exercises the entire body but puts emphasis one muscle group over another on one day and another muscle group the next day. This would exercise the whole body each session with a day of recovery between each exercise session. Periodization within a month includes a cyclic change in intensity throughout the month, incorporating a peak workout at about the same day of every month. Also, weekly periodization can spread varying degrees of intensity. An example is a three-day-per-week training schedule with a light workout on Monday, moderate on Wednesday, and heavy on Friday. When I was a competitive powerlifter, I trained at Western Illinois University and at the University of Alaska where I worked-out with and learned from nationally recognized powerlifters. The athletes that became state champions and made record-setting lifts used periodization by working up to a

higher peak every three weeks, calculating backwards from a competition date so that a peak intensity practice of maximum lifts would fall on the day of winning the event in their weight classes, and that we did.

An isolation exercise, as part of a routine, concentrates on one muscle and one movement. This is most useful for physical therapy and rehabilitation. To isolate one movement using increased aquatic resistance, it is necessary to maneuver the equipment so that resistance is streamlined and minimal on the return to the starting position. Using three-dimensional equipment has a disadvantage because it requires nearly stopping and very slowly returning to the starting position before using velocity in the direction of the isolation. Using two-dimensional equipment with a thin, flat side to it, allows a streamlined return with no change in velocity but with an absence of resistance. An isolated repetition with pulsating resistance that strains a bone is an important method of maintaining bone strength.

Concentric loading, where a muscle contracts with resistance, is the usual type of aquatic exercise since all directions are "positive" in water. You might not think it is possible to experience eccentric loading in a pool and you may not have ever observed it. Eccentric loading extends a muscle with resistance, like slowly lowering a bench press. Pushing up during a bench press is concentric. The prime mover, the pectoralis major, shortens. Lengthening a muscle under resistance is eccentric.

Eccentric loading in water is possible. The Aquatoner® (Figure 181) with an adjustable resistance area and overlapping surfaces, a handle and a foot attachment, is an example of aquatic exercise equipment used against a controlled current of water to facilitate eccentric loading. Controlled water current can be from a portable or permanent swim jet or paddle with an adjustable flow in a swim spa. Most of the pools and tanks with a controlled rate of concentrated

or homogenous water flow, as well as the portable swim spa jets with variable depths, have a flow rate up to 6 mph and sometimes more. That is a lot of water moving per minute. If a horizontal core of water is mechanically forced through a pool for the purpose of swimming against the direction of force, it is also possible to stand next to the area of high flow with the Aquatoner and enter or exit the flow area according to when you want concentric or eccentric loading. An exercise can be in the shape of an ellipse to take advantage of the possibilities for eccentric loading in water against this type of defined flow.

Exercise intensity in water can be measured. The equations are in Chapter 11, *The Kinetics of Water*. Without data input, aquatic exercise is measured only by perceived resistance. According to a person's potentials, they can self-assess it as maximal, moderate, or light effort. Maximal is 100%, moderate is 90%, and light is 85% of maximum maneageable resistance and exercise intensity. Warm-up exercises

gradually increase from 50% to 70% of perceived maximal intensity.

Failure is not possible in water. A single maximum effort with free weights on land means that an immediate second attempt would be a failure and the weight would either drop or not be moved. With a weight machine, the stack of iron and the pulley system would crash to the starting rest position at failure. In water, with the Aquatoner or other large aquatic resistance device, the speed of movement during a perceived maximum effort is slower and slower as the person proceeds to a depletion of energy. The resistance becomes less and less with no failure occurring. It is variable during one single movement by controlling the speed. Using multiple muscle groups and compound movements is preferable to strict isolations. Gravity strengthens tissues, so use gravity to your advantage during aquatic workouts, exercising in the minimum depth of water that still allows the working surfaces of the equipment to be fully submerged.

The illustrations that follow are examples of muscle endurance training exercises using Aquatoners, the AQ-Bar, the T-Bar and the Double T-Bar (Figures 103-116).

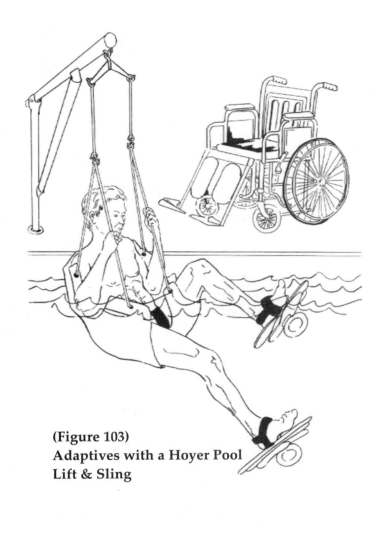

(Figure 103)
Adaptives with a Hoyer Pool Lift & Sling

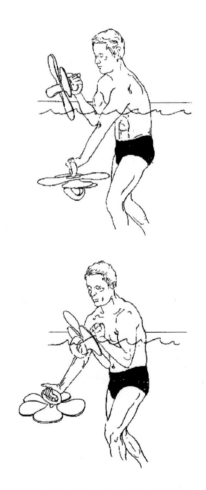

(Figure 104A) "Justice" named by John Hettinger III
"Justice is Blind, Balanced"; Alternate Biceps/Triceps

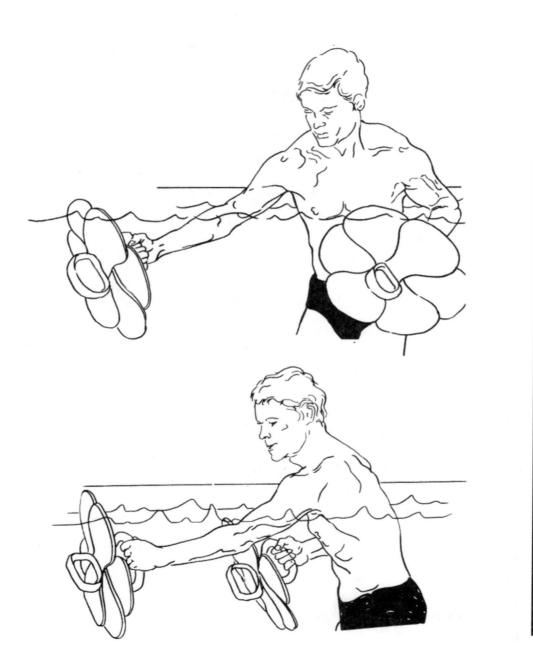

(Figure 104B)
Entire Upper Body
"Boxing"

Nalu: The Art and Science of Aquatic Fitness, Bodywork & Therapy

(Figure 105)
Obliques,
Transverse Abdominals

(Figure 106)
"Bullfighter"
named by John Hettinger III
Lats, Erector-Spinae,
Posterior Deltoid,
Quadratus Lumborum

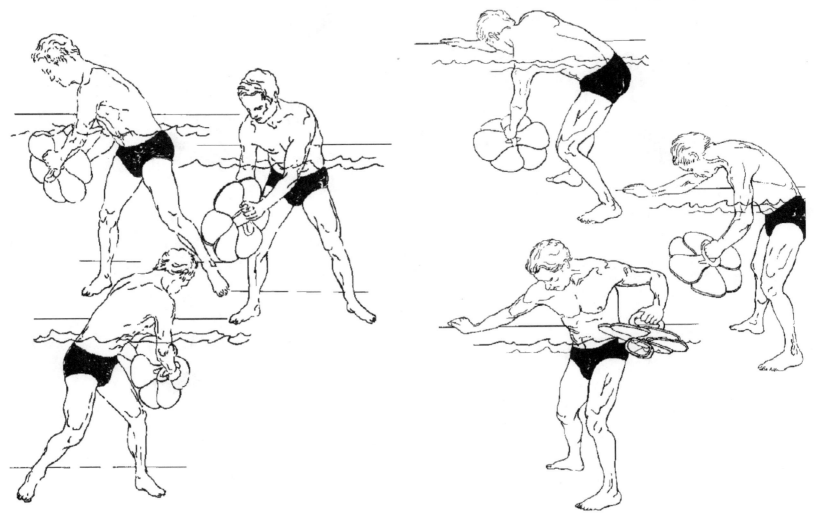

(Figure 107)
"Cymbals"
named by John
Hettinger III
Pectorals,
Anterior Deltoid

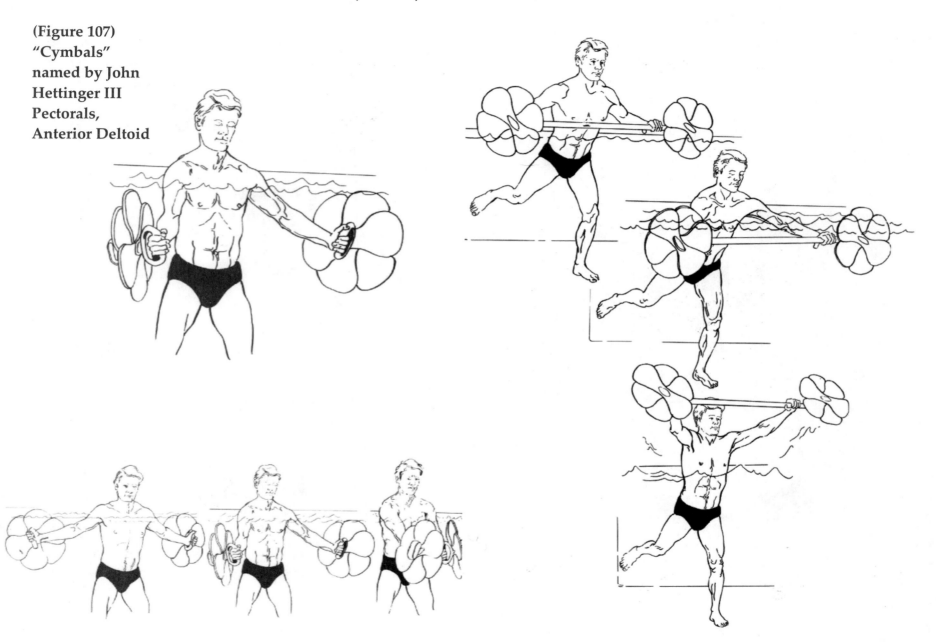

(Figure 108)
Triceps

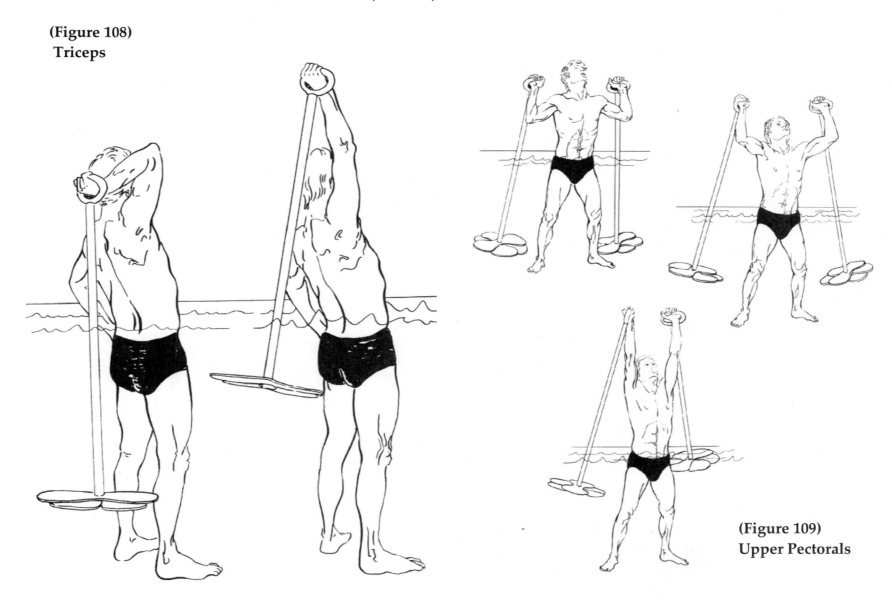

(Figure 109)
Upper Pectorals

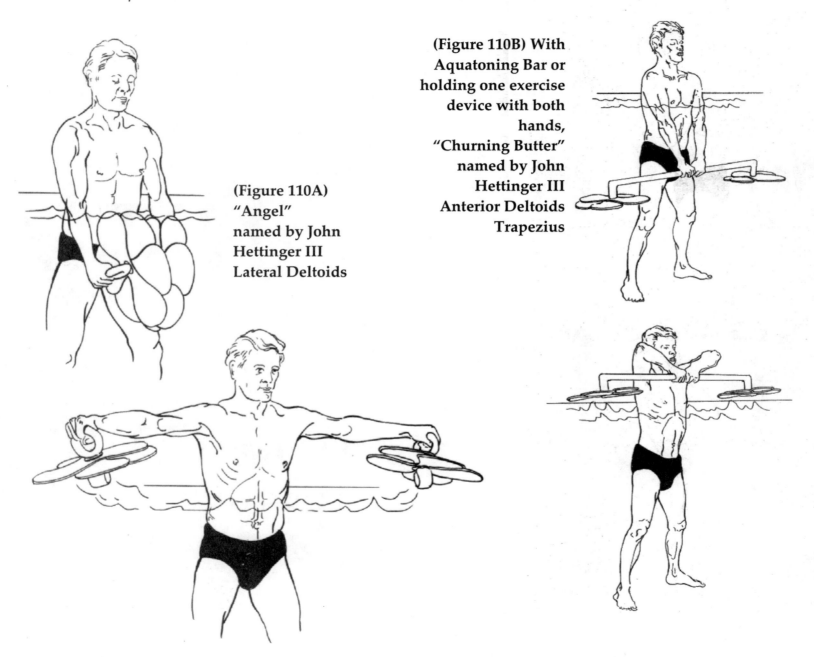

(Figure 110A)
"Angel"
named by John
Hettinger III
Lateral Deltoids

(Figure 110B) With
Aquatoning Bar or
holding one exercise
device with both
hands,
"Churning Butter"
named by John
Hettinger III
Anterior Deltoids
Trapezius

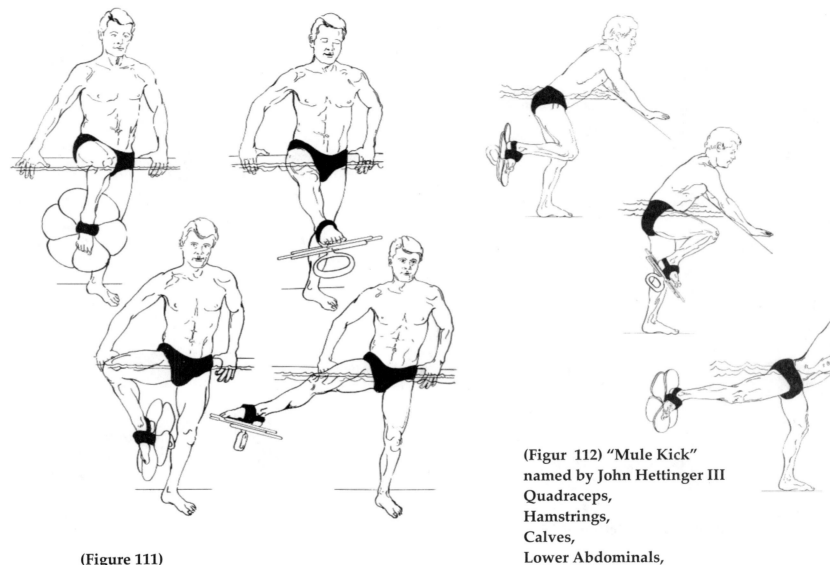

(Figure 111)
"Hinge" named by John Hettinger III
 Quadraceps,
 Hamstrings

(Figur 112) "Mule Kick"
named by John Hettinger III
Quadraceps,
Hamstrings,
Calves,
Lower Abdominals,
Iliopsoas,
Gluteus

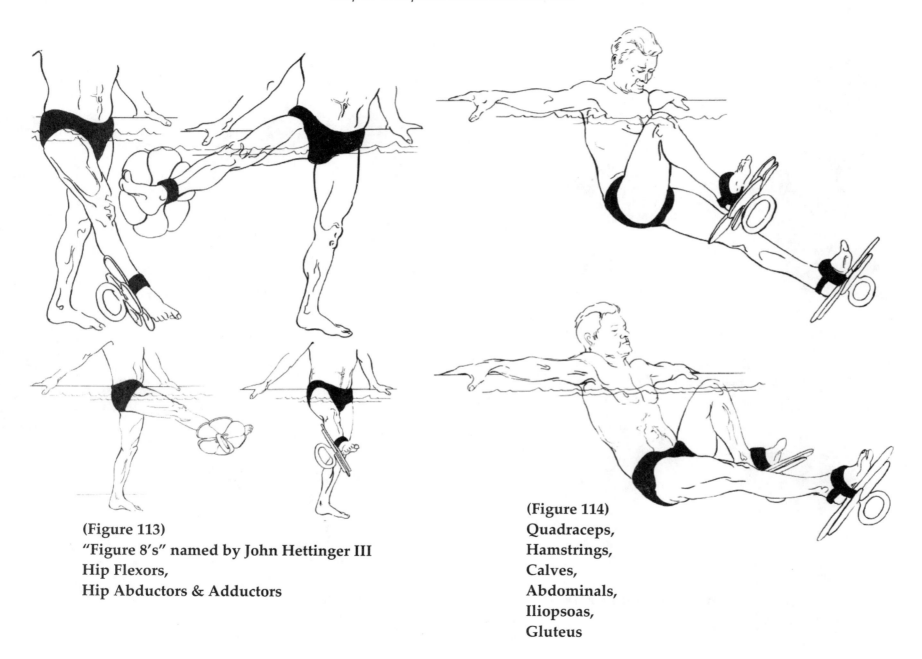

(Figure 113)
"Figure 8's" named by John Hettinger III
Hip Flexors,
Hip Abductors & Adductors

(Figure 114)
Quadraceps,
Hamstrings,
Calves,
Abdominals,
Iliopsoas,
Gluteus

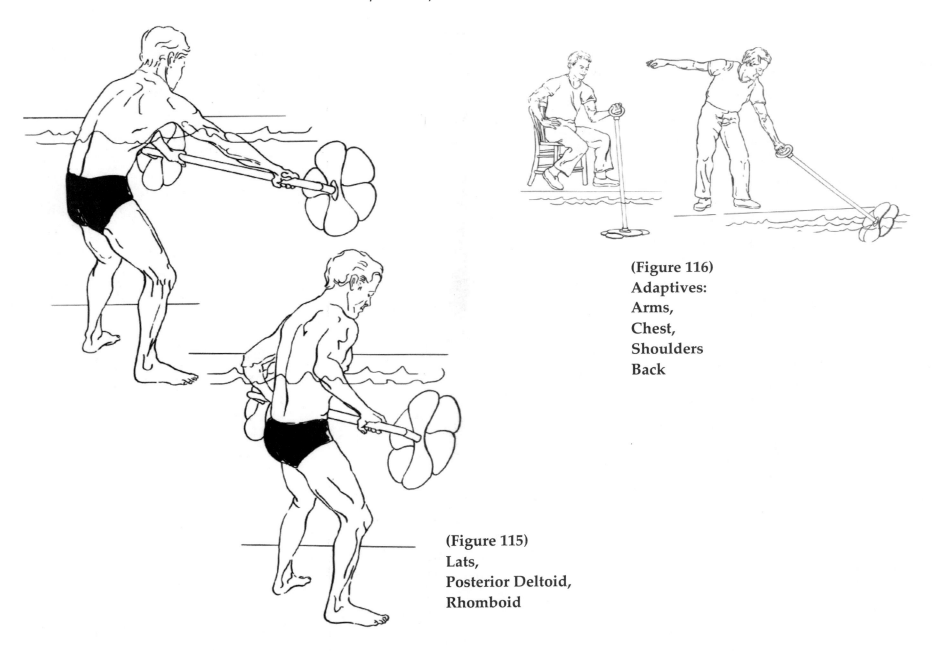

**(Figure 116)
Adaptives:
Arms,
Chest,
Shoulders
Back**

**(Figure 115)
Lats,
Posterior Deltoid,
Rhomboid**

Inactivity and aging

Vigorous aquatic exercise reduces the risk of all-cause mortality. It is speculated by some researchers that exercise increases life-span by increasing the ability to neutralize free radicals. Higher intensity exercise in general reduces the risk of all-cause mortality (Blair, 1989). In other words it increases lifespan. Here is the proof. The Harvard Alumni Health Study at Harvard's Department of Epidemiology studied the effects of many types of vigorous exercise and a variety of non-vigorous exercise on human longevity over a period of many years. Though non-vigorous exercise has health benefits, it did not show a relationship with longevity. Total energy expenditure and energy expenditure from vigorous activities related inversely to mortality in this 26 year study of 17,321 Harvard Alumni males with a mean age of 46 years (Lee, Hsieh, and Paffenbarger, 1995). This high-powered research concludes that exercising vigorously correlates with increased lifespan and a 25% lower death rate. In the longest, most important epidemiological study in medical history, The Framingham Heart Study at Boston University School of Medicine, 5209 adults have been studied since 1948 to investigate diseases and health problems. In the Framingham study on exercise and longevity, those who expended 2,000 calories per week on regular exercise increased life expectancy by two years.

There is less overall physical activity and more mechanized production in the industrialized, developed societies around the world. The decrease in activity has increased death rates from heart disease, cancers, and other causes related to deficient physical exercise. Inactivity has increased the incidence of mental depression (Weyerer, 1992).

In prehistoric times, humans died young of traumatic injuries and medical ignorance more often than from the chronic diseases of old age. Vigorous activities were the norm. We had to climb a tree for fruit and run down a mammoth for food. We had to collect and carry wood for winter fuel and gather a harvest over a large area. We had to carry water. Every aspect of basic survival was often a daily physical challenge. To these ancestors, the more sedentary life today would be equal to living in a convalescent center. Anthropologically, the abnormal circumstance in human history is the reduction throughout many modern cultures in the physical challenges and intensity of everyday activities. It is more logical to express the true statement that certain types of exercise correlate inversely with reduced mortality. Inactivity shortens life-span (Blair, 1989).

Aging beyond 60 years parallels sarcopenia, a decrease in muscle mass at a rate of 3-6% per decade (DiPietro, 2000) with higher loss beyond 70 years old. The physical condition of individuals over 85 years old is commonly frail. Lean body weight declines from disuse atrophy with an age-dependent increase in percent body fat associated with sedentary behavior. Inactivity with aging leads to physiological changes and functional losses (Bortz, 1982). Defects in carbohydrate metabolism and a loss of alpha-motor neurons also contribute to the sarcopenia.

Safe physical activity increases physical function in aging (Haskell, 1995). Structured water fitness is one of the safest forms of physical activity for seniors. In addition to buoyancy and easily controlled resistance for joint comfort, aquatic programs in community pools offer an ideal environment for beneficial socializing that motivates the aging population to maintain an interest in their health.

The Image of Made Belief

By Mark McEachren

I observe life and existence because I am an etiologist of consciousness. If I can understand the causation and patterns of my life I may then influence of my existence. I choose to be the realization of personal, purposeful intentions, therefore, I need to consciously know the appropriate directives that will command specific physical actions. The thoughts that direct our physical actions are often subconscious behavioral responses reacting to the pressures of outside forces. Our Fight or Flight response is a readiness to fight or run away from any situation that posses a challenge. By understanding that the primary responsibility of the body and subconscious mind is to conserve energy our conscious mind may then command "Objective Actions" rather than continually being circumvented by "Behavioral Reactions." This holds true even during willing participation in exercise. No matter how aware or evolved we are, survival and energy efficiency instincts will always remain in the infrastructure in our evolutionary code. This energy economy resonates in our every thought, and consequently manifests in our every action.

These subconscious influences are an essential aspect in understanding the tipping point of exercise success. As a child I expressed my life through athletics. Each physically demanding day was based specifically on practicing, improving, and playing the game. As I look back on this now I see how my youthful perspective willingly funded a limitless account for exerting maximum energy and effort. All I paid attention to was my desire, never my fatigue. I saw the possibilities, not the constraints. This truly is the wonder of youth. Evolving through this life process my youthful orientations inevitably became adult ones. My once-limitless energy pool is now perceived as finite. I tend to mark the daily events of my life on a priority scale, constantly weighing the factors of personal cost and return. The spontaneous joy and exuberance from my youth are far too often replaced by a conservative accountant that rations energy expenditures according to need and availability. This priority scale is like a conscious fulcrum that tilts towards the "Action" of actual physical enhancement, or a "Reaction" that merely allots the minimal energy to animate motions that pantomime a desired outcome.

I am a fitness professional; a fitness enthusiast. I love to exercise, and I spend countless hours of each day professing the undeniable benefits of it. Yet, I still contend with the innate desire to minimize my efforts during a workout. Physical actions tend to be compromised by the energy conservation code of the subconscious mind. I often find myself distracted by the resonating waves of evolutionary emotions and by my in-house energy accountant eagerly suggesting all the possible views of effort reduction. These reactions are simply evolutionary habits. They are part of an automatic survival mechanism that can remain distinct from our conscious view. What we

experience is the contrast of a deeply embedded primal subsistence verses our desire for the higher order of self transcending activity. This is a crucial point in conscious comprehension because the physical success of any discipline may only be achieved by molding and directing the repetitive patterns of our thoughts. The tangible and the empirical are merely a cast representation of the integrated relationship between our conscious and subconscious minds.

Exercise is like an alchemic process where the secret codes and transformative vibrations of a hidden sphere mesh with the apparent world of all that we observe and interact with. Upon opening ourselves we enter the voidless gap where past and present meet. This is like discovering an inception substrate where all physical conceptions are possible. The moment we realize that external developments are a direct result of the thoughts that create them we may then.orient our attention (and efforts) on the "Cause" of our lives rather than the "Effect." Each of our individual

perspectives is offered this panoramic point of view. The choice of "Action" or "Reaction" is either the crystallizing elements of physical success, or the slow drift of good intentions that never transpire. In essence we are the creators of our own reality. Shift your orientation back to the origin of your thoughts. Within this space you will find the platform where physical manifestations begin.

Consciousness is caus— everything that follows is effect. Your body is the Image of Made Belief.

Mark McEachren is a fitness philosopher who has inspired countless individuals in their personal training sessions to reach their goals most efficiently. Nalu is fortunate to have Mark McEachren author the Forward of this book.

Chapter 7
Bone Density and Aquatic Exercise

Weightlessness in Space

When Ruth Sova first conceived of the idea of organizing an Aquatic Exercise Association in the early 1980's she started a monthly newsletter, AKWA. I submitted an article published in one of the first issues titled "Bones in the Pool." Twenty years later, this chapter is a follow-up to that article.

What happens to your bones in a swimming pool? If aquatics is the only form of physical exercise and if the activity in water is only light aerobic exercise, the result would be similar to that of astronauts in space, atrophy of bone mass. To bones it is no different than inactivity because the load is inadequate to build or maintain bone density. Bone density decreases with inactivity and the risk of eventual osteoporosis increases

(Beck and Shoemaker, 2000). Popular water fitness classes create an illusion that all is well. After all, exercise is healthy, right? Not always, not when the real thing is neglected. Compared with swimming or casual water fitness classes, it takes mechanical tension and loading in different directions with higher aquatic resistance forces on the bones for repetitions at higher intensity to maintain or increase bone density. Exercises with higher strain rates are more osteogenic than aerobic exercises (LaMothe, 2003). Gymnasts, for example, have a higher bone mass than runners (Robinson, 1995). Swimmers lose bone density (Stone, 1996).

The weightless environment of space flight, similar in some respects to floating in water, has been researched extensively for thirty-seven years. Twenty-six of the studies regarding bone loss in weightlessness were analyzed by professor Dava Newman at Space Biomedical Engineering and Life Support, Inc. (2001). In summary: there is a significant loss of bone mass, a negative calcium balance,

decrescent mineral density (as much as 2% per month) and a reduction in osteoblast activity while osteoclasts are unaffected. Also found were impaired fracture repair, reduced bone strength and onset of disuse osteoporosis. During long space flights bones become significantly brittle and weaker and fracture more easily, especially in the hips, spine, and wrist. In a 1991 test by Grigoriev, et al, on a long duration Mir mission, one cosmonaut lost 10% of the trabecular bone from L1 to L3. The most severe bone loss is between the second and fifth month of microgravity. Bones loose calcium during weightlessness (Rambaut, 1979; Tilton et al, 1980). Current research focuses on the lumbar spine and the proximal femur, the most critical weight-bearing areas.

Through misty cool clouds
was the place.
A dream it was not.
I was falling through space.

Hooked to the harness of an experienced skydiver, 10,000 feet above the small islands of the Florida Keys, three of us tumbled out of an airplane. For me it was the first time. I needed a break from writing this chapter. I needed that rush of freedom from the burdens of gravity. Yet it was gravity that was pulling so hard at us to return to Earth. There was no escape from it. Air is a fluid like water but 800 times less dense. Evidenced by the roar and its assistance in maneuverability, air viscosity was the only resistance to the fall. Deploying the parachute was the transition. My mind wanted to stay in space but my bones wanted to return to the Earth for a breathtaking encounter with reverse peristalsis.

><((((O>   ><((((O>   ><((((O>

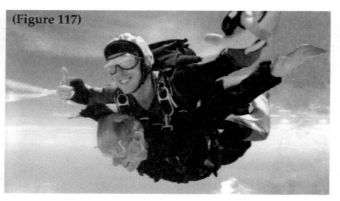

(Figure 117)

The author, free-falling from 10,000′ (3,050m) over the Florida Keys

Back on Earth, the local bone sites that undergo direct mechanical loading during exercise show the greatest increase in bone density. Among tennis players, it was repeatedly confirmed that the playing arm had a 30% greater bone cortex thickness than the non-playing arm (Dalen et al, 1985; Heinonen et al, 1995; Hudleston et al, 1980; Pirnay et al, 1985). In water that means using the proper exercise equipment to enhance and control the forces and directions of tension.

This chapter details how living bone tissue remodels and adapts to the forces of higher aquatic resistance. Data concerning the effects of moderate or light resistance on bone density appears uncertain. Most of the testing is on mice. My investigation of the research indicates that it takes more than moderate aquatic exercise to enhance bone density.

Many "fitness experts" maintain that aquatic exercise cannot enhance bone density. Later in this chapter I will show the data they collected were not specific to the central issue of debilitating bone fractures. The reader will also find a summary of research showing that aquatic mammals have, in fact, higher bone densities than land dwellers. I also present a detailed description of bone remodeling which shows how the greater variation available in aquatic exercise contributes to more comprehensive bone strength. While these opinions, facts and research are not decisive, they do strongly suggest that well-directed aquatic exercise will enhance bone density.

In the beginnings of our lives, earthborn constituents are

nutritionally consumed and used by the body to build tissues, including bone tissue. Initially bones are soft as they grow and lengthen. They adapt to body weight, body mechanics, hormones and exercise. Bones become strong and supportive, increase density and mass, stabilize, and then either maintain density and mass or they can become porous, weak, fatigued and easily fractured. The cortical bone near the medullary canal of an elderly person is riddled with large holes (Smith and Walmsley, 1959). Low bone density causes a high risk for fracture. Eventually, all bones return to the earth and degrade into their original elements.

*S*ince 1942 I never broke a bone…

but it was oh so close to multiple fractures learning how to fly a hot air balloon in Colorado in 1977. Working at the Balloon Ranch, launching balloons mornings and evenings to the tune of Beethoven's Symphony No.9 in D minor op.125 Molto vivace, and chasing airborne, champagne-drenched dudes that stayed at the

ranch for a week or two to get their pilot's license and purchase their own balloons, I wrangled the horses throughout the day, doing carpentry repairs where needed. It was time to learn how to fly. There was an instructor from England willing to teach me to become a balloonist. We flew across the San Luis Valley and back day after day, contouring down along the foothills and rock outcroppings at the west edge of the valley. We ascended to the bottoms of clouds to view Taos and Aspen at the same time. What an absolute thrill. "Ian, what would happen to my passengers if there was a fuel problem at this altitude and the burner went out? I asked." He said that the balloon would descend no faster than about 1100 feet per minute, float down, and land with few or no injuries.

We were at 14,000 ft. (4270m) altitude, the height of the Sangre de Cristo Mountains on the east side of the valley. The valley bottom was at 7,000 ft (2135m) elevation. With the exception of Alamosa and some very small, desolate communities of weathered gray buildings, upside

down rusty remnants of old pickup trucks and a very few ranches, most of the valley was a high desert of windblown tumbleweed, with scatterings of sheep and occasional coyotes. The surrounding snow-topped mountains displayed a spectacular level of golden autumn aspen tress among healthy pines. The bright sunrise, enhanced by our ascent into the sky, was welcome warmth on our backs in the cool, crisp air.

The open question was, should we or should we not experience a fueless descent in the balloon? After all, it would just float down like a parachute. With a mutually agreeable smile the burner was turned off. I pulled down hard on the bridle line that opened the top of the balloon envelope to let out the hot air. In silence we watched the altimeter stabilize at a loss of 1100 ft (335m) per minute as we dropped steadily out of the sky, enveloped and bathed within the stillness of the wind. We were encapsulated in an air current of tranquility. As we approached the planet there was still plenty of time to change our minds and fire up the burner. Onward and downward we went, determined to experience what Ian said would be a gentle parachute-like impact. Fooled by the stillness, we hit the Earth with an immediate horizontal turn of the brown suede-trimmed wicker basket onto its side. It happened so fast we were suddenly face down as the power of the wind kept the colorful rip-stop nylon balloon full of air in a horizontal position, bouncing and dragging us over and through the dirt, sand, rocks, cactus, and sheep dung that began to fill up the balloon basket we were riding in. After nearly a half-mile the basket came to a stop, the balloon collapsed, and there we were out in the middle of nowhere hardly able to walk. Ian and I were both covered with debris, bruised and sore, but laughing, delighted that no bones were broken thanks to high bone density from lifting the balloon and basket in and out of the truck every day. Air, I discovered, is a powerful moving fluid.

⤛⟨⟨⟨⟨O⟩   ⤛⟨⟨⟨⟨O⟩   ⤛⟨⟨⟨⟨O⟩

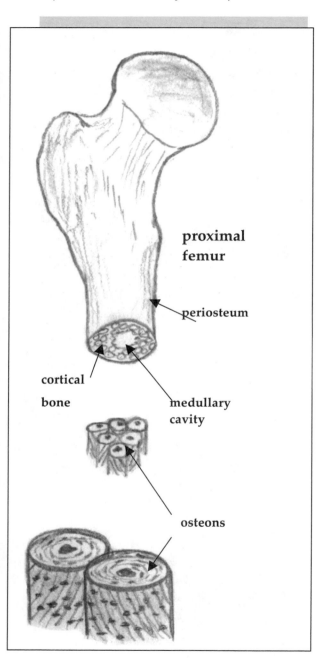

proximal femur

periosteum

cortical bone

medullary cavity

osteons

**(Figure 118)
Osteons in Cortical Bone**

The shafts of long bones and flat bones are called cortex or cortical bone. Cortical bone, sometimes referred to as compact bone, has a central Haversian canal (Figure 119, 120) containing blood vessels, nerves, and a lacunae. The osteons (Figures 118, 119, 120) are arranged in concentric rings called lamellae. Between the osteons are cement lines that separate canaliculi and collagen from other osteons.

Cortical bone is dense for strength and thin to reduce weight and allow space for an inner medullary cavity. On the outside of the diaphysis, the shaft of cortical bone, is the periosteum, a thin covering of high-strength connective tissue for tendon attachment and protection. Perpendicular to the periosteal and endosteal surfaces and the Haversian canals are vascular channels called Volkmann's canals.

(Figure 119) Bone Tissue

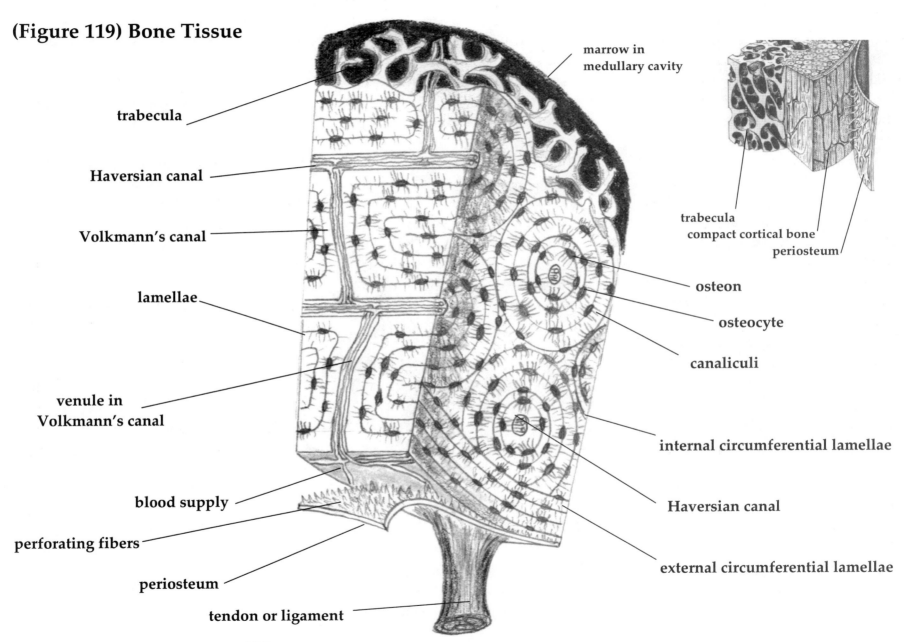

trabecula

Haversian canal

Volkmann's canal

lamellae

venule in
Volkmann's canal

blood supply

perforating fibers

periosteum

tendon or ligament

marrow in
medullary cavity

trabecula
compact cortical bone
periosteum

osteon

osteocyte

canaliculi

internal circumferential lamellae

Haversian canal

external circumferential lamellae

Nalu: The Art and Science of Aquatic Fitness, Bodywork & Therapy

At the larger heads of long bones and along the inner walls of the medullary cavity is the spongy cancellous bone, a porous lattice of mineralized bridges and struts called trabecula that provide great strength with minimal weight. Sometimes called trabecular bone, it is a strong, lightweight lattice of bone tissue that fills the area. The layers in cancellous bone are lamellae and are the architectural pattern in parallel to the long axis of the osteon. Lacunae are the flui- filled cavities along the layer boundaries. The bone cells in the lacunae are the osteocytes. From these cavities that contain the osteocytes are small canals that radiate out, mostly perpendicularly from the lacunae and connect to other lacunae. Cancellous bone does not contain blood vessels. The blood supply is in the bone marrow between the struts. The blood and fluids travel from the marrow through channels.

The numerous canaliculi in cortical bone also transport fluids and ions that act as a communication network between osteocytes. It takes a water molecule 1.24 minutes to travel from a Haversian canal in cortical bone to the farthest osteocyte in the same osteon (Tate et al, 1998). There is a rapid passage of ions and electrochemical signal molecules in this intracellular and extracellular route.

Tooth enamel, a cortical bone tissue, is lower in water content, below 10%, and higher in mineralized matrix. Cortical bone in long shafts is up to 20-25% water as is cancellous bone. 85% of the water is located around the collagen fibers. 15% of the water is located in the canals and cavities that house the bone cells. Increased porosity is associated with aging, and osteoporosis results in higher water content due to an increase in cavities. Normal porosity in bone is 5-30% for cortical bone and 30-95% (mostly 75-95%) for cancellous bone.

Lamellar bone has no central canal or lacunae and spans the regions as thin, dense sheets with circumferencial and parallel oriented fine collagen fibers between secondary osteons. It wraps the concentric rings of Haversian bone and provides high strength from oblique orientation angles and the architecture of its collagen fibers. The structural parameters of the matrix are the angles of wrapping of the lamellar collagen within osteons, ellipticity and angular distribution of the osteons about the bone axis, and the asymmetry of the distribution. Departing geometrically from parallel alignment of osteons and circular-cylindrical symmetry, the true osteonal shape is an elliptical-cylindrical geometry. Geometry is the key to bone strength.

The trabecular lattice pattern in cancellous bone in the ends of long bones lines up parallel to the directions of tension experienced by the bone from external mechanical forces. Weightlessness and buoyancy have a negative influence on bone density. Exercise and bone loading are the major sources of mechanical forces that create strain to strengthen cortical and cancellous bone, altering the internal geometry (Currey, 2002).

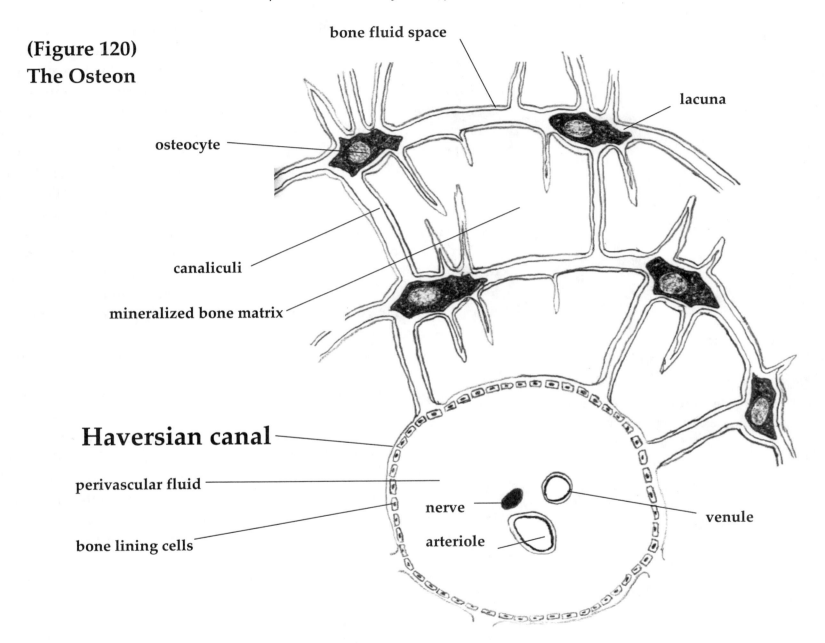

**(Figure 120)
The Osteon**

bone fluid space

lacuna

osteocyte

canaliculi

mineralized bone matrix

Haversian canal

perivascular fluid

nerve

venule

bone lining cells

arteriole

Response to Strain Rate

Strain rate is the rate of bone elongation or deformation divided by the initial length or form before deformation. It represents change with time. Strain is the measurement of the amount of change divided by the initial dimension of the bone before the change, or m/m. It is converted to a percent by multiplying x 100. The unit of measurement commonly used for bone strain rate is %/sec.

Propagated impact to a bone initiates an elastic strain wave (Currey, 2002). The strain wave is partly reflected from the bone and partly transmitted into the bone. The differences are used to calculate a dynamic stress-strain curve. Stresses are linearly dependent on the amplitude of the transmitted wave while the strain rate is linearly dependent on the amplitude of the reflected wave. Strain rate is used in many calculations regarding the properties of bone. Compressive strength of a bone for example is proportional to the square of the apparent density

and to the strain rate raised to the 0.06 power (Carter & Hayes, 1976).

The prevailing demands of mechanical strain, not stress, are partially responsible for determining the architecture of bone (Biewener and Taylor, 1986). Bone cells sense the changes in deformation and initiate deposition and resorption of bone tissue. The continual process of formation and resorption is called "remodeling."

Bone modeling occurs during growth and is different from remodeling. The bones lengthen and change shape. To change shape, osteoclasts resorb in places and osteoblasts form new bone in other places. They work independently for a continuous and prolonged time to reshape diameter, curvature or length of the bone. Modeling is resorptive and formative.

Remodeling, by contrast, is the lifetime process of repair from fatigue micro- damage. Macrofracture from traumatic injury that disrupts bone tissue is also a remodeling process, but in this case fibrocartilage precedes

the ossification just as hyaline cartilage precedes the initial bone growth of skeletal development. In adults the turnover rate of remodeling for fatigue damage repair in large bone shafts is 3% per year (Parfitt, 1983). At times during remodeling the osteoclasts and osteoblasts work together briefly as a team. The team is a basic multicellular unit, BMU. Remodeling does not usually change the shape or size of a bone. It removes part of the older bone tissue and forms new bone in its place to repair microscopic damage that could lead to fracture if not repaired (Currey, 2002). As the BMU tunnels through the bone it creates a secondary osteon (Martin, Burr, Sharkey, 1998). The deep tunnel does not fill completely with new bone because the leading cells at the front of the tunnel need nutrients. Capillaries from the medullary canal or periosteal surface feed the cells at the front through a new Haversian canal. The new bone is a bone structural unit — the secondary osteon.

Osteons accumulate with age (Stout and Simmons, 1979). This causes porosity. In women, the porosity results from an increase in the Haversian canal diameters while in men it results from a greater number of osteons (Thompson, 1980). New osteons can obliterate old osteons as the BMU's tunnel through the bone. There is a big difference between skeletal tissue age and the chronological age of the person. One bone will contain tissue of many ages.

All cells are sensitive to mechanical forces. In bone, osteocytes are the primary mechanosensory cells. Osteons (Figures 118-120, pages 218-221) develop at places in bone where pressures could disrupt the surface periosteum. It takes about a week to produce resorption cavities during osteon formation and about three months to fill them.

The osteocyte is a mature osteoblast among the few left behind during remodeling. It becomes trapped in the mineralized matrix and is then responsible for the maintenance of the matrix (Buckwalter, 1995). Osteocytes communicate through a network of unmineralized canaliculi and through gap junctions, allowing cell-to-cell coupling. Gap junctions are located where cell membranes of two cells fuse together and allow ions to pass between the membranes though channels.

The superficial osteocytes are connected with the periosteum lining that covers the bone surface, and with the new bone-forming osteoblasts on the surface with the periosteum. The thin periosteum surrounds a bone like a smooth envelope. It is connective tissue that merges with the connective tissue of tendons and consequently with the mesh of myofascia that surrounds muscles and muscle fibers. All movements are sensed by the periosteum. Osteocytes are able to adjust their responsiveness to mechanical loading by adaptation of the surrounding matrix and it's porosity. Hormones and the availability of an adequate supply of minerals influence them.

Stress is the applied force and strain is the resulting deformation. In water the forces originate from all directions. With gravity weights or a pulley cable machine the forces originate from just one direction. In water the source is orbital like an electron around a proton. The source, again, is from all directions. The consequence is a more diverse combination of forces than from gravity alone or from land-based restrictive exercise machines.

Bone is alive. Bone is osseous connective tissue. It is vascular, piezoelectric, in constant renewal, mineralized, and responsive to mechanical loads. Bone responds to mineral concentrations in the blood that are needed by the nervous system and other physiological functions. Soft connective tissues, the ligaments and tendons, maintain the assembly as a connected unified system.

Purposes of the bones are: mechanical integrity, locomotion, protection, structural support, production of blood and stockpiling minerals to maintain blood homeostasis. The skeleton is a very complex association of metabolically active cells surrounded by a mineralized matrix. Living bone is 8- 25% water, 70-85% mineral, and the remainder is protein as collagen and a small amount of glycosaminoglycans, which are proteoglycans that cement the various layers of mineralized collagen fibers together. The protein is collagen and the mineral component is calcium phosphate, as hydroxyapetite crystal.

Collagen is the most abundant extracellular protein in bones and is essential for bone strength (Currey, 2002). It consists of a long continuous triple helix, which self-assembles into highly organized fibrils with very high tensile strength for structural frameworks like bone, tendons, ligaments, and skin. Collagen is not the direct nucleator of hydroxyapetite but acts as a scaffold for the nucleators.

Osteoclasts are cells that remove or resorb bone tissue. Oseoblasts build bone tissue. Preservation of bone mass and fabrication of adequate bone tissue by osteoblasts are central to prolonged skeletal integrity. This is perhaps the fullest extent of what you learned regarding bone remodeling in your undergraduate anatomy and physiology classes.

All osteogenic cells are derived from the same place, the cells of sinusoid vessel walls when they are activated by an osteogenic factor in the calcifyable matrix which is in turn formed by maturing cartilage cells (Little, 1973). Osteoblasts are all cells on the bone surface, active or resting. Osteocyte, osteoblast, osteoclast, are not different cell types at all. The names only refer to different activities of the same cell. The most abundant cell of the three is the osteocyte, ten times more numerous than osteoblasts which in turn greatly outnumber osteoclasts. (Parfitt, 1977).

In bone, there is intercellular communication through channels in the sinusoid vessel walls. This communication is necessary for osteocyte survival. In normal marrow only about 10% of sinusoid vessels of varying diameters are open at any one time (Little, 1973). Open sinusoid vessels have thin walls that close when they are in a transverse direction to external forces. When lines of force are altered, the direction of open vessels coincides with the alteration, remodeling proceeds, and the architecture of the new trabecula follows the lines of force. If in the vicinity of bone, granulation tissue differentiates into calcifiable tissue when the granulation tissue proliferates from vessel walls. Woven bone is altered calcified granulation tissue. It is unstable and remodels into ordinary bone.

Nuclear division does not take place in osteoclasts. They develop from fusion of pre-existing cells. In the literature up to the late 1970's it was thought that osteonal osteocytes lived no longer than two days. More recently it has been learned that the lifetime of an osteoclast is arbitrary, that they are an evolving fusion of mononuclear cells with nuclei that enter and leave the cell during the osteoclast's activity. It has been demonstrated that the lifespan of an osteoclast nucleus by itself averages 11 days. Interestingly, there are no reports of the death or transformation of an entire osteoclast (Martin, 1989).

Oganelles emerge temporarily and produce bone-removing enzymes in the osteoclast's cytoplasm. The organelles disappear and the cell disintegrates. The two kinds of osteoclasts are a localized cell from coalescence of osteogenic cells, and a mobile cell produced by the fusion of macrophages. The local cells are active as a result of corticosteroids. The mobile cell dominates when blood flow is hindered. Osteoclasts can go through more than one resorption cycle (Kanehisa and Heersche, 1988). After osteoclasts die, their ingredients are recycled by macrophages and become part of the macrophage cytoplasm.

Osteoblast activity needs a plentiful supply of oxygen. Cell activity is influenced by the partial pressure of oxygen and carbon dioxide in the blood. The presence of excess carbon dioxide favors a change in cell contents from a gel consistency of high viscosity like that of osteoblasts

to a thin consistency of low viscosity like that of osteoclasts.

Anabolism favors osteoblasts. Catabolic hormones coalesce osteogenic cells into osteoclasts while preventing their formation from macrophage fusion.

When vitamin C (Figure 146) is deficient, the sinusoid vessel walls where ostogenic cells are born become weak, hindering intercellular matrix production. Excess vitamin D (Figure 147) weakens the gel structure of the matrices, causing them to readily break down and calcify (Little, 1973). A vitamin D deficiency causes the matrix to be too stable, preventing calcification and hindering resorption. Vitamin D digestive absorption is impaired by an increase in plasma cortisol from stress. Bones can become distorted in shape with a vitamin A deficiency. Vitamin A (Figures 142-144) is necessary for the formation of osteoclasts from macrophages but has no effect on osteoclasts from osteogenic precursor cells.

Hydroxyapetite is the mineralized part of bone tissue. Collagen is the protein part. Bone tissue is a bipartite system. The combination of the two components in the correct proportion creates bone strength. High bone density is a function of hydroxyapetite crystal concentration. However, bone density alone is not an indicator of bone strength in this bipartite system. Collagen provides the high tensile strength and hydroxyapetite provides high compressive strength (Currey, 2002).

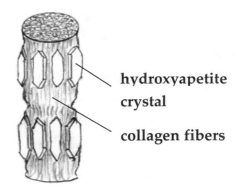

hydroxyapetite crystal

collagen fibers

**(Figure 121)
Bone Collagen**

Seventy to eighty percent of the variance in the ultimate strength of bone tissue is due to age-related decrease in bone mineral density, changes in calcium phosphate (hydroxyapetite) crystal size and shape, and hormonal changes (Yamada, 1970). Twenty to thirty percent of the variance in the ultimate strength of bone tissue is due to altered compositional changes in the mineral portion of the matrix. Collagen does not show qualitative changes in bone with advancing age (Yamada, 1970).

In vivo loading is transduced into a cellular signal. The potential transduction stimuli for bone cell function include changes in hydrostatic pressure, direct cell strain, flow-induced fluid shear, and electrical fields resulting from the electrokinetic effects that accompany fluid flow. Mechanically induced flow of interstitial fluid informs the bone cells about mechanical loading by transporting metabolites through the canaliculi to osteocytes in the osteon.

Electromechanically generated potentials are caused by deformation-induced flow of interstitial fluid within the micropores of canaliculi. not by pressure differences. The fluid shear stress and electrokinetic streaming potentials produce a metabolic response from osteoblasts and osteoclasts for bone remodeling. We will fully explore the phenomenon of piezoelectricity and streaming potentials in a moment.

How does strain on a bone lead to an increase in bone density? First, bone tissue senses the mechanical load that originates from gravity or from the contractile force of a muscle pulling on the interior myofascia. Strain perception is a cellular phenomenon in bone, within and between osteocytes, osteoblasts, and periosteal cells. The mechanosensors initiate biochemical coupling, cellular communication, and effector response. Signals are received through strain- induced alterations in canaliculi fluid and by generation of electrical potentials. The load-sensing cells generate messenger molecules, cyclic nucleotides and prostaglandins.

Basically, mechanical loads are transduced into electrical and chemical signals that cause bone strength to increase. Cells are not sensitive to stress or strain. They are sensitive to the electrical potentials resulting from stress or strain fields.

Within minutes of rythmic load application, the strain field merges with the dense connective tissue of the tendon right to the periosteum. The periosteum covers the bone (except for the ends of it's articular cartilage) and is secured to the bone and canals with perforating fibers. This is where stimulation of glucose 6-phosphate dehydrogenase, G6PD, occurs. The stimulation is a marker for overall cellular metabolism occuring in osteocytes and periosteal cells. At the same time there is a peizoelectric effect in the collagen fibrils from the bone deformation tension that triggers the adenylate cyclase system, circumventing prostaglandins.

Cellular communication from osteocyte to osteocyte through the network of canaliculi directs effector cell proliferation and bone matrix constituent production. Growth factors are released into the canaliculi. There is an activation of genes for cellular proliferation of differentiated functions and regulation of mechanosensitive ion channels in osteoblast-like cells. In cortical bone, mechanical loading stimulates increscent bone formation on the periosteal surface without stimulating an initial resorption phase.

To be an effective initiator of bone remodeling, mechanical stimulation must be dynamic or pulsating (Lanyon et al., 1984). Whalen and Carter (1988) state that load intensity is far more important than the number of cycles performed per minute, that load intensity is first in importance while dynamic character is second. Lanyon et al. (1984) state that the strain rate is the critical factor.

To step back for a look at the issue, stress from the applied force results in strain that deforms the bone. Time is a multiple factor in the process. There is the duration of the applied force. There are cycles-per-minute. One cycle is the stress application followed by a release. This occurs in a rhythmic series. Another time factor is one second. In one second, the applied force strains the bone a given distance. The bone changes dimension. That change is divided by the dimension of the bone before the stress was applied and converted to a percent by multiplying the product by 100. The product is the strain rate.

There would not be load intensity without load magnitude. There would not be a strain rate above zero without the load intensity and bone would not adapt without the strain rate. So all are in the equation and equally important. What can be prioritized is the following:

1) A high strain rate in a rhythmic, cyclic series is more critical to bone adaptation than the duration of the process or the load magnitude.

2) Increasing the load magnitude during a dynamic exercise is a more effective stimulus to increase bone mass than increasing the exercise duration (Van der Wiel et al., 1995).

To restate the research, static deformation doesn't remodel bones. The process of deformation – dynamic strain – remodels them: the actual small motions of parts of the bone relative to other parts of the same bone when it is slightly bent, squeezed, twisted or stretched. A camper can stand all day with a sixty-pound backpack and not initiate bone remodeling. But if the camper hikes with the heavy backpack, then bones will respond. And the greater the speed of the small deformations of the camper's bones, the more remodeling will occur.

Completely immobile hospital patients experiencing hypokinesia rapidly atrophy and loose bone mass in only a few months (Marcus, 1996). Whenever possible, if there is no access to a pool for higher resistance aquatic exercise, people need to walk and exercise every day, as often as they can with as much load as they are able to safely handle. The regularity of resistance exercise is the key to healthy bones.

Micro-architecture of bone, its external geometry, structural integrity, periosteal cell proliferation and bone mineral mass can be salvaged with proper exercise. The effects of the exercise are at localized sites that experience deformation strain (Lanyon et al, 1984). This fact highlights the importance of sufficient loading and variation in resistance exercises so that the angles and directional sources of resistance change almost constantly. Gravity weights and pulley cable machines are one-directional sources of resistance. In water the source is spherical, from all directions, and unlimited geometrical exercise variations are possible because the angle of resistance can continually change in one continuum of movement.

The Integrity of Osteons

Most bone mineralization occurs within about ten days after osteoid deposition between collagen fibers. Sixty percent of the mineralization occurs in the first 24 hours, then the remainder at a degressive rate of

deposition for as long as 4-6 months (Martin and Burr, 1989). The new osteons have different mechanical properties from the old ones.

The six phases of an osteon's lifetime are:

1.activation

2. bone resorption

3. renewal

4. bone formation

5. mineralization

6. quiescence

Activation follows injury or deformation, or occurs at random when BMU's originate and travel along the bone surface. Influenced by vitamin D, estrogens, prostaglandins parathyroid hormone, and growth factors, the pre-osteoclasts are formed from macrophages and merge into multinucleated osteoclasts that resorb

bone for two weeks at any given spot. Osteoblasts are attracted by the self-destruction of osteoclasts as well as by cytokines and growth factors in the activation process. Active osteoblasts fill the cavities with osteoid during bone formation. The layer builds and becomes mineralized with an increase in bone density. The osteoblasts that remain become lining cells that release calcium. Some become osteocytes surrounded by hard bone tissue and canals connecting them to other osteocytes. These canaliculi are where mechanical stresses are sensed during quiescence that follows the active process.

The osteon activation phase frequency is very high in children because bones are softer, more flexible but less elastic, contain more growth hormones, and they temporarily deform from external forces more readily and to a greater degree than the bones of adults. The deformation initiates activation. Rapid growth and faster remodeling in children can produce undermineralized bone.

Effects of Aging on Bone

Slower adult remodeling produces a lower activation rate of basic multicellular units. The activation rate of the BMU's is a function of osteon accumulation and osteon size. BMU activation throughout a full lifespan (Figure 129) shows that the highest rate is at birth. The rate drops sharply down to a low at age 35, increases slightly to age 60, and drops back down again after age 60 (Frost, 1964).

A bone structural unit (BSU) is the quantum of bone formed by a BMU. Old bone is replaced by neoteric bone. A person's bone age and chronological age are different. Portions of bones are always new because they are continually being renewed. There is a large variation in bone tissue age within one bone. The rate of renewal slows in time. Decades of resorbing and forming secondary osteons that traverse through the matrix in all directions strengthen the structure in one way with a more supportive, locked-in geometry. However, the same processes also weaken the structure on account of an increase in fragile lamella boundaries that can more easily separate than those of the secondary osteon interior.

High susceptibility to rapid fatigue increases the potential for bone fatigue damage. The lowest absorption of impact energy and highest accumulation of bone fatigue damage occur at age 60. Over 70 and into senectitude, these effects are compensated for by two changes: crack growth is slowed by smaller secondary osteons, and an accumulation of secondary osteons slows the fatigue processes, resulting in fewer stress fractures (Frost,1965).

Up to the point bones become brittle, osteon maturation is associated with higher mineralization and greater rigidity. The more highly mineralized bone has a higher modulus of elasticity and returns to its un-deformed shape more readily. Attenuated elasticity with higher flexibility in children produces higher strains from a given load because the deformation is greater. Bone's tensile strength is highest at age 20-30, its compressive strength highest at age 35, and its bending strength and torsional strength both peak at age 30. Tensile strength decreases in time more rapidly than the other mechanical properties, followed, in order, by bending strength, compressive strength, and torsional strength (Martin, 1989).

If you are a water exercise class instructor, you must know the abilities and limitations of the participants. Aging increases bone's porosity with decrescent mineralization and accrescent collagen cross-linking. The increased cross-linking interferes with the interstitial flow that would normally initiate activate remodeling.

Cancellous bone has lower shear strength than unidirectional cortical bone and a higher incidence of stress fractures. Cancellous bone has a greater energy storage capacity than cortical bone. Cortical bone can sustain greater stress but less strain, 2%, before failure than cancellous bone at 75% strain. Repetitive loading decreases the load magnitude required to initiate cracks in cancellous bone, yet it increases their resistance to crack growth. Cracks begin in regions of high strain; accumulation is more critical than initiation (Martin, 1989).

Fatigue that leads to bone failure has three stages: initiation, accumulation, and growth. Interference with crack growth prevents failure but damage and accumulation eventually prevail, leading to ultimate failure. The energy needed for full fracture of the femur falls almost 7% per decade. Hopper (1994), in a study of female smokers, found that the effects of smoking reduced bone density and consequently elevated the risk of bone fracture.

The shear plane of the relatively weak cement line interface between osteons (Figure 119) and interstitial bone matrix reduces osteon bone shear strength. Most of the lifetime of a crack is in the growth stage. Initiation is rapid at first, followed by the crack colliding with discontinuities such as poor matrix bonding with weak interfaces and other age-related degenerations. Cracks then branch and split, leading to a dispersal of the stress, dissipating energy and slowing crack growth. Secondary osteons trap the secondary cracks, debonding the osteons from surrounding bone and dissipating more energy.

There is an unusual phenomenon regarding bone cracks. In weakened, aging trabecular bone, cracks start easily but advance with difficulty. The bone's plasticity at the tip of the crack fills and blunts the crack. This is also dependent on fiber diameter. Smaller diameters slow the advance of stress fractures. Osteon diameters vary by species. In humans, osteon diameter decreases with age. The initiation of small, numerous stress fractures in aged bone increases along with resistance to crack lengthening, making it more difficult for a crack to grow (Martin, 1989).

Between the age of 25 and 75 the number of femur resorption spaces increases by 250%. That's a big increase in porosity. The humerus and the femur increase in porosity at the same rate until about age 45 when the humerus starts to become porous more rapidly. The femur porocity begins to level off at age 75 (Martin, 1989).

Avoid abrupt increases in aquatic exercise intensity, magnitude, and velocity with the elderly. Progress should be gradual to allow bones to increase density. Remember the timeframe for adaptation: several months.

Different bones and different parts of bones change at different rates as we age. A bone density test on the heel may not accurately indicate bone quality of a lumbar vertebra and vice-versa. A common place to test bone density is the greater trochanter of the femur, not the femur neck, the most probable location of a fracture. The modern measurement technology today is dual X-ray absorptiometry (DXA). There are local or total skeletal DXA scans over 10 subregions of the body that are somewhat comprehensive, measuring bone mineral content as well as density (Blake & Fogelman, 1996). But there is an inadequacy in DXA scans. They only measure a two dimensional distribution of bone density instead of a three dimensional distribution.

Lower levels of activity in occupation and leisure during youth are reflected in old age by the prevalence of fractures. Many postmenopausal women with hip fractures apparently have had lower levels of occupational and leisure physical activity between age 15-45. High activity during youth, before peak mineralization in the mid 30's, if maintained with continued exercise, will result in fewer fractures in old age.

Immobility under resistive force doesn't work for bone development. It takes movement (Frost, et al, 1984). Ordinary activity is not enough either. For most people, ordinary activity falls between sedentary and moderately active. The greatest opportunity to increase bone mass through increased physical activity that would be of most benefit throughout a lifetime would be during times of growth, during youth.

A decrease in blood flow is a degenerative factor leading to disuse osteoporosis, post-menopausal osteoporosis, and senile osteoporosis. Lack of activity slows blood flow. Stress also blocks the flow of blood through the bone. Small platelet thrombi form and deposit on the walls of minor vessels. Membranes that are damaged cover osseous surfaces. Osteoclasts form, resorbing bone.

There are many exercises that can strengthen an individual bone. The femur is the example used throughout this book. The following list illustrates the points of muscle attachment and beneficial stress from the forces of exercise. Twenty-two muscles attach to each femur (Figure 122). At the proximal end are hip abductors, hip flexors, and lateral hip rotators. On the long shaft are hip adductors, hip flexors, and medial hip rotators. At the distal end are knee flexors, knee extensors, and ankle flexors. The femur is covered with opportunities to respond to a large variety of movements under quick resistive force. The more these

movements differ from an established "routine," the greater is the increase in bone density. \

THE 22 MUSCLES ATTACHED TO THE FEMUR
proximal femur
gluteus medius
gluteus minimus
periformis
gemellus superior
obturator internis
gemellus inferior
obturator externis
quadratus femoris
psoas
iliacus
vastus medialis
vastus lateralis
vastus interemedius
pectinius

long shaft, femur
adductor longus
adductor brevis
adductor
magnus
biceps femoris
   short head
distal femur
gluteus maximus
gastrocnemius
plantaris
popliteus

(Figure 122) MUSCLES OF THE PROXIMAL FEMUR

A. MUSCLE ATTACHMENTS

B. DIRECTIONS OF PULL FROM MUSCLES

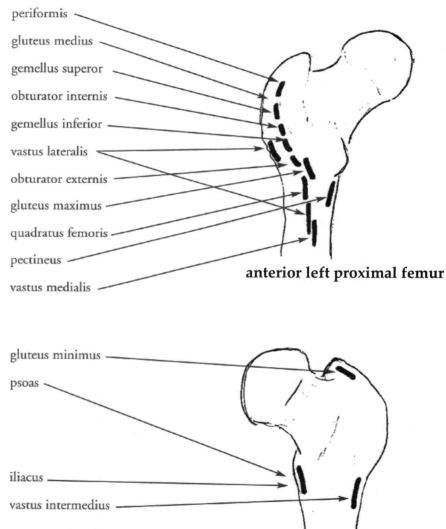

periformis

gluteus medius

gemellus superor

obturator internis

gemellus inferior

vastus lateralis

obturator externis

gluteus maximus

quadratus femoris

pectineus

vastus medialis

anterior left proximal femur

gluteus minimus

psoas

iliacus

vastus intermedius

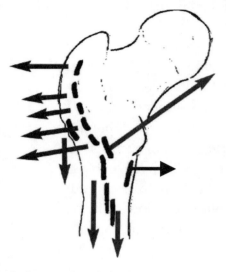

anterior left proximal femur

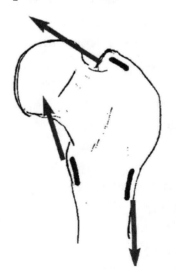

posterior left proximal femur

Nalu: The Art and Science of Aquatic Fitness, Bodywork & Therapy

Cancellous bone has a greater response to mechanical forces than cortical bone. The cortex of long or flat bones survives longer than that of trabecular bone. Trabecula remodels faster and contains sufficient beta-protein at all ages, while beta-protein in cortical bone is only seen in infants and young children. At adolescence there are more stable versions of elongated cells in the fibro-cartilage of the intervertebral disc nucleus pulposus. These cells have greater amounts of sufficiently polymerized rubber-like beta-proteins as a result of steroid hormonal changes and exercise. Trabeculae do not grow when protein is low. These changes in adolescents occur in bone as well as in connective tissues and the matrices of cartilage.

Adequate exercise is necessary for correct maturation of the spine. Exercise reduces elevated blood cortisol stress hormone levels that create undesirable side effects. (See Chapter 16, *Reducing Stress with Water Fitness,* for a long list of the negative effects of cortisol on the body.) Exercise increases oxygenation and blood supply to the bones. Chronically high stress hormones, by anti-anabolic action, cause muscle fiber weakening and reduce blood supply to muscles and bones. Exercise increases the partial pressure of oxygen in the circulating blood. Exercise counteracts the tendencies that lead to osteoporosis and other degenerative conditions.

Thin layers of spirals of collagen fibrils are alternatively turned right and left with the crystallites highly oriented in the direction of the axis of fibrils. When there is an inclination difference between the collagen symmetry axis and the bone axis, this indicates that a bone is inclined to the direction of gravitational force.

On land, bone collagen favors the direction of gravitational force and the direction of muscle pull (Figure 123). In aquatic exercise, bone collagen primarily favors the direction of muscle pull. The effect of gravity in aquatic exercise is reduced proportionately to the body mass that is below the waterline. We know that changes in bone density are mainly in trabecular bone near the ends of long bones, and less in the cortical bone in the hollow shaft. The obvious conclusion that I have reached is that muscles attached to the proximal and distal ends of long bones, as opposed to the shafts, more effectively alter bone remodeling since that is the location of trabecular bone. My deduction here is that aquatic exercises involving forceful contractions of muscles that originate or insert close to the ends of bones are more likely to improve bone density.

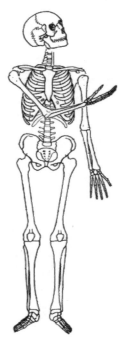

Looking at the human proximal femur again as our example, fifteen muscles attach to it near the trabecular region, eleven on the posterior side (Figure 122). Contractions of these muscles pull on their tendons attached to the bone, resulting in knee extension, hip flexion, lateral and medial hip rotation, extension of the femur at the hip, and hip abduction. Most of these muscles attach to the greater trochanter on down, and others attach to the proximal end of the linea aspera, the anterior and lateral proximal femoral shaft, and to the lessor trochanter. There are numerous exercise opportunities in water to increase bone density at the proximal femur.

(Figure 123)

DIRECTIONS OF FORCE ON PROXIMAL FEMUR

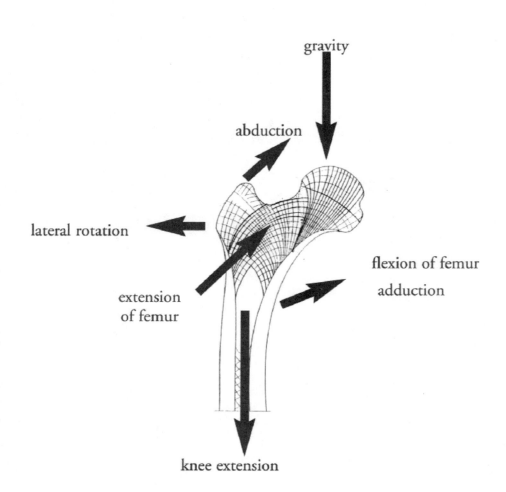

gravity

abduction

lateral rotation

extension
of femur

flexion of femur

adduction

knee extension

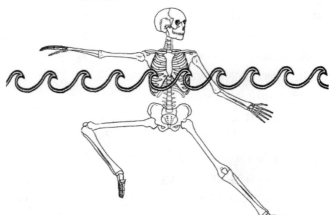

Nalu: The Art and Science of Aquatic Fitness, Bodywork & Therapy

The Hippo and the Rhino

*A*frica is a good place to look for bones of many species of large animals. So is a large metropolitan zoo. But these bones were temporarily obtained from the Museum of Vertebrate Zoology.

I was looking for research that measured bone density with DXA scans of the proximal femur at three locations on different mammal species of equal size, one being more amphibious and the other being more land dwelling. I ☎ contacted professors of zoology, the Field museum in Chicago, authors, researchers, and the Smithsonian Institute in Washington, D.C., where I was directed to Dr. Frank Fish, a leading mammologist in the United States. In our conversation, Dr. Fish discussed research he had published comparing bone density of the same two species that I had in mind, the common hippopotamus (*Hippopotamus amphibius*) and the white rhinoceros (*Ceratotherium*

simum). I planned to compare males of prime chronological age preferably in the wild. My goal was to determine the influence of gravity and of muscle forces on specific points that radiate down from the acetabulum through the trabeculae in the femur by comparing animals that are in the water most or all of their lives with exclusively land-dwelling animals of equal weight and bone structure.

Would the rhino femur head be denser than the hippo from gravity, and would the hippo greater trochanter be the same as the rhino from muscle forces? I could then correlate the data with human bone density scans for weight lifters, swimmers, and astronauts.

>-((((O>   >-((((O>   >-((((O>

The research Dr. Fish led me to is published in Zoomorphology 1991; 110: 339-345 by F.E. Fish and B.R. Stein and in the Journal of Paleontology 1983; 57:197-207 by W.P. Wall.

The research is interesting because it indicates the opposite of my expectations, apparently due to evolutionary adaptation. The bone density at the femur of the white rhino is 1.3-g/cubic cm and the hippo femur is 1.51-g/cubic cm. Fish & Stein reasoned in his paper that the aquatic animal has the higher bone density because it helps with stability in the water. Heavier limb bones counteract torso buoyancy from pulmonary air or thick adipose tissue. An analogy is the weighted keel of a sailboat.

Dr. Wall's dissertation compared limb bone densities of 49 genera of mammals divided into a terrestrial habitat group and an aquatic habitat group. The aquatic mammals exhibited significantly higher bone density than did the terrestrial mammals (Wall, 1983). Natural selection favored high bone density when total body submergence became a habitual part of the animals' lives.

The manatee, living mostly submerged in water, has the highest mammalian bone density with the medullary cavities almost entirely filled with dense, compact bone. The **pachyostotic bone** is solid, without marrow. Both Fish and Wall speculate that the natural selection of these aquatic herbivorous mammals favored heavy bones to remain submerged for feeding and to stabilize buoyancy. The heavy limb bones compensate for breathing and variation in fatty tissue by reducing buoyancy at a level low enough for the manatee to remain effortlessly submerged.

Returning to the aquatic hippo and the terrestrial rhino, I was not satiated with the research because it included cortical femur bone, not exclusively cancellous in the proximal femur head. The research indicates that the hippo femur contains 44% compact bone and the rhino femur contains 25.2% compact bone. The hippo and white rhino are giants. So I searched further into the research of authors Fish, Wall and Stein for a comparison of smaller mammals differentiated by predominant habitat, aquatic and terrestrial.

A femur bone density comparison between the aquatic sea otter (*Enhydra lutris*) and the terrestrial dorcas gazelle (Gazella dorcas), a common Saharan antelope, is in the research. The documented bone density of the Sea Otter is 1.46 g/cubic cm compared to only 1.06 6/cubic cm for the Gazelle (Fish and Stein, 1990). Evolutionary adaptation for land dwelling prey favors light bones for faster flight from predators. The densities of all the limb bones of the aquatic mammals including the humerus, radius-ulna, femur, and tibia-fibula, compared to those of the terrestrial mammals revealed a significant and consistent difference. Aquatic mammals have higher bone density than terrestrial mammals (Fish, 1990). In vertebrates the mechanical and physiological costs of maintaining the skeleton differ according to mode of life and activity level (Curry, 1984) as well as to the constraints dictated by evolutionary history. Stein (1989) hypothesized that greater limb-bone density in larger semi-aquatic mammals was necessary to facilitate support and movement on land and was useful in the evolution of aquatic

mammals to increase density for diving.

Fish and Stein measured all limb bone densities from many samples of mustelid mammal species with a variety of habitats including arboreal, fully aquatic, semi-aquatic, terrestrial, and burrowing. They concluded that in all the species groups, bone density is highest in the radius/ulna, followed by the humerus, the tibia/fibula, and lowest in the femur. Forelimb bones are denser than hind limb bones and distal limb bones have higher density that proximal limb bones.

The normal rate of human bone deposition increases to about age 35, stabilizes, then starts to decline to age 80-85, then stabilizes again(Frost, 1964).

Bones store the calcium and phosphorous used in blood for cardiac function, muscle contractility, cell membrane integrity and permeability, neuromuscular function, and blood clotting. Homeostasis of calcium and phosphorous is regulated by calcitonin andparathyroid hormones. The excretion of Ca and P by the kidneys is hormonally linked with absorption of these in ion form through the intestines. Vitamin D is required in this metabolism while calcitonin inhibits resorption.

In bone regeneration, cells migrate to calcification sites in the organic matrix of collagen fibers. Proteins and polar compounds are the precursors that trigger transcription of hydroxyapetite calcium phosphate crystals. Crystal patterns in bone are specific to each species.

In cartilage, as in tendon, tensional forces elongate flexible cells (see Chapter 4, *Movement/ The Series Elastic Element*). This allows the production of oriented fibrous tissue for greater strength. Compressive or rotational forces on cartilage result in rounded cells with a cartilaginous matrix of unoriented, tangled collagen. Changes in applied physical forces can cause metaplastic changes in tissue structure and behavior. In cartilage, the influence of applied

forces is felt directly by the flexible cells and matrix.

In bone, applied forces cause deformation (Figures123 & 125). Deformation governing bone shape was originally proposed in 1741 by André, but Galileo (1638) wrote about the mechanical implications of bone shape. Monroe (1776), Culmann (1866), Von Meyer (1867), Wolff (1892) and Koch (1917) all illustrated and wrote about the organization of trabeculae in the femur. Examples of proximal femur interior architectual drawings between 1832 and 1892 by scientists Jacob, Ward, Wyman, Engel, Von Meyer and Wolff are depicted in Figure 124.

In an early-recorded description of the porous architecture of bone, Clapton Havers in 1691 observed its organic and inorganic composition. Van Leewwenhoeck preceded him in 1674 and 1678 with details on bone's extensive system of longitudinal and transverse canals. Culmann, a Swiss crane engineer, and Von Meyer, a German anatomist with a grant from the Prussian government to study

skeletal posture, conferred to develop the trajectorial theory of trabecular bone structure.

Another German anatomist, Julius Wolff (1870-1894), further developed the Von Meyer/Culmann theory with his idea that trabeculae were aligned with principal stress directions, but that the orientation of trabeculae could change if there was a change in mechanical stress directions, in other words that bone structure could respond to alterations in stress. Wolff also suggested that bone adapted optimally to changes in stress, seeking to minimize mass to carry the load. Wolff is credited with the general theory of bone adaptation known as Wolff's Law.

> **Wolff's Law: "Every change in the form and the function of a bone or of their function alone is followed by certain definite changes in their internal architecture, and equally definite secondary alterations in their external confirmation[sic], in accordance with mathematical laws."** Wolff's Law is commonly paraphrased as follows: **"Bone remodels in response to the mechanical stresses it experiences so as to produce an anatomical structure best able to resist the applied stress."**

(Figure 124) Historical Representations of Internal Proximal Femur Architecture

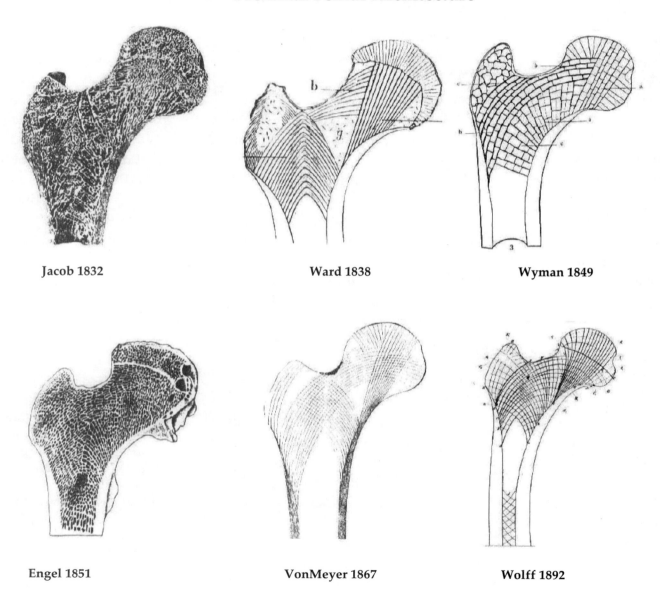

Jacob 1832   **Ward 1838**   **Wyman 1849**

Engel 1851   **VonMeyer 1867**   **Wolff 1892**

(Figure 125) The Response by the Neck of the Femur to Gravitational Force

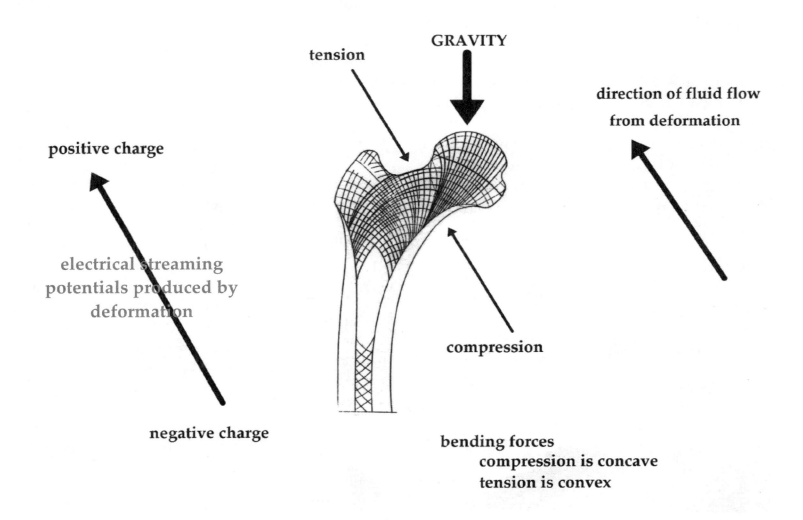

tension

GRAVITY

direction of fluid flow
from deformation

positive charge

electrical streaming
potentials produced by
deformation

compression

negative charge

bending forces
compression is concave
tension is convex

Nalu: The Art and Science of Aquatic Fitness, Bodywork & Therapy

The first suggestion that strain might be the causative stimulus for bone to quantitatively respond to its mechanical environment was made in 1917 by D'arcy Thompson, twenty five years after Wolff's Law of bone adaptation. During the 1950's and 60's, studies substantiated that bone remodeling is a function of mechanical variables. Fukada demonstrated that piezoelectric properties of bone initiated by mechanical forces caused remodeling (Fukada 1957). We will now return to investigate in detail the phenomenon of piezoelectricity in bone tissue.

Electrical Properties of Bone

Piezoelectric refers to electricity is produced by a mechanical force. Bone is piezoelectric (Bassett and Becker, 1962; McLeod and Rubin, 1990). The hydroxyapetite found in bone is a crystal, but it is one of a minority of geologic classes of crystals which are not piezoelectric. The crystals are highly oriented in the direction of the axis of the alternately turned collagen fibrils.

The piezoelectric properties in bone are associated with the collagen, not with the mineral constituent (Korostoff, 1977). The calcium phosphate stored in bone as hydroxyapetite crystals contributes rigidity to collagen fibers. It does not contribute piezoelectric properties. The amorphous non-crystalline type of calcium phosphate accumulates in mitochondria, not in bone.

The formula for non-crystalline hydroxyapetite is

$$Ca_{10}(PO_4)6(OH)_2$$

while crystalline hydroxyapetite is

$$Ca_3(PO_4)3OH.$$

Collagen in bone and mineralized matrix in bone have permanent polarization as well as the ability to acquire electrical polarization upon mechanical deformation, piezoelectric in collagen and streaming potential in the matrix. The collagen and matrix in bone are electrets. The property of permanent polarization results from the hexagonal crystaline structure of collagen molecules consisting of three

twisted tropocollagen polypeptide chains. The structure contains an unequal number of positive and negative charges with a net dipole moment parallel to the long axis (Becker and Selden, 1985). Collagen also has short-range circumferential electric fields that affect nearby cells and the stacking of the molecules in the cells.

Dry bone collagen is strongly piezoelectric, and wet bone collagen indicates the streaming that is the primary source of stress-generated electrical potentials, while fully hydrated tendon collagen is not piezoelectric because of the water it contains (Anderson and Eriksson, 1970). The absence of piezoelectricity in fully hydrated tendon collagen is associated with a more symmetrical structure caused by absorption of water. In bone there is less hydration of collagen fiber due to hydroxy-apetite crystals taking up one third of fiber length. The loss of collagen elasticity from rigid hydroxyapetite being bound to it prevents full structural swelling from hydration, and therefore the collagen still shows a piezo- electric effect. The fibers slip past each other because of the application of shear to the collagen's hexagonal symmetry. The angle between the applied force and bone axis determines the degree of piezoelec- tricity. The piezoelectric maximum per unit length in bone collagen is one-tenth that of quartz crystal and it decays more slowly (Becker and Selden, 1985).

The amplitude of the potential generated in stressed bone depends on the rate and magnitude of bone deformation (Fukada and Yamada, 1957). Polarity of the signal depends on the direction of bending. Compressed areas develop negative potentials that affect neighboring osteogenic tissue. *Piezoelectric* potentials produced by mechanical deformation of bone are sustained throughout the time stress application is causing the bone to change shape. The only association *streaming* potentials have with mechanical deformation is the fact that most deformations cause fluid flow between regions. When a structure contains electrolyte-filled,

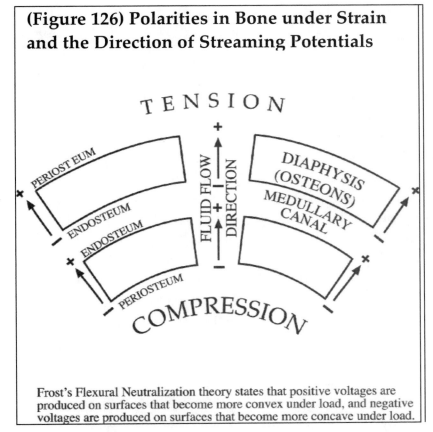

(Figure 126) Polarities in Bone under Strain and the Direction of Streaming Potentials

Frost's Flexural Neutralization theory states that positive voltages are produced on surfaces that become more convex under load, and negative voltages are produced on surfaces that become more concave under load.

inter-connected spaces, deformation then produces streaming potentials are (Little, 1973).

It is known from decades of research studies on the electrical properties of bone that streaming potentials make the chief contribution to the electrical signals produced by mechanical stress, and that the differences in polarity control whether resorption or formation result (Martin et al., 1998). Fluids are forced to flow from areas of compression to areas of tension. **Streaming potentials are the primary source of stress-generated electrical potentials in bone.** What are streaming potentials? Mechanical force causes bone deformation that in turn moves fluid within canaliculi, producing streaming potentials. The walls of the canals have a charged surface. If the surface charge is negative, it attracts positive ions to the canal wall surface. That leaves an abundance of negative ions streaming through the center of the canal, establishing an electric potential from positively charged canal walls to negatively charged fluid. The potentials are directly proportional to the amount of collagen cross-linking in the matrix. Cross-linking in these very small spaces obstructs flow and reduces the streaming potential. Other influencing factors are fluid pH, ion concentrations, and the condition of the collagen, especially collagen elasticity which changes with enzymes (Becker and Selden, 1985). The interstitial fluid viscosity, and the dimensions of the channels and minute interstitial matrix spaces determine the amplitude of streaming potentials. Water moving through a tube has unique properties.

B*efore I learned about the science* of fluids, I was working on a road paving crew in the mountains of Idyllwild, California in 1965. The foreman asked me to locate a water main somewhere in a 5,000 sq ft area of dirt roadway. He knew it was eight or ten feet underground but he wanted to know the exact location and direction it was going. I thought he would have some kind of sophisticated detection device and that he would have to instruct me in how to use it. Maybe I wouldn't be able to do it. Then the foreman, who looked like a giant lumberjack covered in dirt and sweat, handed me two welding rods and walked away as if I knew what to do with them. Now what? I am to find a major water pipeline underground somewhere in a large area using two steel welding rods. I maneuvered over to one of the old timers on the crew who I thought would know everything there is to know in the world. Not saying a word, he motioned me to bend the ends of both rods, hold them in front

of myself like long "L"s straight out from my chest parallel to each other, and walk. Without knowing anything about what I was doing I did that, and we slowly walked and walked the area until finally on their own the rods strongly separated at the ends and swung out wide to both sides. My eyes opened wide as I stood still over the spot and said, "Here it is and it's going in this direction." The magnetic field created by the rapidly moving large volume of water in the pipeline almost instantly lined up the welding rods with the direction of water flow. Moving water is "alive." Does the same thing occur in blood plasma flowing through a capillary? Are we nothing more than bundles of electromagnetic forces in a closed aquatic environment?

✂«(((O>　　✂«((((O>　　✂«((((O>

Streaming potentials are brought about within bone's solid-walled electrolyte filled spaces by deformations that move fluid from one region to another. They are proportional to the rate of change of deformation, the strain rate. When deformation stops or is maintained in one position, no fluid flows and there is no streaming potential. Piezoelectric voltages are also proportional to strain rate and persist for the duration of the deformation process (Bassett and Becker, 1962). Both the streaming potentials and the piezoelectric voltages are transient. This means that static loading does not cause bone remodeling. Cyclic loading leads to bone remodeling (Lanyon and Rubin, 1984). You must move forcefully with repeated flexion and extension in the water with effort to increase bone density.

In cortical bone, sudden muscle contraction blocks venous outflow from the marrow, causing it to fill with blood and to build pressure within the bone. At the end of the contraction, the muscles relax and there is a suction effect on the marrow as the pressure rapidly declines. Over time, the vascular channels through bone cortex become enlarged from osteoclast activity resulting from the repeated muscle contractions. Vigorous osteogenic activity, remodeling, and increases in bone vascularity follow vigorous cyclic or variable muscle action. An increased blood flow stimulates osteonal remodeling for mechanical strength. The cortex of weight-bearing lamellar bone remodels first and is finished soon after adolescence, followed by osteonal remodeling during later development when muscular contractions are strongest.

To summarize the processes of exercise-induced remodeling, muscular contractions apply force to a bone. The electrical potential in bone under stress is dependent on rate and magnitude of deformation. The movement of fluids in bone spaces caused by the mechanical deformation creates streaming potentials. Bone is added on the positive side and is removed on the negative side.

On the compression side of a bending bone are negative potentials and on the tension side are positive potentials in Frost's Flexural Neutralization Theory (Figure 126). The polarity results from the bending direction. The magnitude of the electrical potential manipulates the internal functions, such as DNA synthesis, the functions of osteoblasts and osteoclasts, and bone remodeling.

Cycling, swimming (Taaffe, 1995), and walking without added weight (Cavanaugh, 1988) are not osteogenic. But walking will increase relative muscle strength in the hips and legs and thus help to prevent a fall. Bone mass cannot be maintained in these activities because there is no additional load (Dilsen, 1989). In contrast, there is a pulsating force of gravity during walking with added weight or walking uphill just as there is a pulsating mechanical strain in high intensity aquatic resistance exercise that stimulates bone remodeling. The most osteogenic activities are those with higher site-specific, rapidly placed varying loads on bones. Too much, too fast, combined with inappropriate technique and poor body mechanics can be harmful and cause stress fracture, but, properly paced, these activities can be continued for a lifetime.

(Figure 127)

Forces Acting on Bones

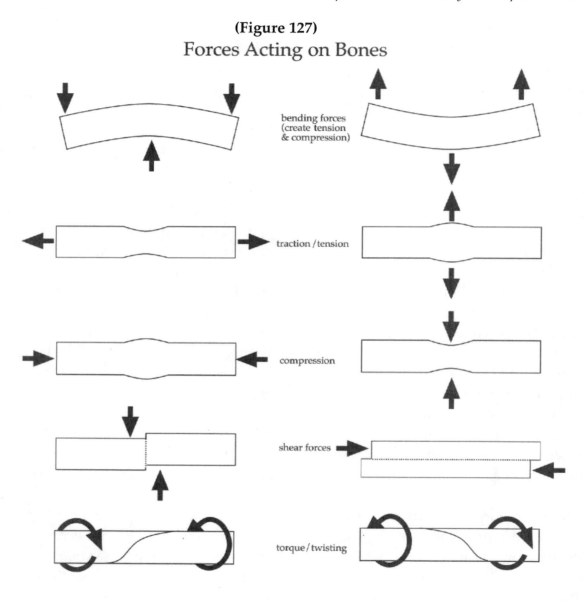

bending forces
(create tension
& compression)

traction / tension

compression

shear forces

torque / twisting

The forces that affect bone are: bending, tension/traction, compression, shear, torque/twisting and their combinations (Figure 127). Tension/ traction pulls bone away from its center. Compression pushes bone together. Bending moves the center of a bone in one direction and both ends in the opposite direction. Shear forces cause contiguous parts to move parallel to their plane of contact. Torsion is longitudinal twisting.

The local points where these forces act on a bone are the areas where the connective tissue of a muscle tendon merges with the thin layer of connective tissue surrounding the bone, the periosteum, and at points created by the forces of gravity. An example of the force of gravity acting on the local points of a bone is walking. The force of gravity, not the contraction of a muscle, applies force to the head of the femur from the weight of the upper body, down through to the ilium and creates tension on the superior side of the neck of the femur and compression on the inferior side.

Osteoporosis

There are no indications of osteoporosis in a medical examination until there is a consequence of the disease, a fracture. How is that for good timing?

Osteoporosis is not osteoarthritis (see *Arthritis Precautions* in Chapter 12, *Floating into Therapy)*. In osteoporosis, affecting 10 million people in the United States and 30% of all postmenopausal women in the world (Kanis, 1994), trabecular bone becomes porous and cortical bone becomes thin. There is a loss of bone mass and a micro architectural deterioration of bone tissue.

Bones can become fatigued and brittle when osteoclastic bone resorption is greater than osteoblastic bone formation. An imbalance between the two causes osteoporosis. Osteoporosis is a decrease in bone density with changes in its architecture that increase the chance of fracture.

A gene has been identified that predicts the two causative factors in osteoporosis. It regulates the peak bone density early in life and the rate of bone loss later in life. The gene accounts for 75% of the total genetic effect on bone density. The gene is in two alleles, one being associated with lower bone density, and codes a protein that enables vitamin D to act on calcium metabolism. Genetics has more of an influence on peak bone mass in a person's life and less on the rate of bone loss. One of the research results predicted that women with low bone density early in life would reach the "fracture threshold" of low bone density 11 years earlier than average and experience a hip fracture rate that is increased by a factor of four (Pocock et al., 1987).

Hip fracture is blamed for 50,000 deaths per year in the United States (Cooper, 1997). More women are susceptible to osteoporotic fractures because men have larger bone size and a higher peak bone mass (Poor, 1995). Men have a higher average dietary calcium intake after age 10 than women (Alaimo, 1994). Racially, African-American females have greater bone mineral density than non-Hispanic Caucasian females (Kleerekoper, 1994). Some degree of long-term care is required for 25% of patients that fracture their hip with an annual cost of $10 billion (Chrischilles, 1992).

Estrogen deficiency, acidosis, corticosteroids and vitamin D metabolites increase osteoclastic resorption while calcitonin reduces it. When mineralization by osteoblasts is inhibited, the result is osteomalacia where resorption cavities are too deep. Trabecular walls become perforated and weak with fewer reinforcing connections. Healthy remodeling, as described previously, replaces brittle bone with a more elastic matrix.

According to the National Institutes of Health, 300,000 people a year in their 70's and 80's experience hip fractures at the neck of the proximal femur in the United States. At a younger age, 1/3 of a woman's lifetime bone loss can occur during the first five years following menopause (Melton, 1995).

Osteoporosis fractures are common to the head/neck of the femur and to the wrist. There are 250% more resorption spaces in the femur at age 75 than at age 25 (Atkinson, 1965). Post-menopausal osteoporosis fractures result from loss of bone tissue. Caffeine makes postmenopausal osteoporosis worse (Harris, 1994). Senile osteoporosis fractures result from weakened dead bone tissue.

The difference between normal and osteoporotic patients is found in the structural variables and not in the dynamic ones. Remodeling abnormalities in established osteoporosis cause loss of trabecular elements. They do not cause a global thinning.Though there is some reduction in trabecular wall thickness, the largest difference is in the amount of separation of structural components. Without indicating a proportionate loss of bone, many struts disconnect and lose attachments. Kimmel (1990) concludes that this is the cause of the porosity, fragility, and the pathogenesis of osteoporosis.

Most conditions that lead to osteoporosis are associated with increased osteoclastic bone resorption with insufficient bone formation. The amount of bone normally resorbed by osteoclasts in 2-3 weeks takes 3-4 months to be replaced by osteoblast bone formation (Ericksen, 1986). In osteoporosis, formation cannot keep up with resorption when there is a high rate of remodeling. This high turnover rate is significant in postmenopausal osteoporosis (Delmas, 1993).

Parathyroid hormone increases the quantity of osteoclasts (Silverberg et al., 1996). There is evidence that estrogen deficiency, hyperparathyroidism, and hyperthyroidism associated with bone loss parallel increased osteoclastic recruitment and resorption. Postmenopausal osteoporosis is characterized by trabecular perforation over time (Parfitt et al, 1983). In hyperthyroidism, trabeculae are thinner but not decreased in number. There are many causes of increased osteoclast number. The mechanical

strain in the bone matrix from the load of cyclic, dynamic exercise may inhibit osteoclastic activity (Hillam and Sherry, 1995). As was stated earlier, sufficient mechanical forces cause bone deformation, creating streaming potentials and consequently stimulating bone formation.

Bone loss leading to osteoporosis can be caused by an abnormality in vitamin D formation or metabolism. Vitamin D, specifically its active metabolite 1,25-dihydroxyvitamin D, facilitates calcium absorption in the intestines, regulation of parathyroid hormone, regulation of calcium in the kidney, and maintenance of bone remodeling (Clemens and O'Riordan, 1995). There is a decrease in circulating vitamin D in older age (Eastell et al, 1991). Most likely the decrease results from dietary inadequacy and less time out in the sunlight. Any gastrointestinal abnormality that impairs the absorption of vitamin D, phosphate and calcium can cause bone loss. Reducing the risk of osteoporosis entails, among other things, consuming 1,000-1,500 mg of daily calcium, using every opportunity to increase bone mass with exercise during the growing years, avoiding eating disorders, following a higher resistance exercise program regularly while not over-exercising, and possible pharmacological therapy at menopause. Exercise is an important part of risk reduction for osteoporosis patients (Beck and Shoemaker, 2000), and carefully controlled exercises (McKinney, 2000) decrease pain and disability for osteoarthritis patients (Van Baar et al., 1999). Physical activity benefits patients with osteoarthritis. Pain in osteoarthritic joints is reduced as strength increases (McKinney, 2000). The Arthritis Foundation (www.arthritis.org) recommends aquatic exercise therapy in the Arthritis Foundation Aquatic Program (AFAP).

Premenopausal estrogen deficiency in women results in increased osteoclast activation with extreme negative consequences. Two examples that cause premenopausal estrogen deficiency are amenorrhea from anorexia or bulimia, and chronic

energy deficit from over-exercising (Beck and Shoemaker, 2000). Osteoporosis among premenopausal female athletes is associated with chronic, intense over-exercise and eating disorders. Circulating hormones are disrupted and bone loss is accelerated despite weight-bearing exercise. Normal bone remodeling depends on the dynamics of parathyroid hormone. Recently PTH has been successfully used as a bone mass-increasing anabolic for osteoporosis (Cosman, 1998). Existing antiresorptives have not prevented new fractures though they do inhibit bone resorption and stimulate bone formation (Reginster, 1999). Too much or too little parathyroid hormone contributes to age-related bone loss. Parathyroid concentrations naturally increase with age (Nussbaum and Potts, 1994).

Qualitative bone changes vary between different cultures with varying diets and activity levels. In men, aging is accompanied by radial expansion of cortical bone in the long shafts as the endosteal surface resorption and periostial surface bone

formation occur at the same time. The wall becomes thinner, with less bone mass but with greater shaft diameter to maintain overall cortical bone strength. Eventually, long bone periosteal expansion fails in women. Also, women have higher mineralization in trabecular bone as they age. There are other differences between the sexes. In women, trabecular (cancellous) and cortical bone density start to decline at about age 35. In men, however, for the bones of the hands, humerus, and the femur, trabecular bone starts to decline at 35 but cortical bone density does not start to decline until age 60.

Different parts of a bone have varying density, as was mentioned earlier. The variations are primarily a result of trabecular remodeling reactions to force. Looking at the trabecular bone content at various skeletal sites, vertebrae is 66-90% trabecular bone, the intertrochanter of the hip is 50%, femoral neck is 25%, femoral shaft is 5%, distal radius is 25%, and the mid-radius is 1% (Einborn, 1996). Let's look at our consistent example again, the proximal femur, and look again at the directional lines of force in it's architecture, the Wolff schematic (Figure 124-125).

The Ascension of Density

Observe the neck of the femur in the figures contained in this chapter and the arrows from sufficient forces that increase remodeling and bone density. Gravity comes straight down, creating compression under the femur neck and tractional tension at the top of the neck. The gravitational lines of force are primarily through the head, perpendicular to the upper surface cartilage, parallel to gravity. Now observe the lines of force from hip extension using the gluteus maximus muscle. The lines arc parallel with the neck, all the way through it. This observation demonstrates to me that the impact of gravity increases bone density in the femur head, but exercising the gluteus maximus increases bone density in the femur neck, the place where most hip fractures occur in osteoporosis.

Not just any kind of exercise will help bone density in the neck of the femur, however. It takes sufficient resistance and velocity, repeated as in the muscle endurance aquatic exercise called "kick backs" in Chapter 6, *Aquatic Endurance Exercise.*

This is not a thesis on zero gravity. Aquatic muscle endurance exercise and gravity are definitely in harmony. Situations involving lines of force through the proximal femur, such as the example above, include the major contribution of compression/tension and the creation of electrical streaming potentials as a result of the deformation of the femur neck from the combination of gravity and movement. Those potentials moving through the bone from bottom to top, from negative to positive, also contribute to bone remodeling. That area of bone is so strong that bending is minimal so the potentials are somewhat low compared to the force from the gluteus maximus on the periosteum where it inserts at the gluteal tuberosity.

Bones need both gravity and muscle action to increase density, not one to the exclusion of the other. They need big aquatic exercise workouts as well as the pull of gravity. Choose the most shallow water depth needed for aquatic exercises. Waist deep is preferable to neck deep. Use gravity in the pool.

In space, astronaut exercise produces muscle growth but bone density still declines rapidly (Tilton, et al., 1980). Would it not be reasonable to anticipate the conclusion of these expensive tests without actually doing them? Do we not realize that our bodies are planetarily evolved and that we are in a permanently intimate relationship with gravity? Healthy bone metabolism needs gravity. Without it there is atrophy. We also need the forceful action of muscles. Intense aquatic muscle endurance exercise offers a diverse modality that benefits bone density.

(Figure 128) THE MECHANISM OF BONE REMODELING
CAUSED BY MECHANICAL STRESS

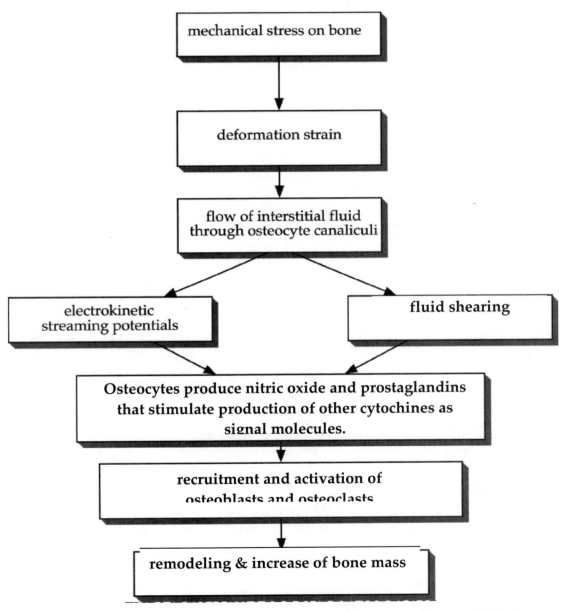

Nalu: The Art and Science of Aquatic Fitness, Bodywork & Therapy

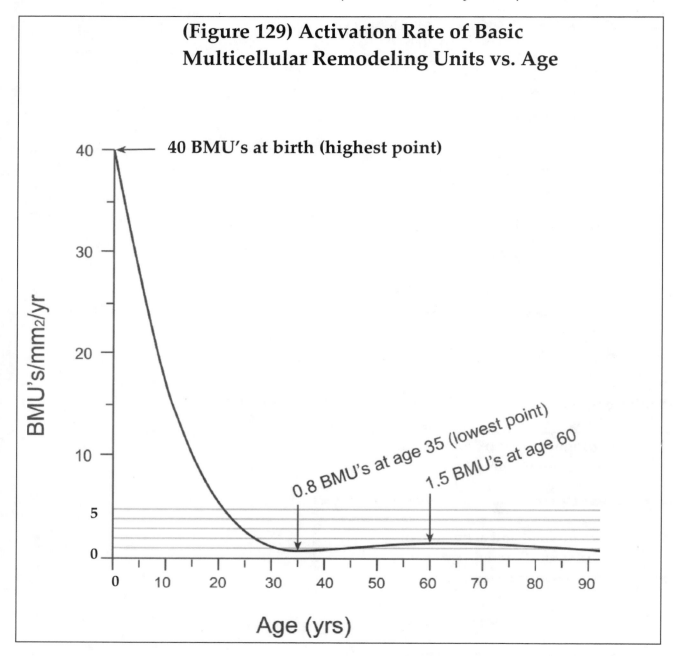

(Figure 129) Activation Rate of Basic Multicellular Remodeling Units vs. Age

40 BMU's at birth (highest point)

0.8 BMU's at age 35 (lowest point)

1.5 BMU's at age 60

BMU's/mm₂/yr

Age (yrs)

Nalu: The Art and Science of Aquatic Fitness, Bodywork & Therapy

Chapter 8
Nutrition for Aquatic Endurance

Essentials

A high fat diet lowers endurance and lowers high intensity performance because the resulting low carbohydrate availability lowers muscle glycogen storage. Regular training, not a high fat diet, increases the availability of fat for fuel. More glycogen is used for fuel with a high carbohydrate diet and more fat is oxidized for fuel with a high fat diet. During regular intense exercise, tissue glycogen levels cannot be restored when diets are low in carbohydrates (Guyton, 1996). Longer duration exercise uses more fat for fuel if carbohydrates are also available, more than if carbohydrates are not available. Using fat for energy is a slow pathway. Using carbohydrates for energy is a rapid metabolic process.

<60% VO2max: fatty acids are used for energy.

60%-85% VO2max: an increasing use of carbohydrates as the energy source.

>85% VO2max: carbohydrate glucose from glycogen is used for energy.

These figures show the predominant sources of energy at different percentages of maximum oxygen volume utilization. Muscle triglycerides, plasma glucose, and muscle glycogen are all used at the same time in varying proportions, depending on exercise duration, intensity, and VO2max.

Participating in high intensity aquatic exercise with maximal use of type IIa muscle fiber is the high road to maintaining the integrity of muscle and bone at any age, as well as restoring lost muscle tissue for the elderly. This type of exercise requires higher overall nutrition. Not everyone can afford expensive superfoods like royal jelly, propolis, bee pollen, blue-green algae, chlorella and spirelina. They are concentrated super nutrition

but still lack fiber and vitamin C according to their supplement fact labels. Nutrient dense foods are recommended. Variety is the key. Using the basic principles of food combining detailed later in this chapter, include vegetables, whole grains, fruit, amino acid balanced protein sources, unprocessed foods, healthy fats, ten or fifteen minutes of sunshine every day, and safe supplements. Most important is cool, pure water. Keep a bottle handy at the poolside. Dehydration is a commonly overlooked problem in aquatic endurance exercise. Dehydration among the elderly is particularly prevalent (Hoffman, 1991).

Digestive distress in a swimming pool is not comfortable. To avoid the possibility of digestive distress and toxicity, exercise on an empty stomach and see the food combining suggestions in this chapter. Most of the dietary information in *Nalu* will be about supplying adequate nutrition for athletic performance and for gains in physical conditioning from vigorous regular aquatic exercise.

To maintain mineral homeostasis, bones become a storehouse for calcium needed not only for bone strength but also essential for muscle contractions (Cooper, 1988). Chemically, crystalline hydroxyapatite in our bones has this molecular structure: $Ca_{10}(PO_4)_6(OH)_2$. The depletion of calcium causes muscle cramps which can also be caused by deficiencies of magnesium, sodium, potassium, and fluid.

The new nutritional numbers published by the National Academy of Sciences are: 1000 mg of calcium per day for 31-50 yr. olds, 1200 mg per day over 51, and 1300 mg for 9-18 yr. olds. Children 4-8 yrs. need 800 mg and 1-3 need 500 mg. (FNB, 1994). Healthy adults, in active physical training that includes incorporating tough muscle endurance aquatic workouts in their routine, regularly need between 1200 mg and 2600 mg of calcium each day.

Calcium is absorbed in the small intestine at a rate of 200 mg out of every 1000 mg consumed in one day by ionic diffusion, facilitated diffusion, and active transport. This rate of absorption diminishes with age to 55-60 years for women and to 65-70 years for men (Fullmer, 1992). Menstruation causes a sharp drop in calcium absorption. Loading up on calcium a week before menstruation helps prevent PMS.

Besides the obvious dairy products, salmon and sardines with bones are high in calcium. Plant foods high in calcium are figs, dark green leafy vegetables like kale and spinach, sesame seeds, peas, sunflower seeds, parsley, almonds, rose hips, and tofu. High protein diets coupled with lactic acid waste from anaerobic muscle endurance exercise decrease blood pH. It becomes more acid with losses in calcium. Severe metabolic acidosis causes calcium loss. That is why anaerobic exercisers need the extra calcium in their diets.

The other mineral in hydroxyapatite is phosphorus, as important as calcium in the strong bone equation. Other functions of phosphorus, besides bone strength, are maintenance of blood pH, carbohydrate metabolism, protein synthesis, transport of fats, insulation of nerve cells with myelin, and the transmission of our genetic code between cells. The need for phosphorus is equal to that of calcium, one to one (FNB, 1994). So the above requirements for calcium apply to phosphorus as well. If they are out of balance there are problems. The development of osteoporosis is accelerated from too much phosphorus and too little calcium (Bronner, 1994). Too much phosphorus degrades calcium absorption. Monitor phosphorus intake to be equal to calcium intake. Phosphorus is found in high protein foods.

Yes, you perspire in the water and lose minerals during a tough aquatic workout, more in warmer water and less in cooler water. Sodium is also lost. However, sodium is abundant in normal diets. Sodium maintains interstitial fluid and electrolyte balance and is a critical component in the transmission of nerve impulses. The minimum daily requirement of calcium is 500 mg and the maximum is 2400 mg per day. The amount of sodium needed for long, hot workouts is at the high end, 1 g/hr (E. Quinn, Exercise Physiologist, www.Sportsmedicine.com). Decreased blood sodium leads to hyponatremia with symptoms similar to dehydration. Over accumulation of sodium by people that don't exercise vigorously and consume too much salt in their diet elevates blood volume and blood pressure by holding water. Hypertension then develops over time (INTERSALT, 1988). Sports drinks contain 50-100 mg of sodium per 9 ounces for re-hydration.

Dehydration during water immersion can be significant. Thirst is naturally suppressed and urine production increased while in a pool (Tajima, et al, 1988; Epstein, 1992). To avoid dehydration in the pool, drink adequate amounts of water before you start exercising. But don't overdo a good thing. Too much water will flush out potassium, a mineral that is the primary electrolyte in the body. Dissolved electrolytes conduct electrical currents, control water balance, control hydrogen ion concentration (acid-base pH), and control the transmission of nerve impulses. Potassium itself is needed in the synthesis of proteins, in muscle contraction, and in heart regulation. Potassium protects against hypertension (FNB, 1994; National Research Council, 1989).

The minimum adult requirement for potassium is 2000 mg per day. For daily aquatic workouts, adults need from 2500 to 4000 mg of potassium per day. Losses occur from dehydration, perspiration, or flushing with too much drinking(FNB, 1994). The best sources of potassium are fruits, vegetables, dairy and to some extent, fresh meat. Examples of foods high in potassium are beet greens, lima beans, carob, figs, and liver.

The best intake ratio of calcium to magnesium is two to one using the intake requirements for calcium above. Magnesium is utilized mainly in the aerobic conversion of glycogen to energy. So cardiovascular exercise of long duration requires more magnesium than anaerobic muscle endurance exercise. Magnesium also regulates heart rate, blood pressure, and is important for muscle relaxation, protein synthesis, calcium metabolism, and as a catalyst for other metabolic reactions. Magnesium is stored in bones.

It is interesting that the giant molecule hemoglobin in blood and the chlorophyll molecule needed in green leafy plants for photosynthesis have identical configurations at their cores (Figure130). The difference is iron with red pigment in the center of the hemoglobin molecule, and magnesium in the center of green chlorophyll. Dark green leafy vegetables are the best source of magnesium.

(Figure 130) Chlorophyll (left) and Hemoglobin (right)

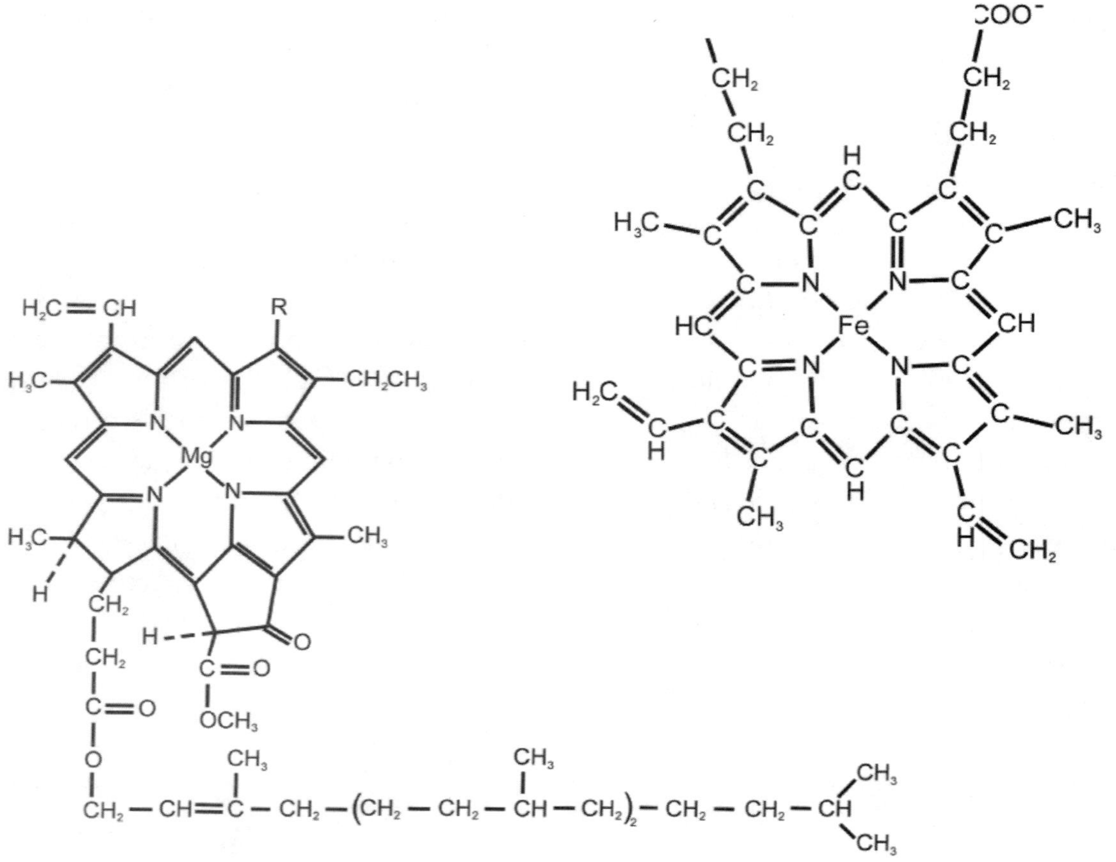

other minerals of importance for exercise performance (copper, chromium, manganese, and iron) besides the trace minerals needed in overall metabolism (zinc, vanadium, molybdenum, selenium, iodine, fluoride, cobalt, and others).

Copper participates in iron absorption and is part of collagen and hemoglobin-forming enzymes. A heavy exercise routine requires twice as much copper as sedentary lifestyles, from 3 to 6 mg per day. When iron is deficient, there is a reduction in athletic performance (Turnland, 1994). Over 30 mg per day causes toxicity. It is found in animal protein, legumes, dried fruit, and green leafy vegetables.

Chromium helps regulate the metabolism of glucose and helps insulin function (Anderson, R.A., 1986). Deficiency in chromium leads to insulin resistance, impaired muscle metabolism, and added body fat (Mertz, 1993). Many athletes consume from 200 to 600 micrograms per day of chromium. However, safe levels recommended by the National

Sulfur deficiencies are unknown in developed economies because it is a component of amino acids in the proteins that we consume. There are

Academy of Sciences (NAS, 1989) are 50-100mcg/day for over 7 years old, 30-60 for age 4-6, 20-80 for age 1-3, 20-60 for age 6 months to 1 year, and 10-40 mcg/day under 6 months. The combination of chromium and carbohydrate ingestion improves maximum exercise performance by increasing anaerobic energy output.

Water is not a nutrient but it is the compound most essential to life. It has such a high polarity that the hydrogen and oxygen ions make water an ideal solvent for many nutritional substances. Chemical substances are either water soluble, oil soluble, or insoluble. Vitamins are classified as either water or fat soluble in the body. The importance of water in the digestion and utilization of nutrients is reason enough to include water in this chapter.

An adult doing normal leisurely exercise only requires one ml of water per calorie of energy expenditure (about 10 cups or 2.5 liters) per day to replace water lost from the skin and respiratory system. But an anaerobic endurance athlete in a hot

environment, like a warm pool, needs as much as ten times this amount. Water is lost for other reasons too. In diets with more protein than needed the excess nitrogen is excreted in the urine with water. Water is a major coolant on the skin to help maintain a delicately controlled body core temperature. High energy athletes in a hot environment need so much more water because they will loose as much as 15 cups (3.75 l) per hour compared to 1½ cups (375 ml) for the inactive, cooler person.

In a warm pool above a thermoneutral temperature, the body overheats and perspiring attempts to cool the body without success. Thermoneutral water temperature is not body temperature. It is the highest temperature that still allows the body to dissipate heat. Water is still lost in the process of the body's attempt to cool itself with perspiration. In a cool pool, the ambient water is the coolant.

Electrolyte disturbances among the elderly are most commonly caused by dehydration due to a reduced sensation of thirst (Chernoff, 1994).

Dehydration symptoms are as follows for the given percentages of body water lost: (1%) reduced VO2max; (2%) early thirst, loss of appetite and loss of endurance capacity; (3%) impaired performance, dry mouth; (4%) vague discomfort, loss of appetite, apathy, impatience, more effort needed for exercise; (5%) slowing pace, increased pulse, increased breathing, difficulty concentrating; (6-7%) temperature regulation impaired, higher pulse and breathing, flushed skin, sleepiness, tingling, stumbling, headache; (8-9%) dizziness, labored breathing, mental confusion, further weakness; (10%) muscle spasms, loss of balance, swelling of tongue; (11%) heat exhaustion, delirium, stroke, coma, difficulty swallowing, possible permanent central nervous system damage, possible death.

To reduce the need for water during anaerobic aquatic muscle endurance training and conditioning, it is suggested that water temperatures feel cool upon entering a pool prior to warming up. This will help to avoid overheating and a burden on the body's cooling system.

Drink mineral water the day before a big pool workout to maintain hydration, 2-3 cups (500-750 ml) of cool water 2 hours before the workout, and 1-2 cups (250-500 ml) of cool water 15 minutes before the workout and ½ cup of cool water with added salt 7g/L plus soluble carbohydrates every 15 minutes during the exercise (Coyle, 1992). After the exercise, drink 2 cups (500ml) of water, with electrolytes like salt, for every pound of fluid lost. The International Marathon Medical Directors Association states in an advisory (Noakes, 2002) that athletes should drink as needed, that blanket hydration recommendations are unsafe, and not to exceed 800ml per hour. The American College of Sports Medicine (Convertino, 1996) recommends that endurance athletes drink as much water as they can tolerate.

Rehydration is the movement of water into intracellular spaces. Re-hydration after pool exercise, with water alone, stimulates urination by increasing blood volume. This decreases thirst and the desire to drink the amount of water needed for full hydration. Electrolytes like sodium chloride and potassium added to post exercise fluids help maintain the drive to drink enough for proper rehydration.

Glucose (Fig.131), added to post exercise fluids in concentrations under 9% helps sodium absorption in the intestines by traveling with it to intestinal microvilli cells. There the mixture separates as the glucose goes directly into the blood (Davis, et al, 1990). The purpose of sodium with glucose is to change the microvilli carrier in such a way that the glucose passes across the membrane by itself from the inner side to the outer side. Potassium then attaches to the glucose as it goes in to the blood circulation. Fructose does not have this ability (Murray, 1987; Murray, 1989).

The thirst response mechanism isn't always activated right away during intense pool workouts when water loss is acute and sudden. Before the thirst mechanism functions in an average adult, nearly two liters of fluid must be lost. The body overheats from fluid loss. Even in water, fluid is continuously lost through skin perspiration and through breathing. Blood plasma volume then decreases and its osmotic action increases. When overheated, hormonal controls begin to maintain fluid balance by conserving body fluids. The kidneys start to hold back the excretion of water. This is controlled by the pituitary gland releasing antidiuretic hormone, vasopressin. Sodium is re-absorbed by the action of the adrenal cortex hormone, aldosterone. Osmotic pressure is then maintained. Therefore it is important to have that water next to the pool and drink regularly, thirsty or not.

During the excitement of tremendously energetic water exercise, dehydration can sneak up on you. Children are at a higher risk of having heat stress so they should drink extra water when overheated from physical activity and the fun of pool exercise.

Carbohydrates come in all sizes (Figures 131-133). Starch and cellulose are large plant polysaccharides made of long chains of monosaccharides, glucose molecules. Starch is absorbed slowly in the digestive tract and broken down to glucose molecules. Enzymes in saliva convert starch into dextrose, an isomer of glucose. The enzyme Amylase in pancreatic juice digests starch into short glucose chains and maltose. Cellulose, a structural component of plants , is a nondigestible fiber that adds healthy bulk to a diet.

Monosaccharides are simple single sugars, saccharides that are quickly absorbed into the digestive tract. Glucose, galactose and fructose are monosaccharides. Disaccharides are a combination of two monosaccharides. Maltose is glucose + glucose. Sucrose is glucose + fructose. Lactose is sucrose + galactose. Disaccharides are absorbed at a rate between that of monosaccharides and polysaccharides.

(Figure 131A) Glucose

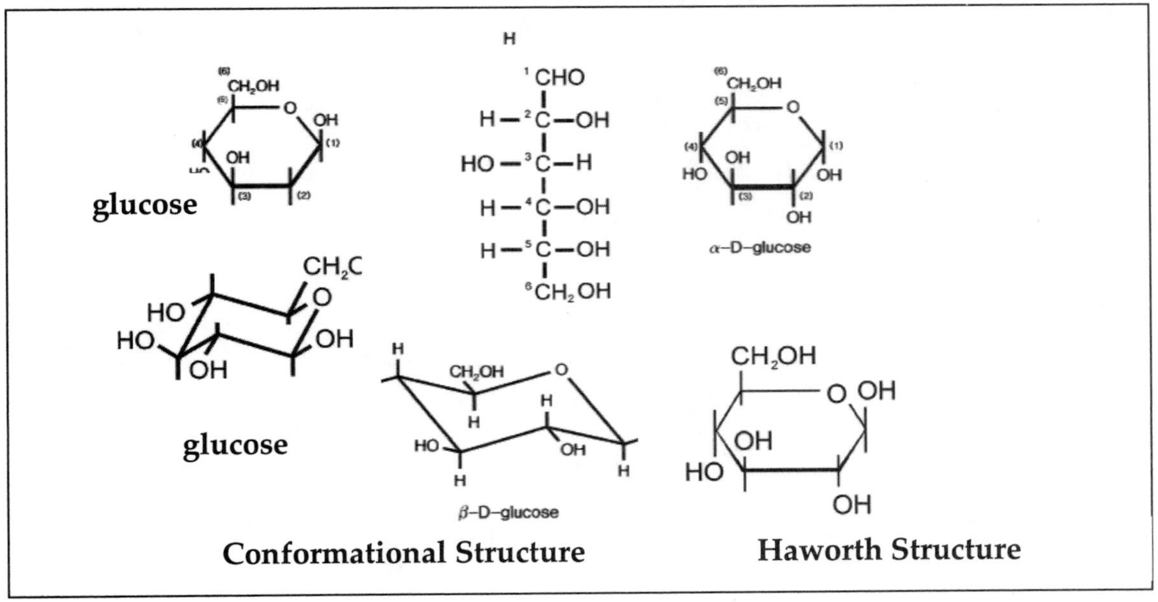

Conformational Structure   **Haworth Structure**

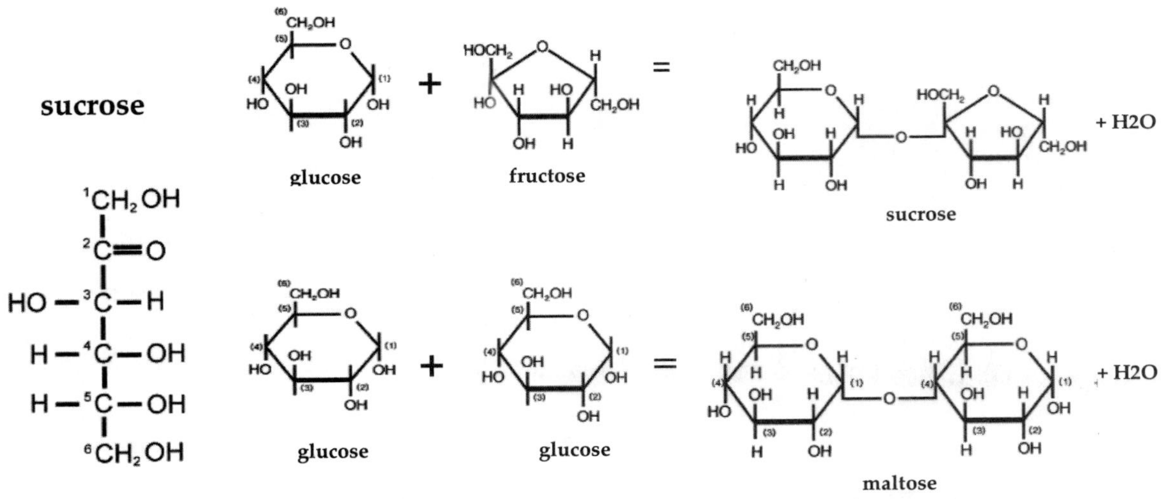

(Figure 131B) Maltose from Glucose; Sucrose from Glucose & Fructose

(Figure 132) sugars

lactose

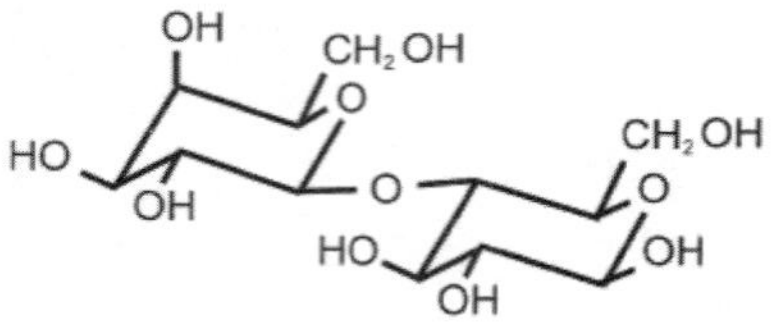

galactose

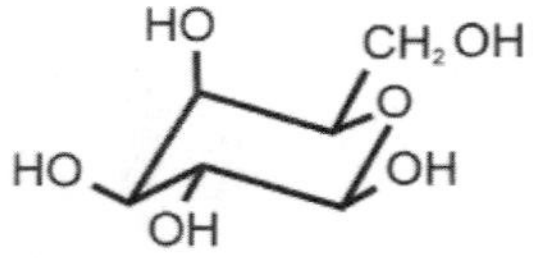

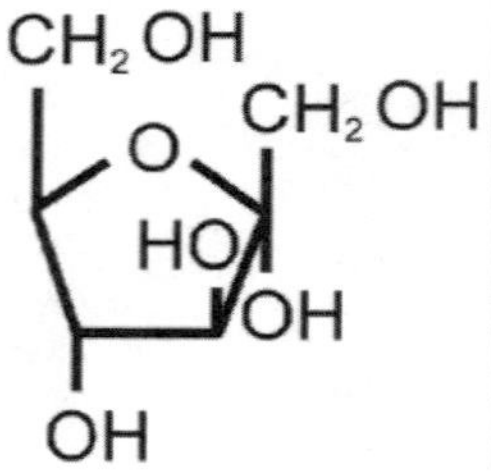

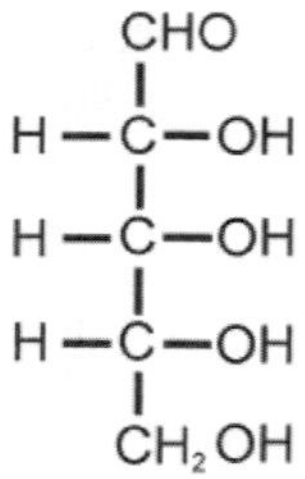

ribose

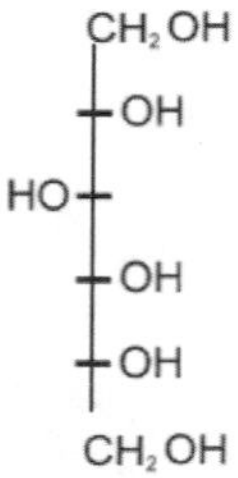

sorbitol

fructose

(Figure 133) Cellulose & Starch

cellulose

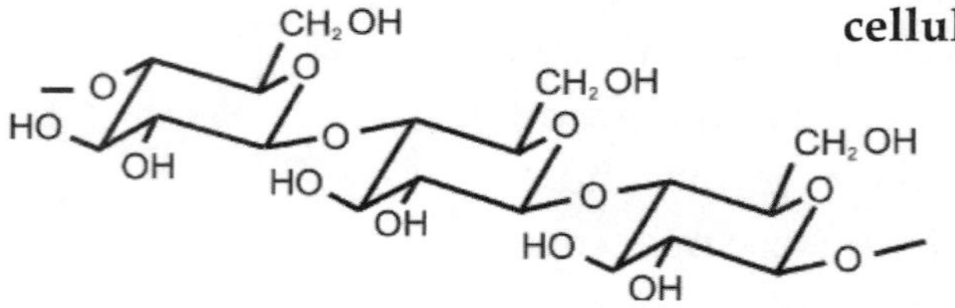

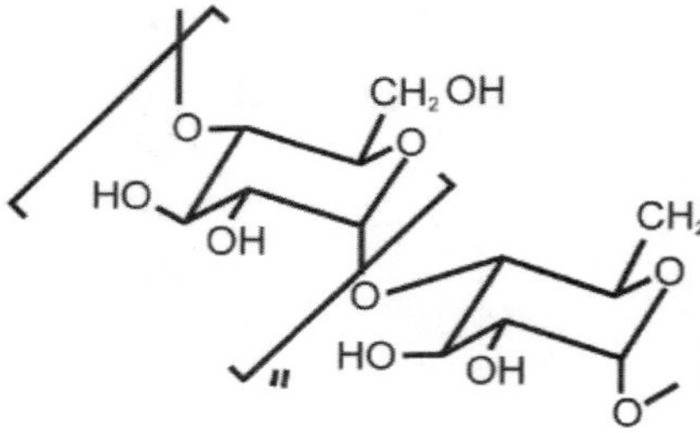

amylose-unbranched starch

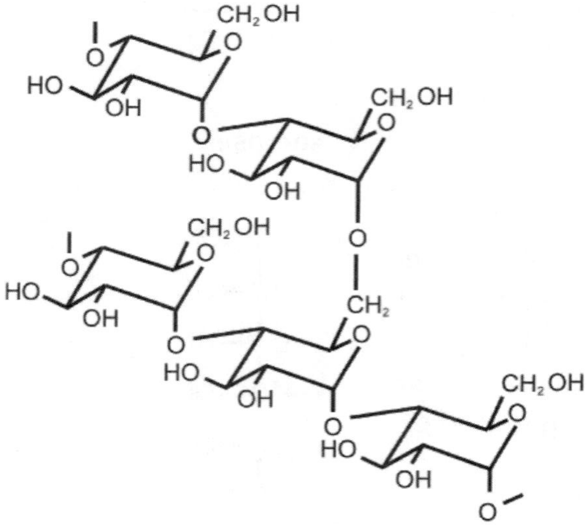

amylopectin-branched starch

High carbohydrate diets, 7-10 g/kg body weight per day, are critical to the high-energy performance of anaerobic exercise. Variation in the carbohydrates is important for balancing the needed nutrients, fiber, and enzymes (Jequire, 1994). Any nutritional deficiencies will decrease performance. Too many carbohydrates close to your scheduled workout will cause sleepiness because serotonin is released in the brain after high carbohydrate consumption (Traber, 1995). 60% of the aquatic muscle endurance exercisers total calories should be from carbohydrates, 25% from healthy fat, and 15% from balanced protein.

Physical fitness is great. But don't neglect the colon. Fiber is the answer and it works well. Rice bran and oat bran are very inexpensive and effective fibers.. High chlorophyll foods help detoxify and clean the colon. Fiber (cellulose) sweeps it out and exercises the intestinal musculature. It is wise to avoid unhealthy fermentation and putrefaction from poor food combinations. Avoiding high fat diets,

harmful chemicals, toxic carcinogens from overheated fats and oils, smoked and pickled foods, pesticides and nitrosamines found in bacon, are some of the preventive measures against colon cancer and other cancers (National Research Council, 1982).

*M*y personal method of maintaining a healthy colon comes from the phrase, "Green is clean." The janitors of the colon are fiber and chlorophyll. At this Caribbean latitude, I own the southernmost vine of *Pueraria thunbergiana* and contain it by keeping the runners up off of the ground and by harvesting the leaves. Normally it requires a dormant winter season but at this location, as the leaves fall, new growth is beginning. Originating in China and introduced to the U.S. in 1876 from Japan, cultivation began in 1902. In Asia it is cultivated for the root as a thickening agent in cooking and for cloth fiber. In the U.S. it was started as a livestock crop and to aid in preventing erosion along new road

construction. Because it got out of control and now covers much of Georgia and the Carolinas, this vine — kudzu— is regarded as a pest; the facts on its high nutritional qualities should be better known.

The powdered leaves of dried kudzu have the mild taste of basil and parsley. They have been a welcome ingredient in my diet for fourteen years.

It is a wise choice to avoid simple sugars. These include honey (fructose, glucose & sucrose), maple syrup (93% sucrose), corn syrup, brown sugar, molasses (70% sucrose), dates and raisins. Cane sugar is often disguised on an ingredients list as cane juice, dehydrated cane juice or Florida crystal. Use large molecule sugars like the combination of maltodextrins, maltose and complex carbohydrates found in brown rice syrup that takes up to 2-3 hours to fully digest, maintaining a steady blood sugar level. A raw carrot is quite sweet, and not much beats the taste of a ripe Hayden mango. But eat mangoes conservatively. Their sugars are not large and digest too quickly causing elevated blood sugar. Too much of anything can cause trouble.

*H*ere is a way to deal with sugar cravings that I pass on to " sweets-addicted" clients: consume a half-teaspoon of royal jelly obtained from a natural food store (pollen that has been digested by bees to feed their larvae), followed by a glass of cool water, then a stalk of celery. It stops right there. The taste for sugar is gone.

ᕈ)))))O>   ᕈ)))))O>   ᕈ)))))O>

Try whole, unprocessed foods, without all the added preservatives and chemicals. Fresh, organically grown raw produce is generally healthiest. However, cooking increases the nutrients available from root crops, especially beta carotene, and increases carbohydrate availability from grains and roots. Whole cereal grains full of many nutrients are far superior to the starch itself that is marketed as white flour and white rice after the nutrients have been stripped from it.

If you eat meat, eat lean for the protein. Eating small fish from clean water is preferable to eating large fish or bovine red meat. Eat nuts and seeds sparingly. They are great nutrition but high in fat. Fats and oils are called lipids. Some are healthy, but for the most part, many kinds of fat are unhealthy in the diet. The unhealthy fats and oils are saturated, hydrogenated, partially hydrogenated or loaded with bad cholesterol (Fig.134). Cholesterol is not a fat but it forms cholesterol esters by attaching to these long-chain fatty acids. The brain needs cholesterol. The common bad fats and oils are: lard, bacon grease, coconut oil, corn oil, "vegetable" oil, palm oil, cocoa butter, cheese, butter, cream, margarine, and any fat or oil subjected to the chemical modifications from heating, frying, or microwave radiation. They become carcinogenic and harmful to health. The best fats are flax oil, borage oil, hemp oil, evening primrose oil and fresh salmon oil. Olive oil is excellent and resists spoilage.

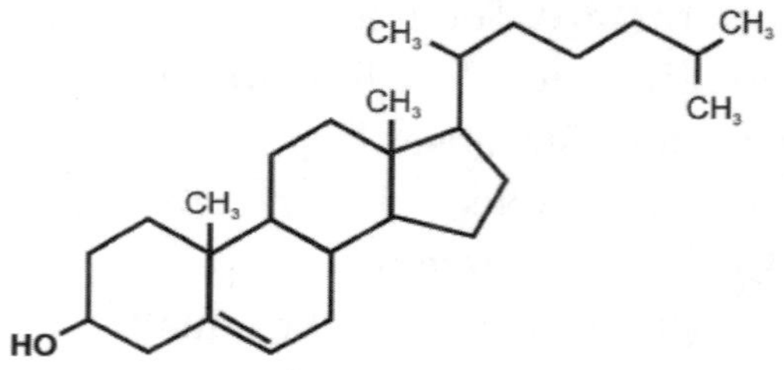

(Figure 134) Cholesterol

Fat is essential. Stored fat has fifty times more energy capacity per gram than carbohydrate. Body fat is used to replace blood glucose lowered during exercise. This protects our muscles from glycogen depletion. Carbohydrates are needed for the complete oxidation of fats. They act together. More fat is used for energy during higher intensity and longer duration exercise. During exercise, the triglycerides within muscle tissue are used first, then the more plentiful energy from fats stored in adipose tissue reaches the muscles. Training and conditioning help the metabolism to use more fat for energy.

In a triglyceride, three fatty acids attach to a glycerol molecule (Figure 135). In general, unhealthy saturated fats are triglycerides from animal sources. They are thick solids at room temperature with an even number of carbon atoms, no double bonds between carbon atoms, and their fatty acids are long chains making them insoluble in water. Saturated fats contain as many hydrogen atoms attached to carbon as possible. Healthy unsaturated fats are triglycerides from plant sources. They are fluid oils with an odd number of carbon atoms and they have one or more double bonds between carbon atoms. The double bonds reduce the proportion of hydrogen by one atom of hydrogen per double bonded carbon atom. Their fatty acids are short chains making them more water soluble. An example of a long chain saturated fatty acid is palmitic acid (Figure 135). You can see that there

are no double bonds between any carbon atoms and it is saturated with hydrogen at every location. It is an ingredient in most waxes. Examples of unsaturated fatty acids are oleic, linoleic, and linolenic acid (Figure 135). Linoleic acid is the only truly essential fatty acid in the human diet. Other unsaturated fatty acids are synthesized from it for important body functions like building cell membranes, transporting cholesterol, and clotting blood. Linoleic acid is a precursor to long chain polyunsaturated fatty acids that act like hormones (prostaglandins) to contract smooth muscle, lower blood pressure, control inflammation, and regulate bodily functions such as temperature and gastric secretion.

Omega-3 fatty acids are long chain polyunsaturated fish oils. The (NIH) National Institutes of Health has credited these with lowering the incidence of heart disease (Anderson, 1987). Many people are confused about what the long names mean for identifying omega-3 fatty acids, names like eicosapentaenoic acid (EPA) and docosahexaenoic acid

(DHA). They look like ominous chemical nomenclatures. What does omega-3 mean?

The letter "omega" is the last letter in the Greek alphabet. It refers to the carbon atom at the very end of the chain, opposite the end that contains oxygen. From the end (Figure 135), count three carbon atoms. That is the first double bond in the chain and where the "3" comes from in the name. Since omega-3's are polyunsaturated, there is more than one double bond in the chain of carbon atoms. Now we will figure out what eicosapentaenoic means. It is all truly Greek. "Eicosa" in Greek, means 20. There are twenty carbon atoms in the chain. "Penta" in Greek, is 5. There are five double bonds in the chain. There it is, eicosapentaenoic omega-3 fatty acid, a long name but easy to understand when you know the translations and what to look for. Observe the location of the first doubl- bonded carbon atom opposite the end of the molecule where oxygen is located in the unsaturated fatty acids (Figure 135).

(Figure 135) Fats and Fatty Acids

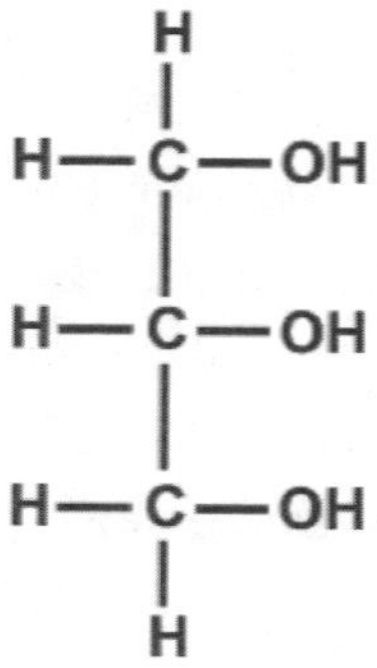

$$H-\underset{\underset{H}{|}}{\overset{\overset{H}{|}}{C}}-OH$$
$$H-\underset{|}{\overset{|}{C}}-OH$$
$$H-\underset{\underset{H}{|}}{\overset{|}{C}}-OH$$

Glycerol

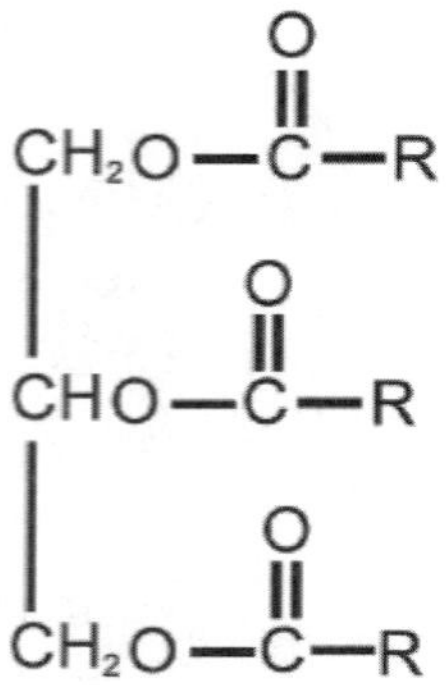

$$CH_2O-\overset{\overset{O}{\|}}{C}-R$$
$$CHO-\overset{\overset{O}{\|}}{C}-R$$
$$CH_2O-\overset{\overset{O}{\|}}{C}-R$$

Triglyceride

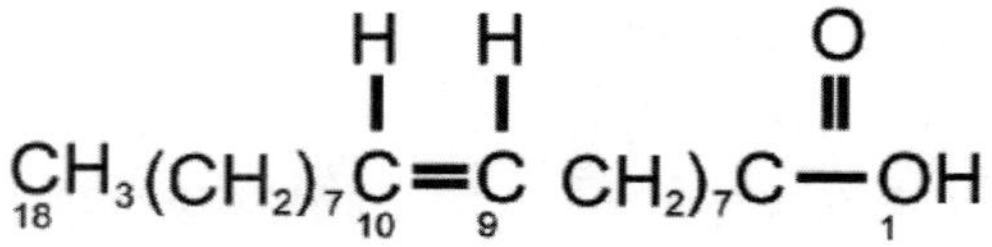

$$CH_3(CH_2)_7\underset{10}{\overset{\overset{H}{|}}{C}}=\underset{9}{\overset{\overset{H}{|}}{C}} CH_2)_7\overset{\overset{O}{\|}}{\underset{1}{C}}-OH$$

**Oleic acid
(unsaturated)**

$$CH_3(CH_2)_4\underset{13}{\overset{\overset{H}{|}}{C}}=\underset{12\;11}{\overset{\overset{H}{|}}{C}}CH_2\underset{10}{\overset{\overset{H}{|}}{C}}=\underset{9}{\overset{\overset{H}{|}}{C}}(CH_2)_7\overset{\overset{O}{\|}}{\underset{1}{C}}-OH$$

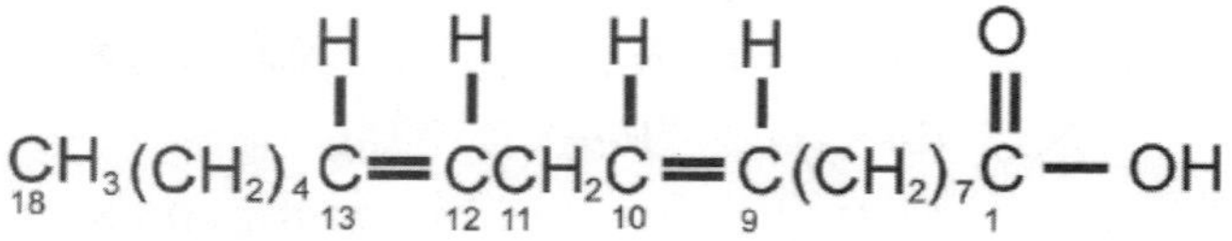

**Lenoleic acid
(unsaturated)**

$$CH_3CH_2\underset{16}{\overset{\overset{H}{|}}{C}}=\underset{15\;14}{\overset{\overset{H}{|}}{C}}CH_2\underset{13}{\overset{\overset{H}{|}}{C}}=\underset{12\;11}{\overset{\overset{H}{|}}{C}}CH_2\underset{10}{\overset{\overset{H}{|}}{C}}=\underset{4}{\overset{\overset{H}{|}}{C}}(CH_2)_7\overset{\overset{O}{\|}}{\underset{1}{C}}-OH$$

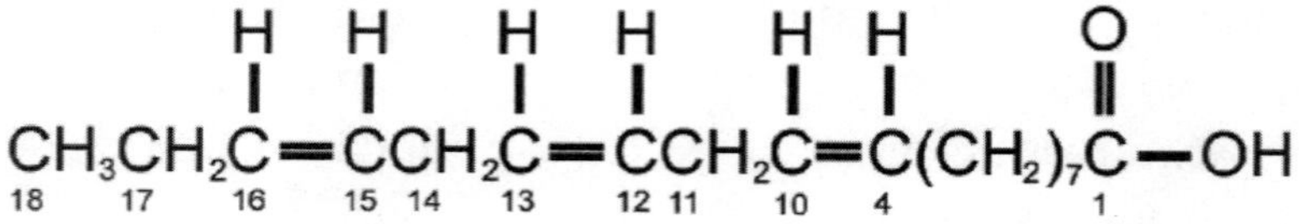

**Lenolenic acid
(unsaturated)**

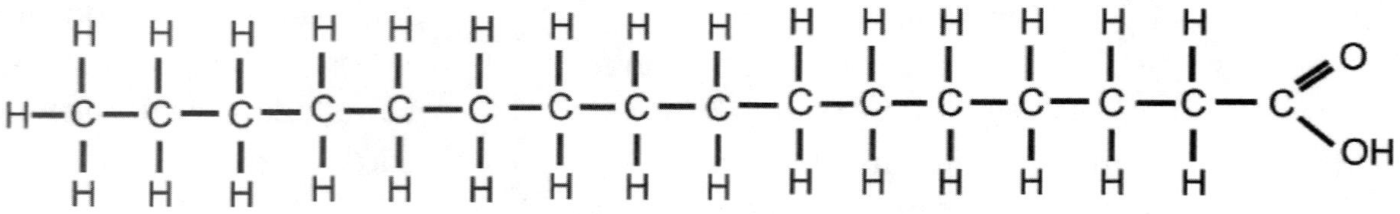

$$H-C-C-C-C-C-C-C-C-C-C-C-C-C-C-C-C\overset{\overset{O}{\diagup\!\!\!\!=}}{\diagdown_{OH}}$$

Palmitic acid (saturated)

Nalu: The Art and Science of Aquatic Fitness, Bodywork & Therapy

Fats are used less and carbohydrates more during faster high intensity anaerobic exercise, while fats are used more during aerobics. Sherman (1987) reaffirms that the most effective diet for aquatic muscle endurance exercise is high in carbohydrates.

Pushing exercise to the limits requires protein for tissue healing and repair. Actin and myosin, the contractile units in muscles, are proteins. Proteins are combinations of amino acids (Figure 136). The body synthesizes most of the needed amino acids but there are several that are derived essentially from dietary sources that must be proportionately balanced for building proteins (Figure 137). Aerobic endurance at 75% VO2max requires protein just under 1g/kg body weight per day combined with adequate energy intake from carbohydrates. This should be ten times the amount of protein, in grams. For heavier anaerobic endurance workouts such as those with aquatic exercise equipment adjusted for high resistance, protein needs are a little higher at 1.5g/kg (Meredith et al., 1989).

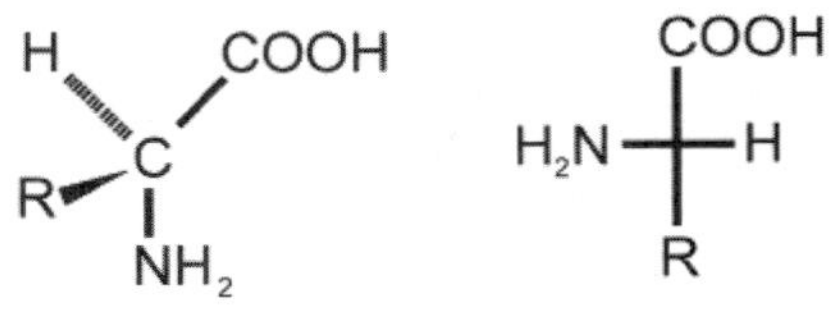

(Figure 136) Amino Acid

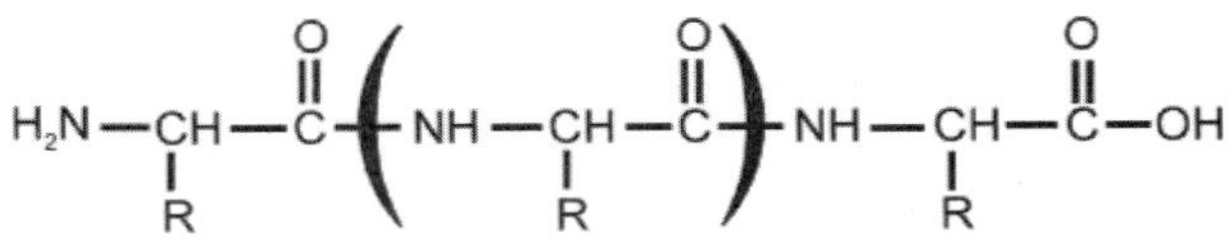

(Figure 137) Protein

In one way, humans are inferior to other mammals. For example, herbivorous cows eat grass. That's all they have to eat to get nitrogen from the cellulose (Figure 133) so their bacteria can make all the amino acids they need to grow and produce milk. But the inferior humans have to eat a mix of everything we can get our hands on to find complete amino acids ready-made by plants and animals. These are the nine essential amino acids we can't make ourselves from dietary nitrogen and carbohydrates. And we don't have the kind of bacteria it takes to digest cellulose and produce amino acids from it. The human appendix may have been a long lost evolutionary antique that at one time was the place for cellulose digestion in lower animals, that second stomach.

When more nitrogen is taken in as protein and less is excreted, there is a net growth in tissues. The opposite causes cannibalism of one's own muscle tissue. This relationship is the nitrogen balance. Digestibility, or net protein utilization, is different for various individuals and dietary protein sources. Whey from milk and albumin from egg whites are easily digestible proteins for most people. Some are allergic, however. Most meats supply all the essential amino acids (Figure 138) in ideal proportions, although eating red meat is controversial in terms of optimal health and longevity. Wheat germ is nearly 20% protein.

Essential Amino Acids (Figure 138)

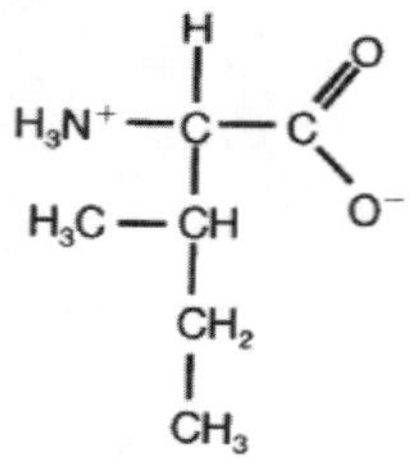

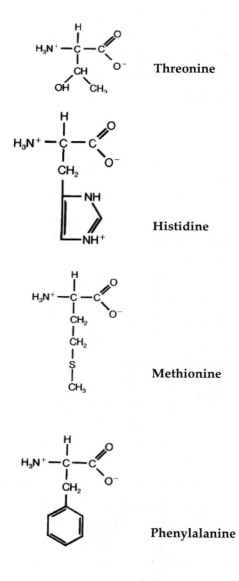

Isoleucine

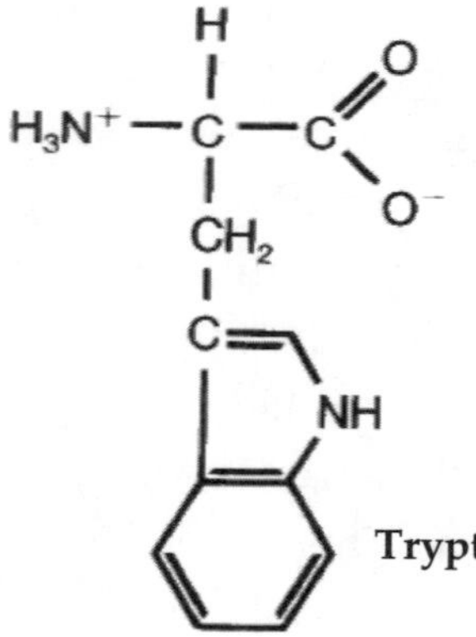

Tryptophan

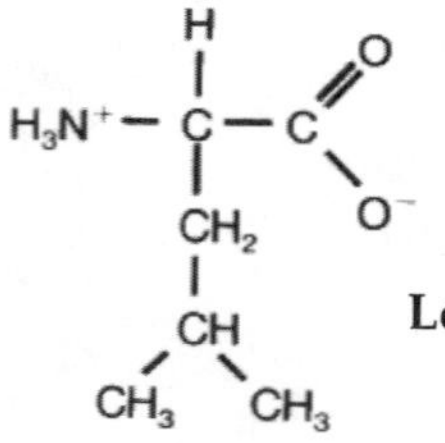

Leucine

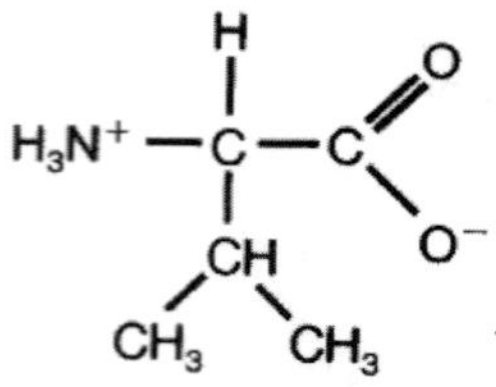

Valine

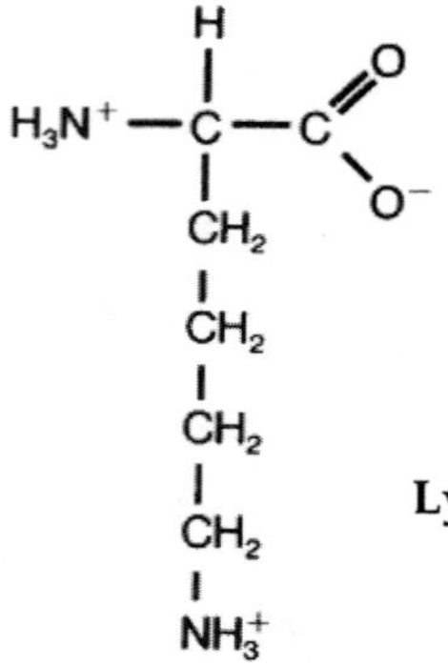

Lysine

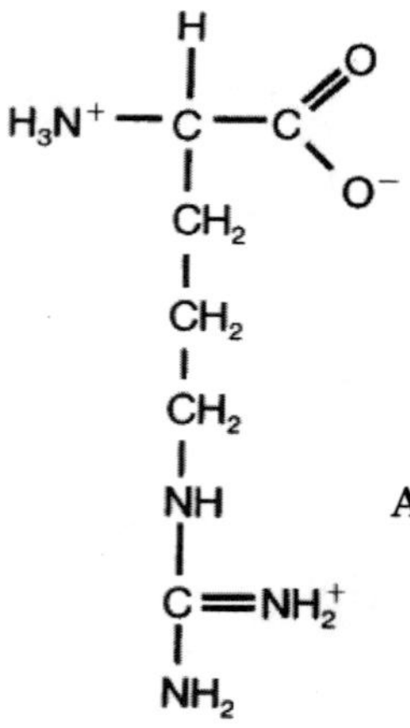

Arginine

Threonine

Histidine

Methionine

Phenylalanine

Non-essential Amino Acids   (Figure 139)

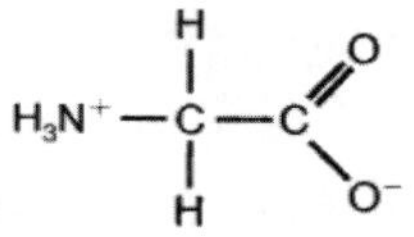

Glycine

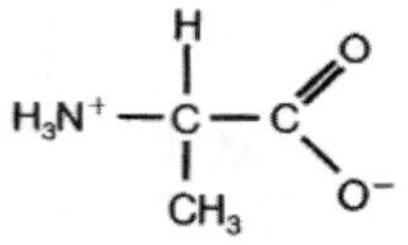

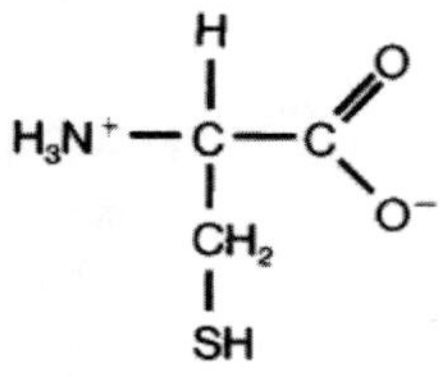

Cysteine

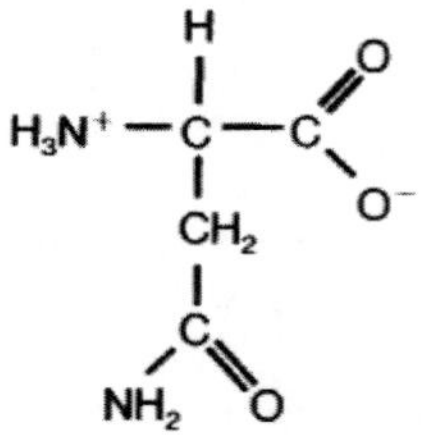

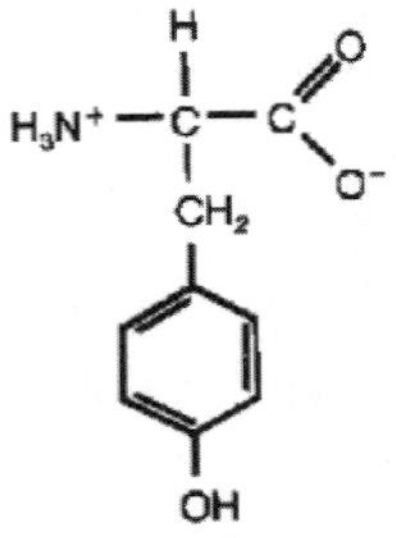

Tyrosine

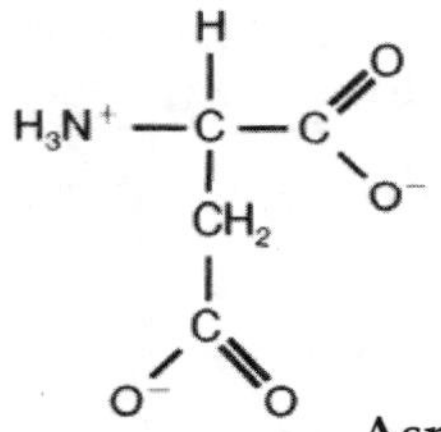

Alanine

Aspartic acid

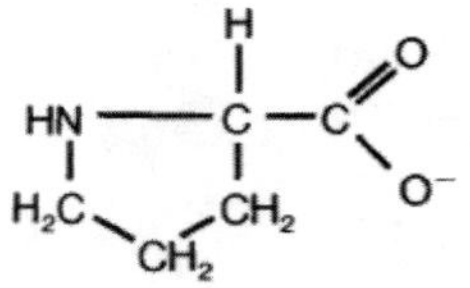

Proline

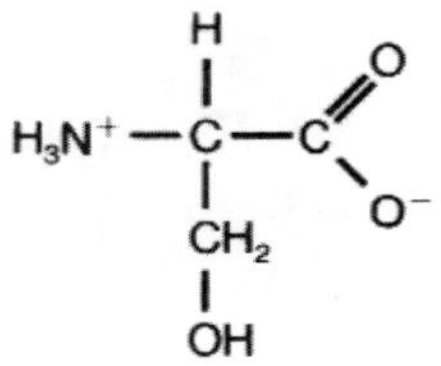

Asparagine

Serine

Glutamine

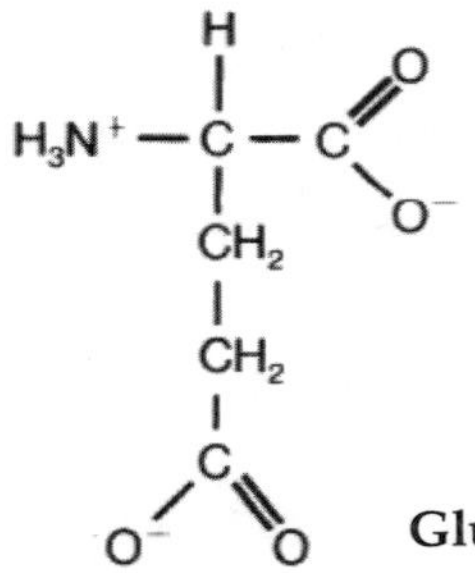

Glutamic acid

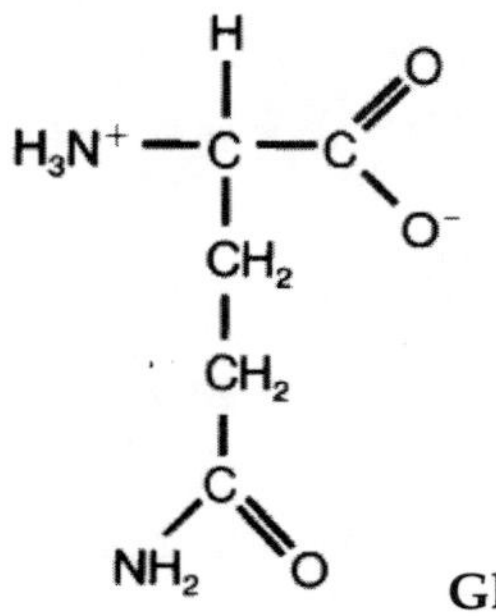

Nalu: The Art and Science of Aquatic Fitness, Bodywork & Therapy

Soybeans are exceptionally high in protein but for some they could be difficult to digest. Powdered protein supplements are excellent sources if they are well balanced in essential amino acids and a quick meal is needed. Natural sources are always best. Overconsumption of protein is unhealthy and expensive. It is a burden to store it as fat and to eliminate the added nitrogenous waste. Urea (Figure 140) is the nitrogenous waste carrier produced in the liver. The process of urea production requires energy from ATP at several points during transamination reactions and also during oxidative deamination which is the breakdown of protein into amino acids, to glutamate, and finally to nitrogenous waste.

$$H_2N - CO - NH_2$$

$$NH_2$$
$$|$$
$$C=O$$
$$|$$
$$NH_2$$

(Figure 140) Urea

*T**his is how I became a vegetarian.*

In 1969 I drove a VW Bug from Illinois all the way up the unpaved, muddy, rutty, rocky Alaska Highway to Fairbanks. The one book I had was "How to Stay Alive in the Woods: A Complete Guide to Food, Shelter and Self Preservation" by Bradford Angier. The exciting forest fire fighting adventure I had not anticipated there lasted for the following five years interrupted by some winters in Hawaii and Jamaica or back in school at Western Illinois University. I learned that termite larvae were one of nature's most concentrated protein sources, at 76% with a good balance of amino acids for humans. Some years later, with that knowledge, a carpenter partner and I were building a cedar log house in Banff, Alberta and accidentally came across a new nest of bees on the roof framing. The bees fled from the vibrations of our pounding hammers. There they were, a handful of larvae waiting to be tasted for the first time.

You know they actually had quite a wholesome protei-rich sweetness.

During one of my last winters in Alaska, I earned a 1400 pound share of fresh moose meat by backpacking the quarters from a kill site for two hunters from Pennsylvania. They had hired a hunting guide friend, Ron Long, to fly the three of us to his primitive camp at the base of the tallest mountain on the continent. I carried nearly two hundred pounds of the fresh meat per trip through September snow to a small landing strip just north of Mt. McKinley. We flew with it all to Fairbanks in an old four- passenger airplane that had been used by "bush pilots" to bootleg whisky into Eskimo villages. Two years before that I had built a prospect site cabin in Goldstream Valley, several miles outside of Fairbanks. I carried the meat on my back to this site where I had built a log cache to keep it from the wolves whose hungry howling echoed throughout the valley. Here on my "homestead" that I later named "Happy Creek Wildlife Sanctuary," formally Bedgood Association Mining

Claims, my Eskimo girlfriend and I dined on moose meat cooked on a wood burning stove twice a day until spring, then gave the remaining several hundred pounds to friends around Fairbanks and to local hippie communes before the Spring thaw when ice broke up and quickly rumbled down the rivers. I have been a vegetarian ever since.

>‹(((O>   >‹(((O>   >‹(((O>

For exercise, the adult human body requires 1.0-1.5 grams of balanced protein per kilogram of body weight per day (FNB, 1994). This amounts to 10-15% of the calories in the total diet. Fat should be less than 30% of the diet. The only essential fat is linoleic acid for heart muscle energy. Excess calories are stored as fat regardless of their source. Carbohydrates are the major nutrient for energy support for exercise (Jequier, 1994). They should be 50-70% of daily caloric intake for exercise energy needs. As stated earlier, 65% is ideal for the intensity of resistance exercise proposed here for aquatic conditioning.

Efficient digestion of meat requires proper choices of the other foods eaten with the meat. When a person eats meat and starch at the same time, digestion is poor. It is slow. The best digestion is a fast process. What happens in the stomach and intestines? When meat and potatoes are together they produce fermentation and putrefaction at the same time. Digestion stops until something gives, until the pH swings one way or the other. The meat putrefies because the pH is not acid enough for digestion due to the presence of starch (Fig.133) which requires a high stomach pH. The starch ferments because it remains in one place waiting for the pH to go up for its digestion, but the stomach fluids attempting to digest the meat are too acid to digest the starch. There you have it, hunger over mind, indulgence over reason, the cause of poor digestion, very poor utilization of food, and toxic products in the intestine from the conflicting, rotting processes.Proper food combining is a simple science. Eat concentrated proteins and heavy starches separately at different meals or far

apart during a meal. Eat the protein first. Non-starchy vegetables can be consumed with protein. Dairy products stop all other digestion. Eat or drink dairy alone. Sweets stop digestion of everything else until they move through the intestinal walls into the blood. Sweets will interrupt a smooth flowing fast digestion until the simple carbohydrates are out of the way. It is healthier to use the larger, more complex carbohydrates than simple sugars. Read all the ingredients on food labels. Drink unfiltered fruit juices diluted, fifteen minutes or more before a meal. It is unhealthy to dilute food by drinking abundant liquids with the meal. If you wash down the food it dilutes the pH and digestive environment.

Concentrated foods are basically a majority of one food type with the exclusion of most of the others. Nuts, meat and soybeans are examples of concentrated protein. Potatoes, roots, corn and other grains are examples of concentrated starch. Avocados, oils and cream are examples high in fat. Dates, honey and cane are examples of concentrated simple sugars.

Food Combining

* Symptoms of improper food combining include flatulence, gastrointestinal distress, loss of energy, stomach cramps, "heartburn," lack of motivation, irritability, and hours of general discomfort.

* Toxins are produced during incomplete and inefficient digestion.

*Eat foods of concentrated proteins or concentrated carbs/starches separately and at different meals. Eat vegetables with either concentrated food.

*Eat fruit alone, not mixing acid and sweet fruit or either of them with melons that decompose very rapidly. Sub-acid fruit is compatible with sweet or acid fruit.

* A natural combination of unseparated, concentrated food found in nature is digestible. Examples are grains, nuts & legumes.

* Different concentrated starches can be mixed but not different concentrated proteins.

* The digestion of food and the elimination of toxic waste can take more energy than physical exercise or athletic activities.

* Fermentation and putrefaction in the digestive system are unhealthy and toxic.

* Fermentation results from carbohydrate digestion being slowed by a lowering of pH from ingesting concentrated proteins that require an acid environment for digestion.

* Putrefaction results from protein digestion being slowed by raising the pH due to the ingestion of concentrated carbohydrates and starches that require an alkaline environment for digestion.

Dairy products create coagulated curds that adhere to intestines and inhibit absorption of nutrients. They are acid forming, mucous forming, and clog mucous membranes. It is a waste of calcium to have to neutralize all the acid formed from dairy products. Are you weaned yet? If you must have it, consume dairy by itself. Most all nuts, seeds and vegetables contain calcium that is easily assimilated.

To put it simply, don't eat protein and carbohydrate in the same meal (Figure 141). Generally, eat fruit alone on an empty stomach and wait 20-30 minutes before a carbohydrate meal or an hour before a protein meal. Sprouts are an exception and can be mixed with fruit. Avoid fruit for 3 hrs, after eating other foods. Acid fruit with sweet fruit is a poor combination. Sub-acid fruits can be eaten with sweet or acid fruits. Eat melons alone. Wait two hours after a protein or carbohydrate meal before eating fruit. Eat proteins or fats with vegetables. Eat carbohydrates with vegetables. Do not eat concentrated proteins with concentrated fats. Wait three hours between different meal types (protein, fat, or carbohydrate).

Proper food combining reduces the work of the digestive system and conserves energy.

Only eat when hungry and stop before you are full. Don't drink fluids that dilute digestive juices when eating food Avoid fried, canned or processed food. Room temperature is best for food being eaten. Extreme food temperatures damage digestive enzymes.

Most supplements used as meal replacements may be convenient but lack fiber (Anderson, 1994). Examples are: Nutrament, Ensure, Balance, SlimFast, Boost, and others.

(Figure 141)

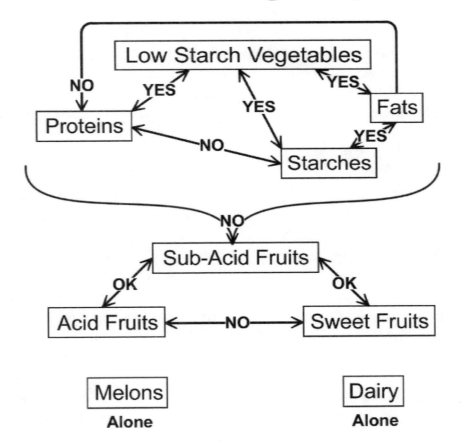

Exercise increases the formation of the free radicals that can damage healthy tissues (Jackson, 1987). Free radicals are unstable portions of compounds that come loose and search for electrons to become stable again. They accelerate aging, weaken the immune syste and cause vascular disorders, cancer and other diseases. Different types of exercise produce different free radicals from different sources. Pool aerobics can increase oxygen utilization 10 to 20 times higher than at rest and this generates many more free radicals than at rest.

Hormones released during anaerobic exercise affect nerves, release stored fat, and cause glycogen to be transported to muscles. Free radicals form during the oxidation of these hormones, epinephrine and norepinephrine. Aerobic exercise increases the population of mitochondria, which in turn increase ATP production and oxygen metabolism. The resulting increased oxidation forms free radicals. The prolonged deep breathing of aerobics in polluted air combines the oxygen with nitrogen oxide and ozone, forming more free radicals.

What can be done to counteract the free radicals resulting from strenuous exercise? The answer is vitamins. There are at least eleven vitamins needed for healthy metabolism and healing. Some are of particular interest here because they are most helpful as antioxidants to protect against free radical damage. Along with its role   in the synthesis of connective tissue during recovery from strength workouts, vitamin C (Fig.146) is a major antioxidant that protects muscles against free radical damage (Gohil, 1986). After exercise, vitamin C also lowers the stress hormone cortisol, which would otherwise weaken the immune response. Vitamin E reduces muscle soreness after intense exercise by reducing toxic waste products from muscle activity, leading to quicker and more comfortable recovery. It protects against free radical damage, oxidative injury and acute immune response changes (Meydani, 1993).

Beta- carotene, an antioxidant, is a precursor for vitamin A and transformed into vitamin A after ingestion. It lowers the risk of cancers and heart disease. Endurance athletes need extra beta- carotene. Vitamin D is needed in the absorption of calcium and availability of phosphorus for bone development. A vitamin D deficiency allows the departure of calcium from bones causing osteoporosis. Assuming there is sufficient direct skin exposure to sunlight to produce a daily vitamin D quantity of 200 IU or 5 micrograms, up to age 50 adequate daily intake of vitamin D is an additional 200 IU or 5 micrograms. From there to age 70, adequate daily consumption increases to 600 IU (Beck, 2000).

The vitamin B complex is needed in higher quantities for active endurance exercise participants. The B's and C are the water-soluble vitamins.   The B's include:

B1   Thiamin   B5   Pantothenic Acid
B2   Riboflavin   B6   Pyridoxine
B3   Niacin   B12 Cobalamine

The B vitamins serve as the functioning part of coenzymes in energy cycles. Extreme aerobic athletes, vegetarians, and the elderly need extra vitamin B12. (Clementz, 1990). It is the only vitamin that contains a mineral. It contains cobalt. Higher plants like fruits and many vegetables do not contain B12. It is manufactured by the beneficial bacteria in our intestines, but much of the vitamin does not make it into our blood. We need them to help digest our food properly and even to survive. We are full of intestinal flora, beneficial microorganisms in our intestines. They are part of us. We are one symbiotic multi-organism, including our mitochondria.

Vitamin B5, pantothenic acid, becomes part of enzyme activity for carbohydrate utilization and hormone creation. It also protects muscle tissues, nervous tissuies and hemoglobin. An average diet includes less than 20 mg of B5 per day, but vigorous regular exercise requires up to ten times that amount. The big workhorse among nutrients is vitamin B6 which releases other nutrients and energy from food (Leklem, 1994). B6 transfers amino groups to other amino acids to synthesize new amino acids. It has other critical functions too like conversion of tryptophan into a chemical brain messenger, serotonin. Higher protein intake requires a higher vitamin B6 intake of about ten times the recommended daily allowance for inactive adults. B6, B1 and B2 are needed in similar quantities. B1 and B2 should be ingested in quantities proportional to carbohydrate intake since they help release energy. B3 —niacin— participates in sugar and lipid metabolism. The RDA of B3 is about 10-13 times the RDA's for B1, B2 and B6. The B vitamins, like vitamin C, are water-soluble so if you consume more than is needed, the excess is quickly excreted.

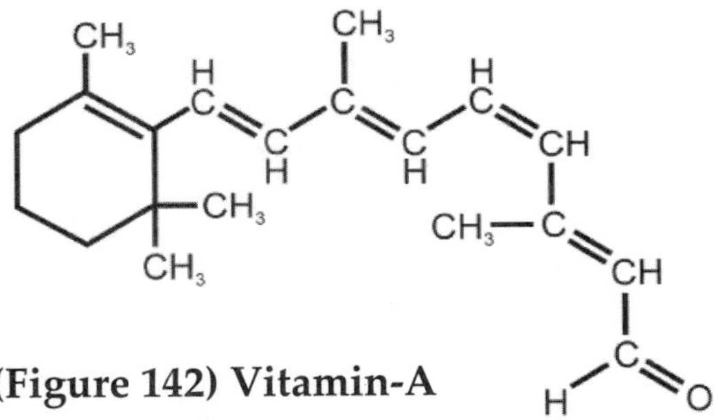

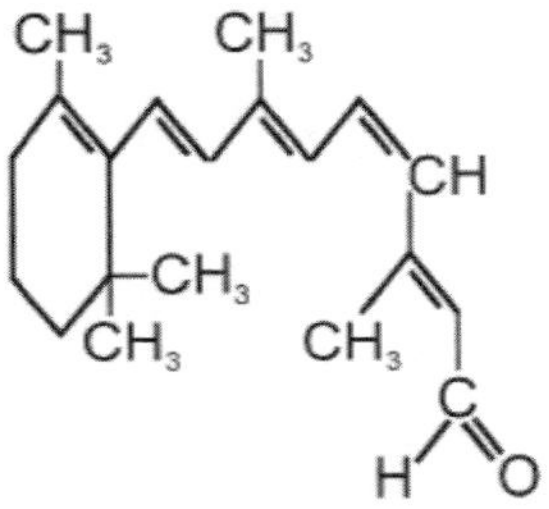

(Figure 143)

Retinol

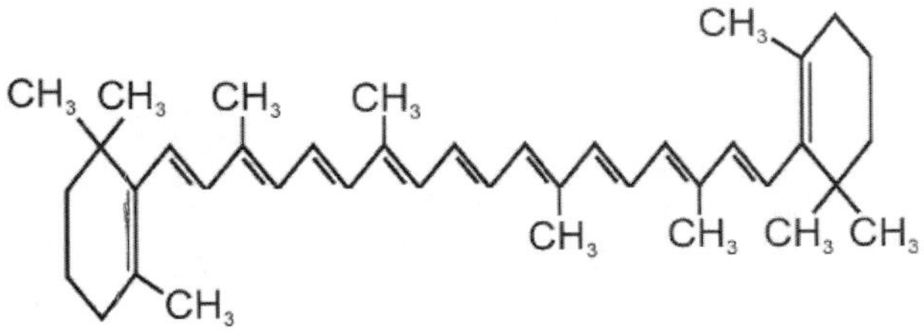

(Figure 144)

Beta carotene

(Figure 142) Vitamin-A (retinol derivative)

The Vitamin B Complex　(Figure 145)

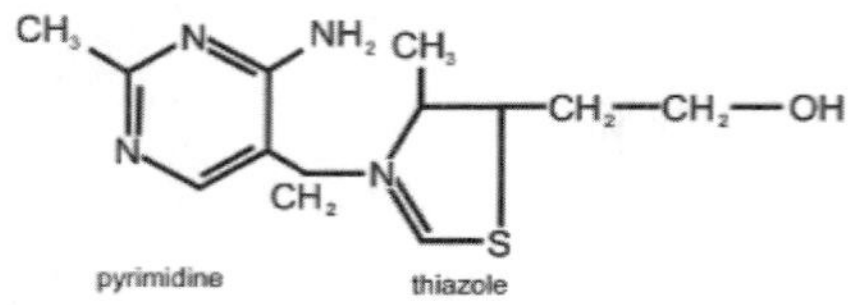

Vitamin–B1 (Thiamin)

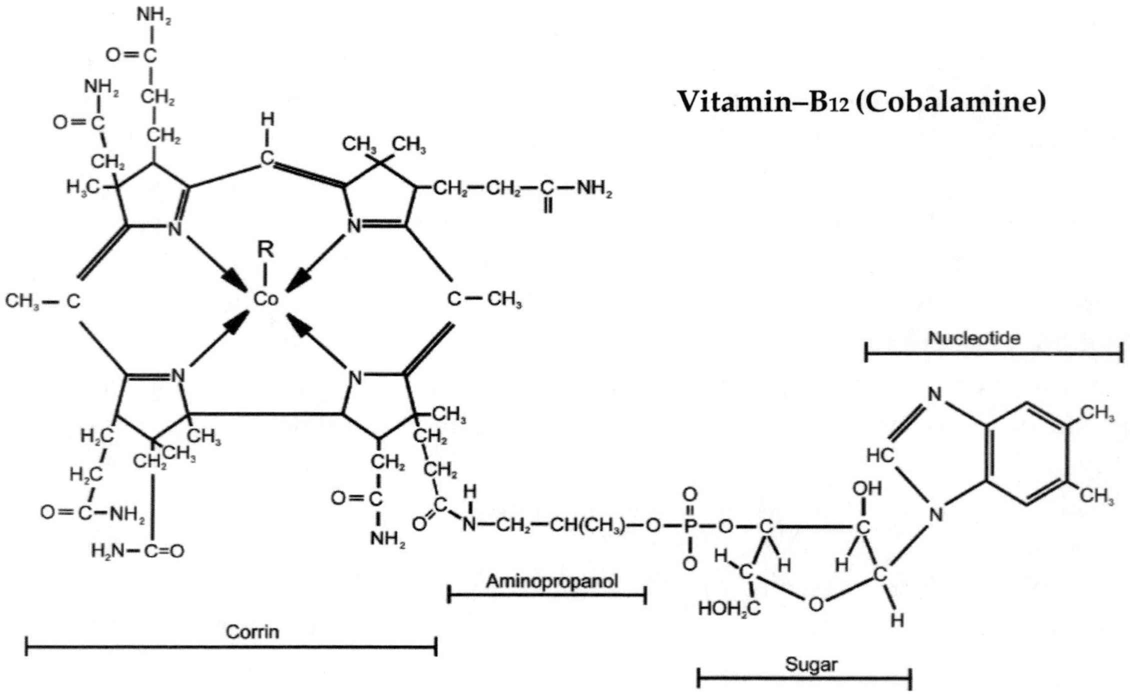

pyrimidine　　thiazole

nitric acid

nicotinamide

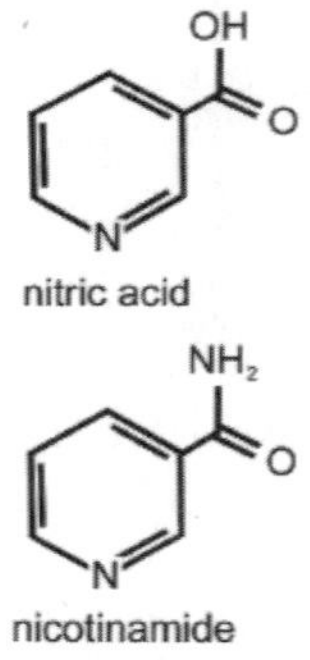

Vitamin–B3 (Niacin)

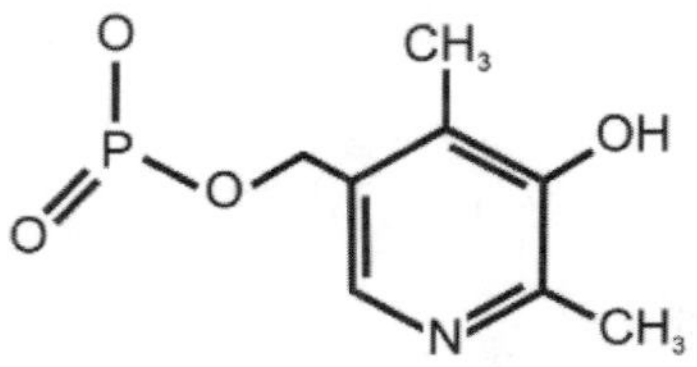

Vitamin–B6 (Pyridoxine)

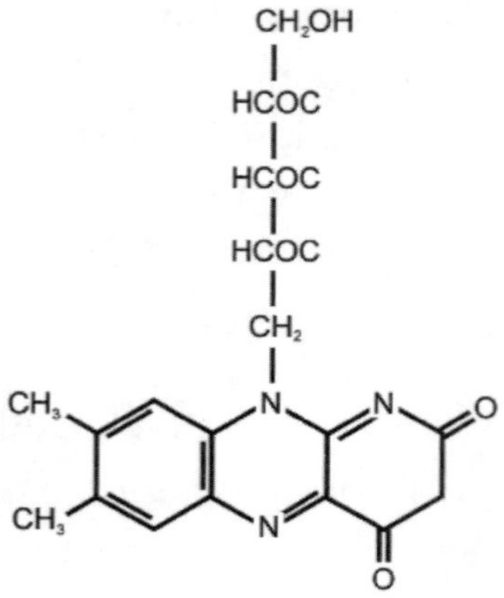

Vitamin–B12 (Cobalamine)

Corrin

Aminopropanol

Sugar

Nucleotide

Vitamin–B2 (Riboflavin)

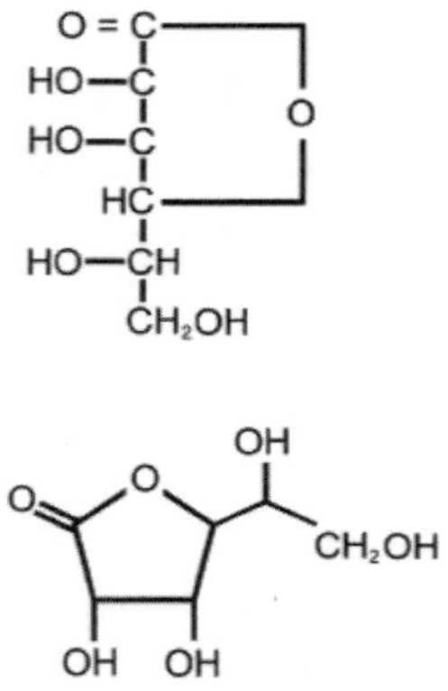

(Figure 146) Vitamin C (Ascorbic acid)

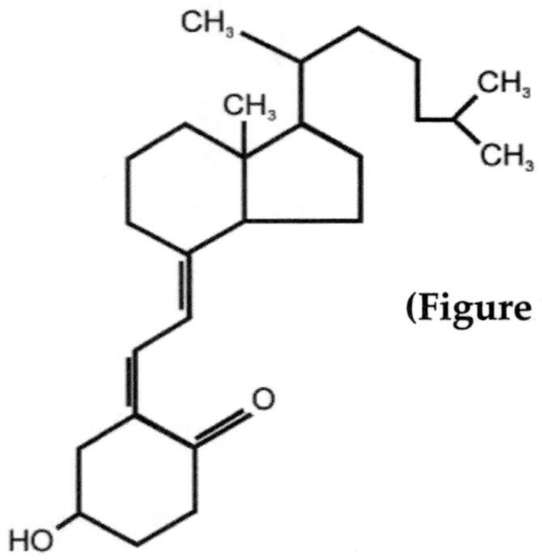

(Figure 147) Vitamin D

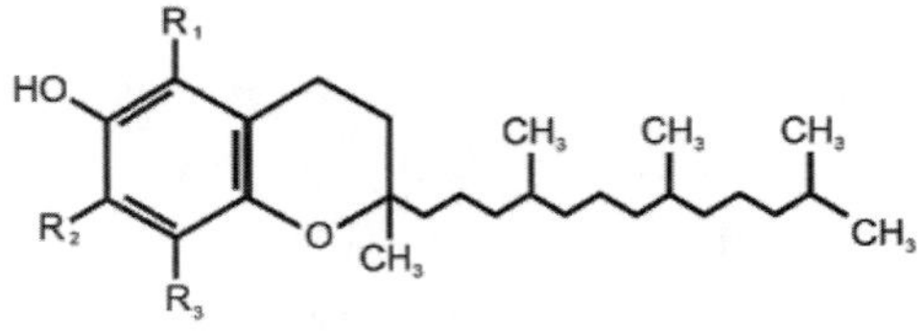

(Figure 148) Vitamin E

Breathing, digestion, growth, blood coagulation, reproduction, they all require enzymes and there are thousands made in the human body. An enzyme shortage caused by stress, illness, chemotherapy, aging, or a habit of eating dead foods void of functional enzymes requires us to get them from outside sources. Enzymes break apart specific molecules when needed for metabolism. They work with small coenzymes as a team (Figure 149).

Dead food refers to food with enzymes destroyed by microwave radiation, food processing or lengthy storage. Inadequate digestive enzymes result in poor digestion similar to the results of improper food combining. Enzymes fight destructive free radicals. Some illnesses indicate an enzyme shortage. Commonly used enzyme additives come from papaya, pineapple, barley malt, and figs. Mixtures of enzymes are more effective than individual enzymes in diet therapy. Enzyme categories are:

hydrolases, isomerases, ligases, lyases, oxidoreductases, and

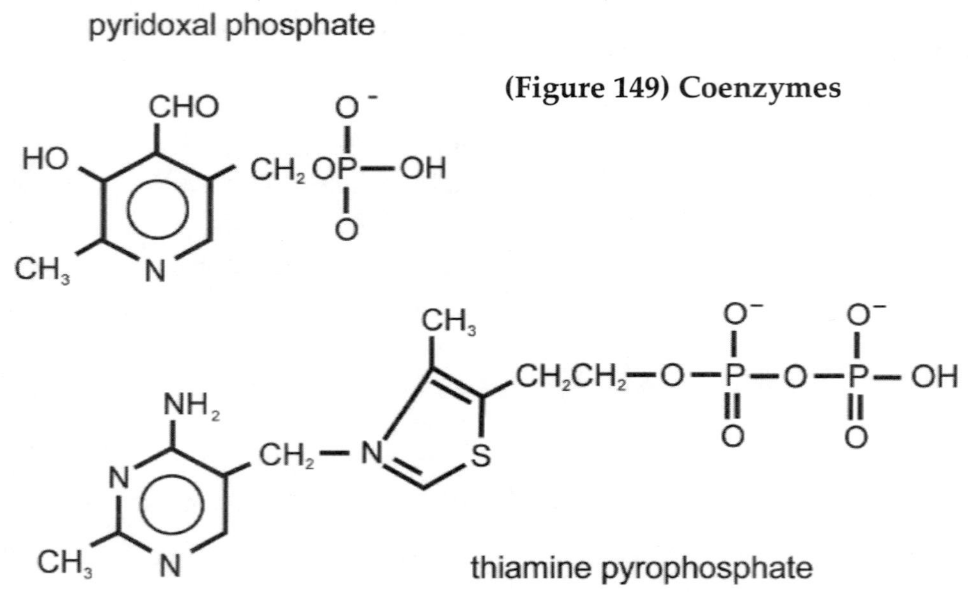

food into it's constituent parts during digestion. Taking supplemental enzymes is prudent.

radicals, ginseng to reduce stress and increase vitality, gotu kola to increase endurance, turmeric as an anti-inflammatory, garlic to fight infection, and ginger to energize, just to name a few. There are books on herbalism at health food stores.

(Figure 149) Coenzymes

pyridoxal phosphate

thiamine pyrophosphate

transferases. Each catogory includes hundreds of enzymes normally made in our bodies for catalyzing chemical reactions, transferring chemical groups from one molecule to another, moving a chemical group to a different part of a molecule, assistance in bonding together separate molecules, and for breaking down of

The investigation into herbs is worth an investment of time. Standardized herbal supplements in conservative small quantities not only provide immune strength but also stimulation, homeostasis, and vitality for the needs of extreme activities like aquatic power aerobics and aquatic anaerobic exercise. Some examples include ginko as a scavenger of free

Be very careful when considering steroid hormone sports nutrition products. Better yet, don't consider them at all. Prostate health is at risk as well as female reproductive health. Untested products with no clinical history are unsafe until proven otherwise. Experimenting with mixtures of new sports-enhancing products is also unwise and a risk to good health. The most effective results from an aquatic exercise program occur when you know your nutritional needs and establish healthy eating habits.

The most important dietary improvements to general health are the elimination of harmful substances and proper food combining. Dietary improvements that most affect aquatic endurance are adequate hydration and healthy fuel sources.

Chapter 9
Kealawai
(The Path of Water)

This Chapter is different. It is an open door with no literary rules so you can expect some interesting divergence from the subject.

The islands of Hawaii are the very tops of huge volcanoes in the middle of earth's largest ocean. In the language of the island we follow the path of water, "kealawai." Prepare for a wild canoe ride, from the birth of water, through its history, into a structural molecular analysis. We will meet Neanderthals at the Rock of Gibraltar, meet wolves in the Alaska wilderness, and dive out of the canoe into hot springs with Native American shamans into deeper realities than you may have experienced ever before.

In the Beginnings

Where to start is not a place or a time. As humans, most of us feel limited in our comprehension of the beginnings of things. We ask why, when, how? Truth is ever-present and knowledge can be infinite. To some it is unacceptable for a story not to have a beginning or an end. The discomfort arises from the insecurity of not knowing. We want to know. That is what makes us distinctively human. We want to know the past, explain the present, and predict the future.

The past we want to know now is, "Where did water come from?" It sounds like a child's question.

Going to the beginning, the emergence of water's highly polar constituents was preceded by unorganized matter, radiation fields, and initiated by a singularity of infinite density that modern theoretical physicists call supersymmetry. All this was preceded by potential. There was the potential for a hydrogen-based universe to come into existence and the potential for oxygen to develop from the subatomic particles of hydrogen. So it did. Eventually potential becomes manifest. Potential precedes everything. Theoretically, expansion of unorganized, initial radiation fields, was quite sudden, in and from every direction and away from every point in space, not from a central source. Waves of oppositely charged subatomic particles are thought to have preceded light and gravity. Random protons and electrons captured each other to form neutrons. The passage of time and a lengthy reduction in heat produced condensations of swirling galaxies, massive dark matter, and stars (Hawking, 1990).

Electrons travel as waves in atomic orbits at nearly the velocity of light, approximately186,000 miles per second. That is over 670 million miles per hour (1.08 billion km/h, 300,000 km/s). The theory of physicist Carl Segor, www.orbits.00space.com in a paper dated November 2, 1999, is that mass in today's universe is accelerating while the speed of light has been decelerating over time. He states that gravity is the result of a decline in the speed of light.

All is still in motion, spinning, rotating, and precipitating from gasses to liquids and eventually into some solids. The masses generally keep moving away from each other, yet there are pairs of attractions on a galactic scale. Stars sometimes have partner stars. Galaxies dwell in pairs. Could there be another universe? Don't be confused. The best of nature is reborn out of chaos.

In astrophysics, all known natural elements are formed from the nuclear reactions on stars, reactions that change hydrogen to helium as a more stable structure for further development of heavier elements like oxygen. In space, where radiation rules, carbonaceous molecules that permeated the solar system easily formed from our sun's reactions and became the source of Earth's carbon. Our planet seems to be a spheroid of recycled space debris. Our star, the sun, is the birthplace of water's atoms just as supersymmetry is the birthplace of the stars.

I have seen the solar wind

from the latitude of the Arctic Circle, looking straight up at the winter sky. Ft. Yukon was the place and infinity was the background. It started as a small, faint ripple of light that grew to curtaining waves of iridescent colors moving at incredible speed while expanding slowly to the entire horizon, filling the night sky with a silent and unforgettable light show. Wearing many layers of clothes, I looked out from the fur that surrounded the tightened opening of my parka hood. You might say that the sight took my breath away but, in reality, the vapors of my breath froze onto my eyebrows and to the protecting fur. The sight of the Aurora Borealis was too spectacular for me to move any more than in a small circle in the snow to take in the full view of the sky.

>–((((O>   >–((((O>   >–((((O>

The scientific consensus is that the sun is half gone and dying, that all life in this solar system is mortal. According to biologists, half of the long existence of our planet was devoted to the waiting game, waiting for conditions to change so that primitive molecules could organize into primordial life. The environment had to cool down and water was needed for life to begin.

We now arrive on the early planet Earth in this story, in a solar system traveling a half million mph around the galaxie, a planet that had a long wait for water in the liquid form and for life. Geologically, radiation of the interior Earth sent heat and gasses up to the surface from a molten mantle that never did completely solidify. Water vapor, nitrogen, carbon dioxide, sulfur dioxide, sulfurous gasses, and rare gasses were all erupting, adding to the volume of the atmosphere. Minute quantities of volatile nebular gasses clung to surface dust.

Where is water? There is water throughout the cosmos, according to astronomers. Some planets are nothing more than solid water, ice.

There was water before the Earth condensed from exploding solar gasses. You could say that water was already in the soup. It was buried in the solid material. Out of present day volcanoes come water vapor, carbon dioxide, and nitrogen, among other materials. Surprisingly there are even small amounts of methane and ammonia in volcanic gasses. The early Earth tells its story in these eruptions.

Unlike other planets and moons, Earth was so rich in oxygen that some of the iron bonded to it in silicates, remaining on the surface mantle. The core is iron and nickel. Corrosive gasses from volcanoes combined with water to produce strong acids, sulfuric and hydrochloric. Heavy atmospheric pressure from other gasses enabled the accumulation of a high volume of water vapor which condensed rapidly into liquid to form the vast ocean that covered the solid mantle. Dissolved calcium in the water bonded with carbonates into true limestone. This is a chemical sediment, calcite, formed when decreased carbon dioxide reduced the amount of calcite that could remain in solution (the limestone later formed from organisms is an organic sediment). The acidic water eroded volcanic minerals and became salty. In areas where the water was alkaline, calcium and magnesium precipitated forming dolomite that started to absorb carbon dioxide. For millions of years, water continued to increase until the Earth was totally covered with it and the hydrosphere was created (Zumberge, 1963).

The air was high in nitrogen and low in carbon dioxide. There was no free oxygen in the air. How did it arrive? Out of the billions of years covered on these few pages, oxygen shows up in abundance only in the last half a billion years and very slowly before that. The conclusion is that terrestrial life began as plants. During photosynthesis they released the oxygen that began to infiltrate the atmosphere.

Before terrestrial life, when the Earth was covered with water, two long molecular chains bonded together with links of amino acids into the shape of a helical spiral called deoxyribonucleic acid or DNA (Figure 62). In the right conditions, suspended in water, it was able to duplicate itself. The DNA, in the shape of closed circles, led to the first unicellular bacteria. DNA helical spirals in the shape of long chains became larger multicellular plant beings three and a half billion years ago, creating organic sediment limestone. The first multi-cellular animal, an arthropod trilobite, appeared only six hundred million years ago. You can see that it took considerable time to get to that point because it took that long for the air to be sufficiently oxygenated for respiration by cellular mitochondria. Reptiles were born. Many became extinct. Mammals finally appeared only one hundred million years ago. Primates and then man, the newcomer, appeared several million years ago, perhaps more. On the Discovery Channel program "Human Evolution," July 2003, it was estimated that all primates are expected to become extinct five million years from now. Our moment in time is brief. Water is the survivor, the continuum.

We are ready to look more closely at water. How long does a molecule of water take to complete the Earth's water cycle? This could be uncommon knowledge to many. Follow that drop of rain or the dripping water as you exit the pool or the hot springs. In the atmosphere, that drop of water with the mini-waves on its surface stays an average of 11 days. On a continent, water that is not confined in underground caverns stays 100 years. In the ocean, the reservoir of our hydrosphere, water remains on average for 40,000 years. Evaporation from the sun removes 208 cubic miles of water from the oceans each day (Ball, 1999).There appear to be large uncertainties in calculating the hydrological cycle. Unesco.org estimates are 2500 yrs in oceans, 1400 yrs as groundwater, 8 days in the atmosphere and only several hours as biological water.

My view is that water came from the broken supersymmetry when the cosmos cooled enough for radiation to reveal itself as having what I call dynamo mass. This is a quality of change with so much force behind it

that electrically charged particles of energy organized themselves into clear identities whose variations sought balanced combinations, attracting opposite polarities. The organizing particles led to an escalation in subatomic construction, then to multiples of the first complete atom, and then to the coming opportunities for complex combinations of atoms. Initially hydrogen waited as a pair of atoms and eventually parted from the association of its bonded twin to become available for chemical reactions. It could have been the nature of the universe from the beginning, to change in order to have the opportunity to explore other possibilities in the vast arsenal of "potential." This may be the basic law of nature: that change through infinity guarantees progress, in other words there is no limit to the quantity of failure leading to a successful alteration in quality. So, as I see it, hydrogen reached out with an attractive force of instability for a big partner with an opposite electric quality, one in the same condition of need for neutrality, different than that

of a twin. Hydrogen and oxygen, one of the first pairs of elements to meet in highly attractive polarity, became a stable compound molecule. Water has been around ever since that glorious association.

Studying water more closely, the atoms of hydrogen and oxygen bond through their orbital electrons. Two atoms of hydrogen and one atom of oxygen bond in a polar equilibrium. Nuclear stability is an endowment of neutrons that have the freedom to grow in number beyond that of the protons that are forced to cohabitate by the neutron's binding and insulating properties. Neutrons keep protons from repulsing each other. This quantum electromechanics reveals that one element can have different masses due to the different numbers of neutrons in the various forms of the element, while still maintaining the same chemical properties. These variations are isotopes. Hydrogen and oxygen both have isotopes.

The Water Molecule

Unlike what you may have learned in high school chemistry, a water molecule is not in the shape of a 'V.' You can construct a model of the water molecule to help visualize its form. The materials needed are a sheet of paper, a pencil, a ruler and adhesive tape. Draw a large equilateral triangle on the paper. Draw another triangle inside the first one so that the vertices join the center of each side of the outer equilateral triangle (Figure 151A). Cut out the large triangle and fold on the lines of the smaller triangle, bringing the vertices of the large triangle together into one point. Tape this shape together. It is a tetrahedron, the true shape of a water molecule. In the very center of the water molecule is oxygen. Two of the outer corners are hydrogen atoms and the other two corners are lone pairs of electrons. This tetrahedron shape enables all four peripheral entities to be as far away from each other as possible.

Now we will suppose that the paper is somewhat elastic. The two lone pairs of electrons have stronger charges and need to be separated from one another as if each had intolerable body odor. Identical polarities repel each other just as opposite polarities attract. The isolated pairs of electrons position themselves accordingly so that their repelling nature causes the hydrogen atoms to move slightly closer together at an angle of 104.5 degrees (Figure 153) instead of the 109.5 degree angle of a perfect tetrahedron.

Four degrees might not seem important. After all, it is just a slightly smaller angle. What difference does it really make? But wait! We will stop the canoe for a moment and take a closer look at the water still.

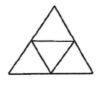

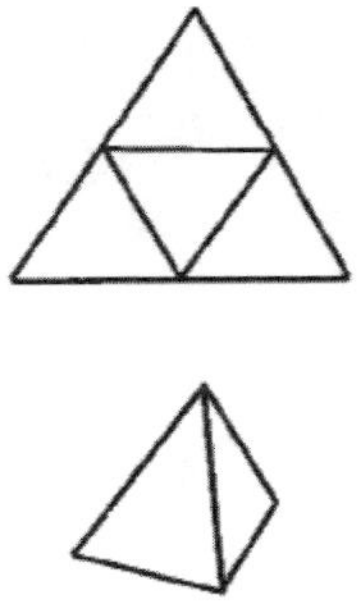

(Figure 151A)
Tetrahedron

(Figure 151B)

Representations of a water molecule from symbolic to realistic

H_2O HOH H   H
                    O

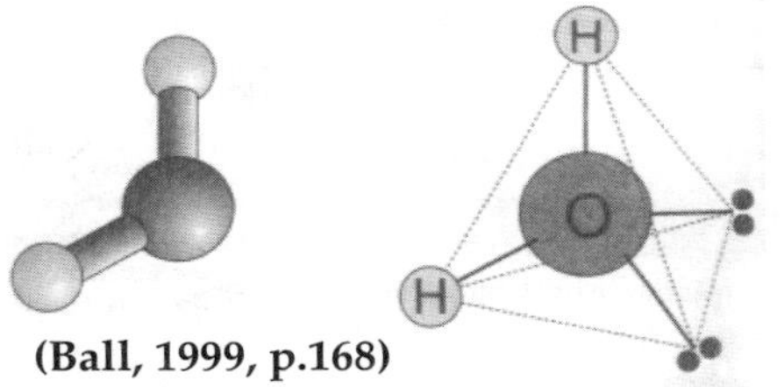

(Ball, 1999, p.168)

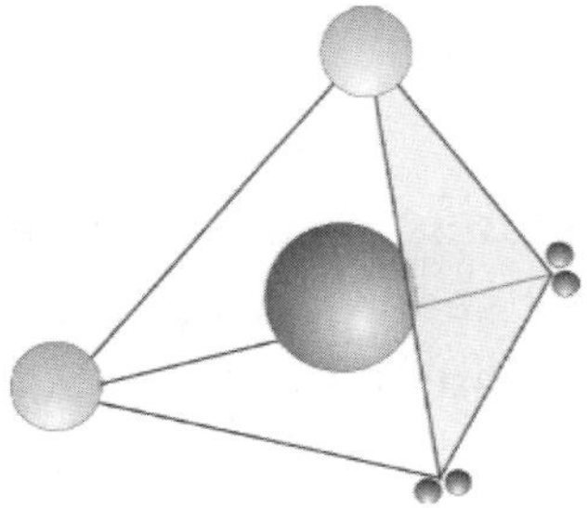

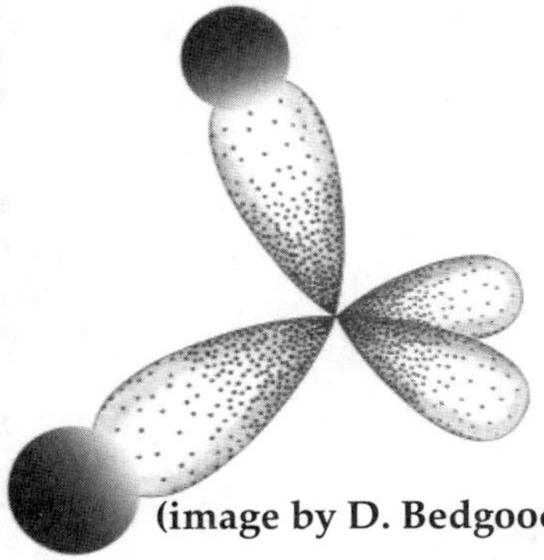

(image by D. Bedgood)

(Figure 152) Realistic Stationary Electron Waves in a Water Molecule

Dot concentration represents relative probabilities of electron location.

spherical electron wave for hydrogen atom with central nucleus

a 3D pedal or tear drop shaped electron wave for oxygen atom

Electron bonding area where orbits are shared and attracted simultaneously by both nuclei of oxygen and hydrogen

orbital waves for electron pairs, with opposite spin

oxygen nucleus

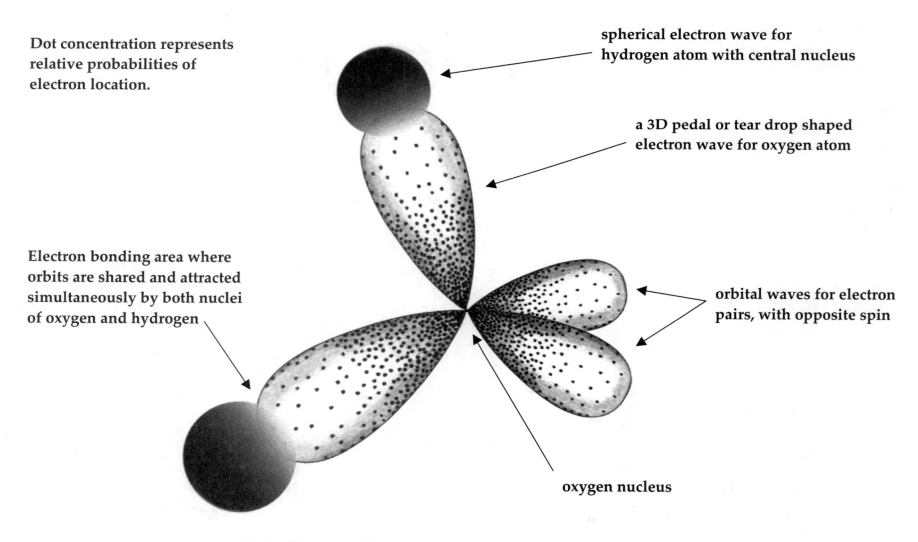

A water molecule undergoes constant rapidly changing distortions. By itself, a water molecule spins like a top at a rate of a million billion turns in one second (Salem, 1987). Electrons are wave functions because they have wave properties, stationary peaks and troughs. The diameter of an oxygen atom is 100,000 times larger than its nucleus. The electron waves of oxygen reach out in long, conical, pedal-like shapes (Figure 152). In a water molecule, the two lone pairs of electrons are satisfied because each electron is spinning in an opposite direction from its partner. But the two electron waves at the other two corners of the tetrahedron are single electrons seeking a partner with an opposite spin and they are found in the two hydrogen atoms. The shape of the single electron wave in hydrogen is spherical. The electron waves of oxygen and hydrogen overlap, allowing them to share electrons in their orbits as they are simultaneously attracted by both nuclei.

When water molecules are not isolated, this transparent liquid has a random, dynamic and disorderly network of hydrogen bonds that connect all the water molecules together, a bonding that spans the volume of all the oceans in the world, including all the rivers that drain the land and empty into the oceans. No other liquid has this ability to be hydrogen-bonded throughout its entire volume (Ball, 1999). Now that's one big, happy family of molecules, with each one holding the hands of four others.

In most other liquids, repulsive forces arrange the structure of the molecules (and repulsive forces arrange the structure *within* a water molecule) but it is the attracting forces of the hydrogen bonds that arrange the liquid water molecules with respect to other water molecules. The forces create orientation preferences. Like King Kamehameha sitting on his throne on Hawaii's ancient Big Island, the oxygen atom sits at the core of the tetrahedron network of bonds with his two advisors in two of the four corners and two pairs of military subordinates that don't get along in the other two corners. As it is in the imperfect tetrahedron shape of a water molecule, the two corners that contain hydrogen (the King's advisors) are closer together than the electron pairs (the military subordinates) in the other two corners. The hydrogen atoms also reach out away from their oxygen to establish bonds with other oxygen atoms in nearby tetrahedrons, forming ionic bonds throughout the body of water that connect all the molecules in the shape of tetrahedrons with each other, like the King's advisors establishing bonds with other Kings creating a unity across the entire culture.

(Figure 153)

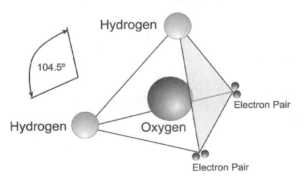

WATER MOLECULE
Showing tetrahedron structure and HOH angle.

Hydrogen

104.5°

Hydrogen   Oxygen

Electron Pair

Electron Pair

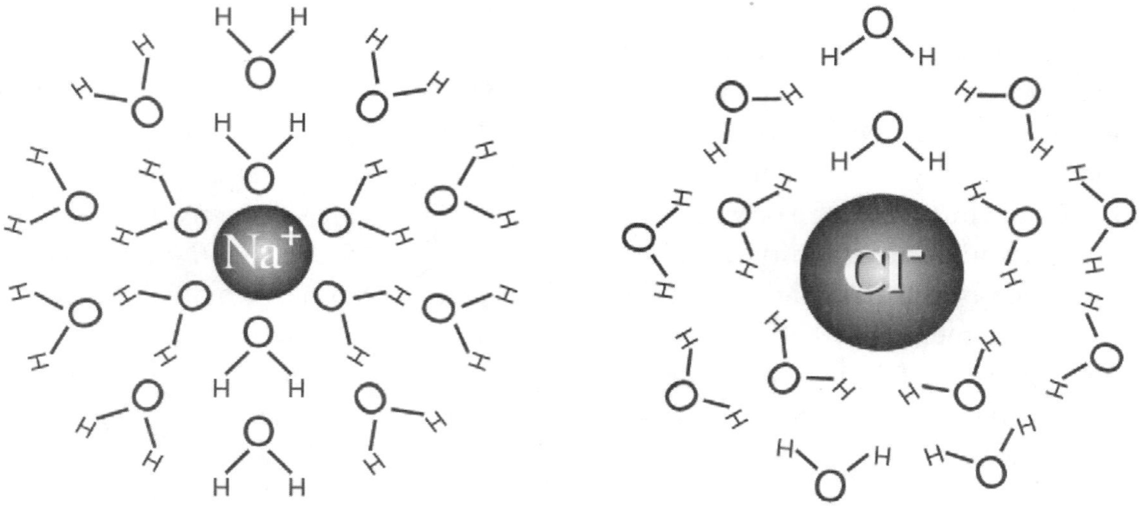

(Figure 154) The Effect of Ions on Water Molecules

Water molecules can become quickly organized as a solute when ions like sodium and chloride are introduced (Figure 154). The analogy here would be an army surrounding or imprisoning its enemy, or it could be compared to an elite guard protecting royalty. Opposite polarities attract and

re-orient the water molecules as shown in the illustration of a salt water solution, H+ to Cl⁻ and O⁻ to NA+.

The water molecules in ice have an arrangement with large voids. In fact, the structure of ice crystal molecules takes up more space than the liquid structure because in the liquid, random molecules fill the spaces to a

higher density. So that is why water expands in volume when it changes state from a liquid to a solid.

Water crystals are a natural work of beautiful art. There are different perspectives on the origin of their geometric forms. René Descartes (1596-1650), French physicist, physiologist, mathematician and one of the most important philosophers in the past few centuries, stated that these phenomena of matter are merely a series of vortexes in space. Space or air at the time was referred to as the ether. Thomas Hobbs, 1588-1679, theorized that "all things have but one univeral cause which is motion" (Calkins, 1948). Physicist Dewey B. Larson is confident in his hypothesis that physical theory explaining crystalline geometric growth or any other physical reality or physical theory is based on a universe of motion. He states that these physical phenomena are not just caused by motion but that motion is the sole constituent of the physical universe (Larson, 1979). Larson summarizes theoretical physics into four types of theories.

Three are based on uncertainty: the relativity, kinetic, and nuclear theories. The fourth is reciprocal which is fully integrated. Larson describes his theory as reciprocal: V=S/T, or "velocity equals space divided by time." One doesn't exist without the other. There are no assumptions and no uncertainty, only a numerator and a denominator as two reciprocal aspects of motion — space and time only occur in association as motion. In the Larson hypothesis, all physical realities are manifestations of motion or a combination of motions such as electric charge, gravitation, radiation, and all wave phenomena. Albert Einstein is known for his relativity theory, a mathematical fourth dimension of space-time, generally accepted by physicists worldwide because mathematically it is successful. But mathematical agreement is no guarantee of conceptual validity. There are defects in the relativity theory due to invalid assertions (Larson, 1979).

There is another theoretical perspective shown in Chapter 1, p. 84 in this wide spectrum of hypotheses. It associates philosophical meanings and intent in the form of tangible, human communication of affect and consciousness as an influence on water crystal structure. See Emoto(2002). Masura Emoto, who expresses this idea, has an under- graduate degree in International Relations and a background in alternative medicines. Mr. Emoto founded a company that photographs crystals made from distilled water on a petri dish at one moment during their growth and has published the photographs in his books, although their dendrites are much shorter than water ice crystals found in nature. His attractive books are sparkling with crystals. The interepretations appear to be unscientific but as we wait for confirmation and repeatability on his results we can certainly admire the beauty of water crystals.

Another perspective is that ice crystals in snowflakes form in an enormous variety of hexagonal dendritic geometries by random

chance, more than any other known substance.

Ambient temperature during formation, humidity, and unstable facet surface irregularities are the main influences on water crystal growth patterns. Philip Ball PhD, who arrives at this conclusion (1999), is a consulting editor for Nature Magazine with a degree in Chemistry from Oxford and a PhD in Physics from the University of Bristol. He has authored several other scientific books including *The Self Made Tapestry: Pattern Formation in Nature.*

According to Dr. Ball, the slightly off-balanced angle of water's tetrahedral molecular shape gives it an occasional imperfection resuling in a fragmented bond in 1 out of 500,000,000 molecules. The hydrogen bonds can rearrange themselves to relocate the broken bond, creating the ability to move any attached ions from place to place. That is enough to have major implications in chemistry. Water's uniqueness includes the ability to provide hydrogen ions or hydroxide ions and act either as an acid or an alkali. That rare fragmented bond acts like a superhighway for ion movement and electrical conduction.

Subtle, off-balance adaptations in nature, demonstrated by a simple water molecule, have been the key to the formation of the universe and to subsequent evolutionary processes. Imperfections are opportunities to alter direction. The imperfect tetrahedron demonstrates that the only survivable universe is one where destiny is not immune to change.

What are we looking at in a drop of water? It is mostly empty space just as we are. If a proton in a hydrogen atom were the size of a pinhead, the proton and the electron would be ten miles apart. Consider the power of the electric charges that keep them in an invisible association over that relatively phenomenal distance. The electrons of oxygen spin in several orbits at various distances from the nucleus. You can visualize that most everything is empty space and waves of energy. We are looking mainly at emptiness. That heavy iron shotput that you pick up, well, it isn't much more than nothing. It is no wonder that cosmic rays from space travel right through our bodies, non-stop through the earth and out the other side. Water did not come from some magical process on the Earth. It did not come from the Earth. From what I have learned and concluded, water came *with* the Earth. Water indeed is older than the rocks. Have a drink. It's older than you think, as we exercise in its antiquity. Our ancient water molecules are older than the Earth itself.

Aquatic Adaptations

Water is our protector, our feeder, and our mother, the very being in our membranes which contains us. The human fetus is floating, bathed in water, immersed in its amniotic fluid. The vertebrate brain and spinal cord are suspended in a flow of cerebrospinal fluid. Water carries nutrients in and toxins out of our cells. Cells are aquatic containers for nuclei and organelles to function. We live entirely in a self-contained aquatic environment surrounded by skin. Water enters. Water exits. It moves throughout the cosmos. We move our bodies, human "swimming pools," to dwell on the land. All living plants and animal share this commonality. Dehydration signifies dormancy, death, a loss of interstitial transport or a change away from life.

One of the first major challenges for life was to be able to make its own fuel for energy. Chlorophyll and bright sunlight found a way and in the process that yielded the by-product, free oxygen, pairs of oxygen atoms were turned loose in an ocean of water. Animal life was only inevitable after photosynthesizing chlorophyll released oxygen for billions of years and after unicellular beings found a way to extract free oxygen from the water. Finally multicellular animals slowly emerged in more recent times including the trilobites, then on to fish. Our earliest heritage is aquatic.

The next major adaptation took place after rising masses of tectonic plates, the earth builders, formed land amidst the ocean of water. It was the opportunity to adapt to the utilization of oxygen derived from the atmosphere using lungs, foreign from the aquatic origins of life. After multitudes of species failures, amphibians crawled up onto the land from the warm waters. Failures and extinctions continued for millions of years but there were always some successes, enough for progress and adaptation to environmental changes and progress. As land dwellers and a unique species of mammals and primates we are only one of the very

few survivors. To comprehend this with our own intellect is an understanding that we alone possess.

Life is an aquatic phenomenon. Water is our home. What makes us distinctively human is aquatic. To explain my hypothesis, make a list of interesting human qualities such as: sensory iconic and echoic memory, short term memory, closure, episodic and semantic long term memory; higher metabolic functions; higher brain systems, functions, and structures like the complexities within our hyppocampus, hypothalamus, and amygdala; problem solving; our genetic blueprint; language; child pretend play leading to adult creativity; learning capacity; cognition including knowledge and judgment; communication, speculation, future prediction. Now consider them as a whole being and visualize a body of water surrounded by a membrane that contains all those items on your list. Inside the bubble are smaller compartments of water surrounded by freely moving water. There are substances and molecular structures within the water that give it

organized and distinctively differentiated properties in the aquatic compartments. All these qualities originate in this bubble, some as electrical discharges voluntarily controlled, or responses and impulses created by external stimuli activating synapses that modulate behavior. Communication via chemical neurotransmitters across a synapse to receptors increases the dendrite network and new protein production to establish the complexities of memory and creativity. All this and more are all in our aquatic container.

*W*ater viscosity in a boundless sea, how can its resistance against a moving object be measured? This question emerged one early frosty morning in the mountains of North Carolina on the Cherokee Indian Reservation in the mid 1980's. I was living in an open barn in the Appalachian Mountains with 10,000 Aquatoners. The thunder of horses' hooves was the early morning alarm clock that woke me. My telephone line was strung along the frosty tall weeds by the fence line that flanked the narrow dirt road down the steep hill to the barn. A call to Dr. James Liburdy at the Clemson University, Chair of the School of Engineering's Department of Fluid Mechanics, was the start of a lesson in the hydrodynamics of the Aquatoner ☎.

My question was: how can a physical therapist know the force being exerted in water by a patient using the adjustable resistance area of an Aquatoner? What I had in mind was to develop a handheld, computerized, digital timer/calculator that collected and graphed data throughout the course of a patient's entire rehabilitation and throughout one session in a therapy pool. The intent was to create a means for physical therapists to measure and record every resistive movement in the pool using the Aquatoner. There was a need in clinics for accurate progress documentation in aquatic sessions to facilitate insurance reimbursement. Dr. Liburdy's department needed a research grant and a large container to

answer the question. I drove fifty beautiful miles to the Granger farm supply store in Asheville and purchased a galvanized cattle watering trough, eight feet long, two feet wide, and three feet high. Dr. Liburdy needed it to be five feet (1.5m) high. Strapping it to the top of my Subaru, I hauled it to a welder who added two feet of aluminum to the height, then drove south to Clemson for the delivery (Fig. 155). Dr. Liburdy and his graduate students carried out the research measuring force versus time and measuring energy dissipation rates for various oscillation amplitudes, frequencies. and effective diameters. You will find the equations in Chapter 11, *The Kinetics of Water*, and the results in the Appendix.

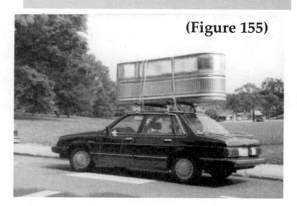

(Figure 155)

W*est of Hawaii*

in 18,000' deep Pacific turbulence, swimming from an escort boat to replace a paddler during a long-distance outrigger canoe race, I realized that water has no boundaries. Down in the valley, between the wave giants, was a remote and isolated underworld of it's own. Up on top of a crest, multiple rainbows to the east, a feeling of infinite freedom prevailed.   Beyond description was the blue blackness opposed by the bright skylight. This was a magical moment.

>-(((((O>   >-(((((O>   >-(((((O>

Shamans and Springs

Springs attract human habitation. Hot springs, and spring-fed limestone sinkholes that are not fed with hot water but are a collection of rainfall percolated into aquifers, have been used for healing practices for much of human history and are used for healing purposes throughout the world today. Cold springs bubble up from underground rivers and permeable aquifers in porous limestone cavities and tunnels that are essentially the ground water reservoir in a zone of saturation. Originating as rain, the water accumulates minerals during its infiltration down through the absorbent limestone. Limestone is primarily calcite, calcium carbonate. Impurities can be present like silicon dioxide in chert, magnesium carbonate in dolomite, and other combinations.

Another kind of spring is called a "perched" spring when ground water seepage occurs at a location where there is sandstone over shale. The permeable sandstone is a mixture of various sizes of sand grains and is very porous.The underlying layer of shale is impermeable compacted silt and clay. The spring is found where a slope exposes the contact point between the two layers. If there is no impermeable rock layer above the saturated stratum, the aquifer is unconfined. If the aquifer is capped with an impermeable layer, the

aquifer is confined and remains under pressure.

Filtration springs are mainly found in France, Germany, Great Britain, Eastern Europe, Korea and the Northeastern United States. They are rain-water percolations through higher altitude fractures in hard rock down to the source of heat near magma, sometimes over a mile deep. The water is heated 100°F (38°C) for every kilometer it descends as it leaches minerals from the rock formation (Altman, 2000). Pressure from heat expansion forces the water up fault lines. One cycle can take thousands of years.

Saratoga Springs in New York yields water from the melting of the Ontario Lobe of the Wisconsin ice cap, a Pleistocene Age glacier that existed for 70,000 years. A layer of shale prevents rainwater from mixing with the ancient mineral water trapped below it. The cool water at Saratoga is 55° F (13°C).

Hot Springs, Arkansas has 47 filtration springs yielding 1 million

gallons (3,800,000 liters) per day of highly mineralized water at 143°F (62°C). The water percolated down to a depth of 6,000 ft (1.8km). over 4,000 years ago. The system of hot springs across Europe extending from France to the Czech Republic is similar in geology to Hot Springs.

Primary springs are associated with volcanic activity where magma is closer to the Earth's surface. They are typically located in western United States, western Canada, Italy, Taiwan, Japan, and New Zealand. Super-heated water reservoirs under pressure are many miles below the volcanic rock. The water, containing antibacterial sulfur as hydrogen sulfide and sulfurated alkaline metals, rises through small fractures in the rock as steam and as it approaches the surface it cools to liquid water that is very hot, flowing constantly from these hot springs. The primary hot springs at Harbin Mountain in Northern California are above a dome of hot magma that is thirteen miles (21km) in diameter and 4 miles (6.4km) below the surface.

Florida's limestone aquifers produce one of the highest concentrations of cold springs in the world — over 350. For a reason unknown to science, there is a species of blind crayfish living in Florida's underground water caverns 100 years, five times the average lifespan of surface crayfish. Alligators are older than the dinosaurs. Was it the healthy water? Did Ponce de Leon really find the Fountain of Youth?

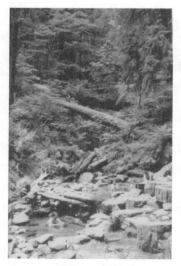

(Figure 156) Undeveloped Hot Spring in Oregon

There are thousands of hot springs worldwide, mostly at fault lines where tectonic plates meet. They are geothermal sites where, as was described earlier, water from precipitation enters the earth and descends to the hot mantle to be heated and then expanded up a nearby fault usually through small fractures in impermeable quartz or granite. The mineralized water has touched the earth's hot pulse.

In his interesting "Healing Springs – The Ultimate Guide to Taking the Waters," Nathaniel Altman cites the many names for springs in their locations. In Greece the thermal pools are called "ayiasma" or "sacred water." There are over 10,000 hot springs in Japan where they are called "onsen." Kyushu Island alone contains over 3800 primary hot springs with a combined flow of 9,200 gallons per minute. In Italy they are "terme." In Poland a hot springs site is a "Zdroj." In Germany the thermal baths are for "Kneipp cures" named after Sebastian Kneipp and the developed springs are "Kneipp Cure Towns." In Nepal they are "tatopani." In France healing springs are places of "thalasso therapy." In Belgium is the city of "Spa" where the term for their hot springs originated. "Bad Ragaz" aquatic therapy is named after the spa in Bad Ragaz, Switzerland where a hot springs is a "bad." There are thousands of medicinal waters in Eastern, Central, and Western Europe. Karlovy Vary in western Czech Republic is a spa with a concentration of over 130 springs that produce 180 tons (163,440 kg=163 metric tons) of mineral salts per year for commercial and medicinal use (Altman, 2000). Along the river at Budapest are 520 thermal and mineral springs known since ancient Roman times. The spas in Europe are operated under medical supervision. The Tuscany Provinces of Northern Italy are comparable to Northern California in their concentration of thermal springs.

Classification of a spring as "mineral" requires a concentration of various minerals in the water of at least 1,000 mg/kg (Fabiani, 1996). Most springs are classified further as thermal, bicarbonate, sulfate, sulfite, chloride, sulfur, iron, or lithium. A sulfate spring, for example, contains over 1,000 mg/kg of a sulfate of calcium,

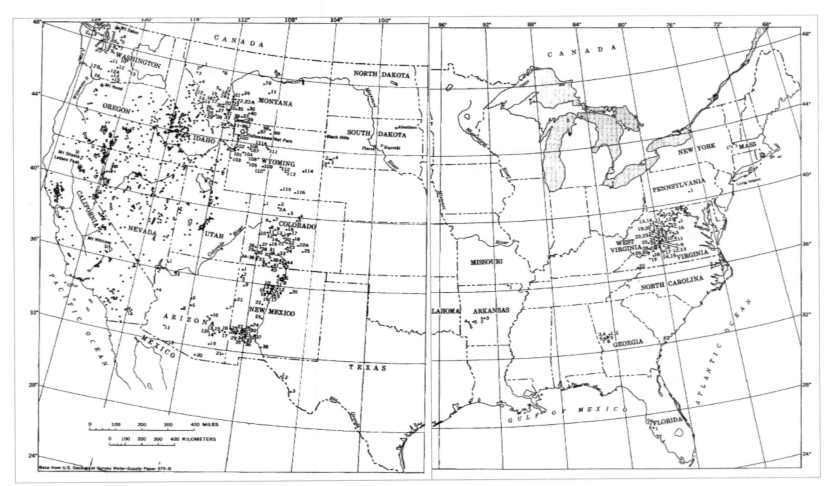

(Figure 157)
Hot Springs in the U.S.

sodium, or magnesium. Springs are thermal when they are over 77° F (25°C). Most hot springs are over 100° F (38°C).

Springs are considered medicinal when they are either hot or cold, when they contain sulfur as alkaline hydrogen sulfide that raises the pH or when they contain acidic hydrogen sulfate that lowers the pH. Chloride and sulfate ions are stimulating. Medical indications are also used today to classify mineral water at natural springs. For example: anticatarrhal mineral water contains hydrogen sodium sulfide. Reconstituent mineral water contains ferrous ions. Diuretic mineral water contains a high ion content of sodium, calcium, chloride and sulfate ions. Alkalizing springs contain large amounts of sodium, calcium, bicarbonate and chloride ions. Stimulating waters are high in sodium, chloride and sulfate ions (Barron, 1995).

Listed geographically and prominently known for medicinal qualities that relieve the discomforts of chronic joint diseases, these are some of the mineral thermal springs developed as treatment centers and healing resorts (Altman, 2000):

Australasia
Australia: Daylesford, Hepburn Springs, Moree
New Zealand: Rotorua, Hamner Springs, Miranda Hot Springs

Eastern Asia
China: Huanqing
Japan: Atami, Beppu, Dogo, Hakone, Ibusuki, Ito, Katsuura, Kusatsu, Narugo, Nikko Yumoto, Noboribetsu, Shiobara, Shirahama, Tamagawa, Unzen, Yugawara
South Korea: Bugok, Onyang
Taiwan: Peitou, Chipen, Wulai, Yangmingshan

Central Asia
Russia: Bashkiria, Pyatigorsk, Repino, Sochi

Middle East

Israel: Hamme Zohar, Tiberias
Eastern Europe
Slovakia: Bojnice, Piestany, Trencianske, Teplice, Ciz

Slovenia: Catez, Dobrna, Moravske Toplice, Smarjeske Toplice
Croatia: Lipik, Topusco
Czech Republic: Frantiskovy Lazne, Jachymov
Hungary: Budapest, Bukfurdo, Eger, Hajduszoboszlo, Heviz
Poland: Busco-Zdroj, Ciechocinek, Cieplice Slaskie-Zdroj, Potczyn-Zdroj

Northern Europe
Iceland: Hveragerdi

Southern Europe
Bulgaria: Velingrad, Pavel Banya, Kyustendl
Greece: Aedipsos, Icaria, Loutraki, Thermopylae
Italy: Abaon Terme, Acqui Termi, Asnano Termi, Bagni di Lucca, Castrocaro Terme, Ischia Terme, Montegrotto Terme, Salsomaggiore Terme, Sirmione Terme
Portugal: Caldas da Rainha, Furnas, Curia, Cucos, Luso, Sao Pedro do Sul
Romania: Baile Felix, Baile Herculane, Calimanesti, Geoagiu Bai
Spain: Alhama de Aragon, Archena, Caldes de Montbui, Caldes de Malavella, Fitero, Jaraba, Ledesma

Turkey: Bursa, Izmir-Cesme, Pamukkale, Yalova

Western Europe
Austria: Bad Aussee, Baddeutch-Altenburg, Baden bei Wien, Bad Gastein, Bad Gosern, Bad Schallerbach
Belgium: Spa
France: Balaruc, Neiderbronn-les-Bains, Bourbon-Lacy, Dax, Bagneres-de-Bigorre, Bourbonne-les-Basins, Bourbon-l'Archambault
Germany: Bad Griesbach, Baden-Baden, Bad Nenndorf, Bad Wildbad, Bad Kreuznach, Wiesbaden, Wiesenbad
Great Britain: Bath, Buxton, Harrogate, Leamington Spa, Llandrindod
Ireland: Lisdoonvarna
Switzerland: Bad Ragaz, Bad Schinznach, Baden, Leukerbad, Rheinfelden, Yverdon-les-Bains

South America
Argentina: Cachueta, Los Molles, Pismanta, Banos de Copahue
Brazil: Araxa, Caxambu, Lambari, Pocos de Caldas, Sao Pedro, Serra Negra
Chile: Termas de Chillan, Termas de Huife, Termas de Puyehue
Columbia: Paipa, Tabio
Ecuador: Baños, El Tingo, Guapan, Papallacta
Peru: Banos del Inca, Monterrey, Yura
Uruguay: Termas de Arapey

Venezuela: Las Trincheras, Aguas Calientes

North America
Canada: Banff, Fairmont Hot Springs, Harrison Hot Springs
United States:
Saratoga Springs, NY; Berkeley Springs, WV; White Sulfur Springs, WV; Hot Springs, VA; Hot Springs, AR; Calistoga, CA; Glenwood Springs, CO.
Mexico: Agua Hedionda, San Jose de Purua, Ixtapan de la Sal

Caribbean
Cuba: Ciego Montero, Elguea, San Diego de los Banos
Jamaica: Milk River

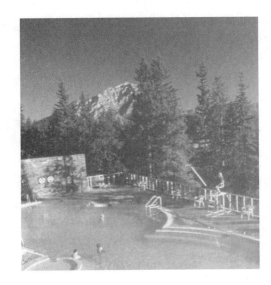

Banff Hot Springs (Figure 158)

It is not possible to know what humans called the hot springs around the world during the Pleistocene epoch or more importantly, how hot springs were used. Soaking the feet in warm water naturally felt good and relaxing. It is speculated that springs have been used for healing purposes for many thousands of years. Homo habilis, early hominids, were present from 2.3 million to 1.8 million years ago. Homo erectus, with its larger brain, inhabited Africa, Asia and Europe starting 1.9 million years ago and became extinct less than one million years ago. They both had an average lifespan, determined by dental analysis of fossils, of 20-30 years. *Homo sapiens neanderthalensis*, named Neanderthal after the Neander Valley in Germany, with an even larger brain size than Cro-Magnon today, lived in the Middle East, the western portion of Asia, and throughout the forested, temperate areas of Europe from 120,000 years ago until the peak of the last ice age less than 40,000 years ago. The first Neanderthal skull was discovered in 1848 on the Rock of Gibraltar, not in Germany's Neander

Valley, but it was not publicized, so the second discovery eight years later in Germany is credited with the name (www.gib.gi/museum/p74.htm).

Cro-Magnon people, *Homo sapiens sapiens*, emerged in Africa at the same time Neanderthals emerged in their habitat. There were vast differences in mitochondrial DNA between the two species. The Cro-Magnons migrated north through today's Egypt and Israel, merging with and absorbing the cold-adapted Neanderthal people as the ice shelf receded (Johnson, 1983) so that both of the human species eventually inhabited the grassland of the middle east and southern Europe at the same time. Like the Yavapai Indians of Arizona, native Cro-Magnon tribes of the European savannas transitioned from hunters/gatherers to settled agricultural societies 10,000 to 20,000 years ago. Then perhaps there was time to soak in the hot springs after a long day working in the fields. Of all our predecessors in the genetic family Hominidae, we are the only survivors. We are the Cro-Magnon people who peacefully bred with the

Neanderthals. In the many thousands of years that Neanderthals and Cro-Magnons cohabitated in Europe, there has not been any archeological evidence that there were any large battles or conflicts between the two.

The individual life expectancy of Neanderthals was not very different from that of the modern inhabitants in parts of Africa today. The life expectancy in Zambia today is 37, Angola is 38, Mozambique is 38, and in Botswana it is 39 (Map Quest, 2004).

Anthropologists can see what happened to the Neanderthal by evaluating the evidence underwater along the Mediterranean coast of France and Spain southwest all the way to the small, 2 ½ mile long Gibraltar Peninsula. In this far corner of Europe the last of the pure Neanderthals died out in the Jurassic limestone caves and rock shelters at the base of the 1400' Rock of Gibraltar. They ended their 60,000 year occupation on the Rock during the Middle Paleolithic period 31,000 years ago, very late in the overall lifespan of

the species. As the polar glaciers melted, the sea level came up a long distance, burying Neanderthal cave homes along the Mediterranean Sea. With modern diving equipment, the caves are now being discovered and explored by archeological divers. Exposed and excavated caves at sea level on the north and east sides of the Rock of Gibraltar have revealed skeletal remains, food processing activities, hunting tools and other lithic artifacts of the Neanderthal families (Barton, 2003). Ten thousand years before Neanderthal extinction, *Homo sapiens sapiens* was building canoes to paddle to Australia. The Neanderthal people were advanced hominids but never did they ever discover how to make a craft that floated on water. If they could have constructed rafts or primitive canoes at Gibraltar, there is a possibility that some families could have easily escaped the disruptive cooling temperatures of the approaching glaciation, the quickly changing seasonal biomass, and the Cro-Magnon encroachment on the last of the pure Neanderthal species. They could have crossed the short 14 miles to the tip of present day Morocco that is in view from the Rock. They could have occupied Africa where they might have survived among the many mineral and hot springs of Morocco and remained our cousins. Was it just a fear of deep water? Was it fear of the unknown? For 60,000 years they sat on the Rock and looked at Morocco but they never crossed the Straights and they are now gone, melted into our species. Late Neanderthal skeletons with Cro-Magnon traits have been found. Have you ever seen anyone that looked somewhat Neanderthal?

Today, the Rock of Gibraltar is inhabited by 2 packs of "Barbary Apes" with no tails, the only wild monkey in Europe.

Neanderthals had rituals and religious belief systems, evidenced by their "afterlife" methods of burial (Jordan, 1999). They could have had their medicine men or herbalists and probably did.

We are *homo sapiens sapiens*. Our cranial capacity was a couple of hundred cubic centimeters smaller than our strong Neanderthal cousins, but they did not use as much of their potential intelligence. We were more intellectually creative and aggressive and we put information to greater use. We could build boats. We could fabricate intricate hunting tools and efficient weapons. We could communicate well linguistically. We could express ourselves through art and music. We could and did develop therapeutic remedies at the healing waters around the world.

In the American past, springs were the places for tribal inhabitants to recover from chronic diseases, illness, and injury. Despite an average lifespan under 45 years, there were many elderly native Americans at the high end of the range. Infant mortality was high. From a paleopathological point of view, there is extensive research evidence demonstrating the prevalence of degenerative joint disease in pre-Columbian North America (Bridges, 1991). They include vertebral arthritis (Bridges, 1994), spondylolysis (Bridges, 1989; Rothschild, 1992), rheumatoid

arthritis (Rothschild, 1990; Short, 1974; Domen, 1981), symmetrical erosive arthritis (Rogers, 1989; Woods, 1988) and calcium pyrophosphate deposition disease (Rothschild, 1993). It is hard to imagine that sufferers of these diseases would not have sought relief in the healing waters of the springs.

Hot springs were places for shamans to practice among the Kutenai Indians at Banff; the Cahuilla at Palm Springs; the Esselen and Costanoan tribes at the thermal waters near Big Sur; the Cherokee at Hot Springs, North Carolina; among the Athapascan tribes at Banff, Radium Hot Springs, throughout Canada and Alaska; and among most of the native cultures on the Continent. At Harbin Hot Springs, California, the Pomo Indians called the healing waters "atawyomi" or "the hot place." The peaceful Miwok, who called themselves "koocako" for people, that migrated to Harbin Hot Springs and established villages in the area. Their shamans or "yomta" were the true heads of the villages. The chief or "hoypu" was merely a politician that settled disputes. The yomta was the religious, ceremonial, and medical leader of the community (Klages, 1991).

Hot springs provided a venue for shamanism as a conduit for spiritual and divine communication. They were also places of solitude to fast, bathe, purge the body and to cleanse and purify the soul. These were the requirements to be acceptable by the supernatural powers, to influence them and acquire one of the powers as a guardian or personal protector (Narby, 2001). The springs were entirely natural places to secure strength from higher deities, places equal to drumming and dance where one "called" to become a healer could train to become a shaman. To the shaman, illness was caused by external, tangible sources or by an absence of the soul. Hot springs, waterfalls, cliff edges, unusual rock formations, old trees, mountain tops and other natural locations were thought by the Native Americans to be portals to the spiritual world, spirits could be visited at their domain to restore the soul. A shamanic state of consciousness is a

nonordinary reality in special locations where deliberate, serious intent are the source of power (Harner, 1990).

The first use of the word "shaman" came from "saman" in a 1661 description of a Tungus native diviner in Siberia by Avvakum Petrovich, a Russian clergyman. Samans was only used by the Tungus, Buryat and the Yukat native tribes of Siberia. Elsewhere in the world there had been similar members of indigenous tribes and communities for many generations. The medicine men, healers, pagan doctors, diviners, conjurers, sorcerers, communicators with the supernatural, communicators with good spirits, communicators with evil spirits, future predictors, protectors who possess guardian spirits, ministers of magic, jugglers, those that cast spells and curses, those that practice sacrifice, those that induce convulsions or hallucinations in themselves by consuming or smoking herbal substances to experience extrasensory perception, hypnotists, those that speak in tongues unintelligible in any

language, those that believe they are the interpreters of gods, sorcerers, wizards and witches, those with supernatural powers, mediums, those who control mental imagery and consciousness -- they are all shamans. There were and are good ones and bad ones.I am referring to the good healers. They were called many names in many cultures. The following are some of them (Narby, 2001). Note the linguistic similarities between some of the cultures.

Siberia – shaman, saman
West Africa – boboro
Alaskan Eskimo – angakoq
Iroquois Tribe – angakkut, arendiouannens
Indians of S.Mexico – curanderas
Venezuela – wisiratu
India – lhapa
Lake Miwok Tribe - yomta
Japan – miko
French Guyana – piage
Amazon – piai
Vaupa Tribe, S.America – paye

Harbin

The Lake Miwok (Indians) at Harbin Hot Springs northeast of San Francisco called their springs "eetawyomi" from the Pomo language. It was a gathering place for Native American shamans for centuries. A real estate grabber named Archibald Ritchie took it upon himself to possess the springs in 1849 because they were next to his land grant. The Lake Miwok neighbors brought Ritchie to their sacred springs and apparently Ritchie thought he could presume ownership just by verbally and illegally claiming the land, but he never formally owned the land or the springs.

Harbin was actually the name of a squatter, James Harbin, and his son James "Mat" Madison Harbin both from Tennessee. Young Mat arrived in California in the first group of westward pioneers that successfully crossed the Sierra Mountains with their wagons. One or both of the James Harbins built a squatter's shack on the land they didn't own after Archibald Ritchie's death in 1856 and lived there at times during the following nine years. James Harbin the father became a successful Napa Valley businessman and died in 1877. His son, Mat, became a hermit in Mexico, returned to California for his last three years and died in 1900 (Klages, 1991).

In 1865 the springs became legally owned for the first time and were developed as a resort called "Harbin Springs," later bought and sold many times over the next century. The buildings were destroyed by a major fire in 1894. The property became a boxing training camp in the early 1900's and then a health promotion enterprise. Harbin Springs, as one business or another, managed to survive the Great Depression. In 1943 it was partially destroyed again by fire, then converted from a health cure destination to a resort in the 1950's. Then there was deterioration and foreclosure. There was another fire that completely destroyed the main hotel and the land was put up for auction. New owners with residential development aspirations renamed it "The Golden Spa" and built a golf course. Loans defaulted. There was another auction. Briefly the thousand-acre property was converted to a gay community called Harbin Springs Club in 1968. In 1969 Harbin was occupied by Harbinger University and a non-profit commune of homeless transients on LSD called Frontiers of Science. Suddenly the Hot Springs were polluted and contaminated to near oblivion by thousands of San Francisco hippies on psychedelic drugs. The next year a force including the county sheriff and state narcotics agents totally evacuated the entire property.

Next came a holistic and New Age church community called Heart Consciousness Church whiling away its time on long-term internal disputes. The 1970's ushered in the arrival of massage therapists as the place became associated with Shiatsu and Esalen massage. Bodyworker Harold Dull purchased the Niyama School of Massage at the springs from Phil Lutrell in the 1980's and started Watsu, the aquatic bodywork he taught to my co-author Alexander Georgeakopoulos in 1990. Still an intentional community associated with Harold Dull's Watsu, Harbin and nearby Middletown are now the headquarters of the Worldwide Aquatic Bodywork Association.

I *can relate to James Harbin,* the squatter on public land at the sacred waters of the Miwok, remembering how I drove my '68 VW up the muddy, rutty, rocky Alaska Highway in 1969 to fight forest fires for the Bureau of Land Management for five seasons. I first lived in a small, abandoned squatter's cabin near the Alaska Railroad out from Sheep Creek Road 15 miles west of Fairbanks. While there, I researched the history of public land in the area and located a nice place to make a claim and initially staked it as an 80 acre prospect site. The property, situated in a valley, included three creeks merging into Lake Killarney and one creek coming out of the lake. The valley was bounded on two sides by hills of birch and spruce. Beyond the hills were valleys totally destroyed in the past by gold mining dredges. I wanted to protect the land. To do so I had to find gold and own a claim to the mineral rights. Two years later I found just enough placer gold to file two adjacent 40 acre mining claims. The following summer, using only simple hand tools, I constructed a unique and well-built two-story cabin with gables and, piece by piece, carried in and assembled a large and handsome wood-burning stove; and constructed and installed a stained-glass skylight and a fancy outhouse. I called the 4" thick solid wood door with huge iron hardware "the bear door" because it could keep them out. No bears ever visited but there were moose, beaver and wolves. That side of Fairbanks had the Goldstream Valley wolf pack echoing their songs throughout the long winter nights under the aurora borialis. There was a large brass bell inside the cabin attached to a very long nylon rope that meandered through the trees for several hundred yards to a swinging log gate across the path (Figure 159) so I would know when visitors arrived. These would be friends from one of the three communes around Fairbanks or the other cabin people living farther out around Ester Dome, some passing through on dogsleds to buy groceries in Fairbanks with their food stamps. The sleds around Fairbanks have more than likely all been replaced with snowmobiles or off-road vehicles today. I cleared the boundaries around the 80 acres and named it "Happy Creek Wildlife Sanctuary." For parts of two winters I returned to Illinois to finish a degree in Health Science. I departed Alaska to live in Idyllwild, California in 1976 and allowed a graduate student in the Environmental Sciences Department at the University of Alaska to live in the cabin for free as long as he performed the annual boundary clearing and filed the necessary papers every year with the State of Alaska Department of Natural Resources to maintain the active status of the mining claim. There was never any mining performed on the land. There it sat for 17 years until the now-Environmental Scientist neglected to file the papers one year. The State of Alaska was eager to gain possession of Happy Creek Wildlife Sanctuary, formally called "Bedgood Association Mining Claims," because of its proximity to Fairbanks and that they did. It may be developed land by now.

⤙⫷⫷⫷O⫸   ⤙⫷⫷⫷O⫸   ⤙⫷⫷⫷O⫸

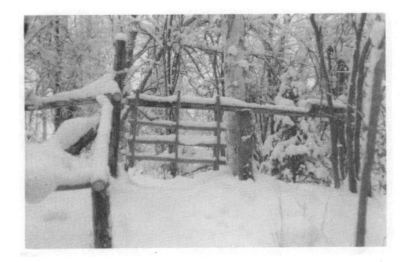

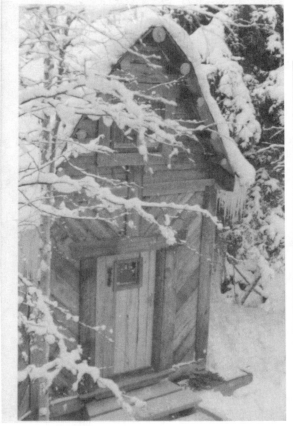

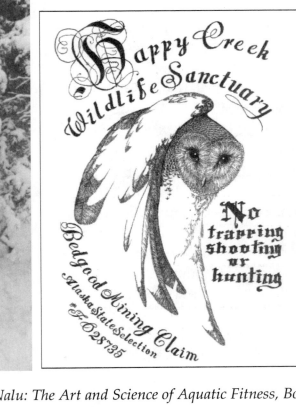

(Figure 159) The Author's Abode in Alaska

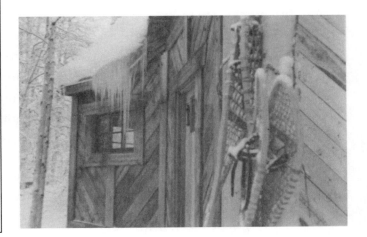

Chapter 10
Aquatic Exercise and the Laws of Physics

All the oceans, all the mountains, all the cities of concrete, all the dirt, all the trees, all the people, all the whales, all the granite, all the polar ice, the vast inner sea of molten basalt and the liquid metallic core – all these are some of the massive components of our eight thousand mile diameter planet. indeed, but how much does it all weigh? There is no need for complex calculations. It all adds up to nothing. That's correct. How is this possible?

Jump up and down. What are you doing when you are coming down? You are falling. You are being pulled down by the Earth's gravity. That same pull attracts the moon towards the earth but the moon has it's own acceleration. It is in motion as it is acted upon by the earth's gravitation and simultaneously falls towards the earth, captured indefinitely in a suspended free fall. The earth,

similarly, is free falling towards the sun as the earth moves along its elliptical orbit. True free falling objects are weightless. The weight of the earth is zero.

Many laws of physics apply to aquatic exercise. They are laws related to motion, vibration, gravity, fluid mechanics, weight, inertia, mass, thermodynamics, force, and more. We will explore some of these properties and their laws.

First I will reveal that water has its own laws different from those for other liquids. One example is that water contracts as temperature drops, until it is reduced to 40° F (14.4°C), then it expands until it freezes. So you see, water in a liquid state is not at its highest density when it is at its coldest temperature. This little phenomenon has profound meaning to our planet since the water flowing under polar ice sheets that float above it dissipates heat from tropical currents in the Earth's circulatory system.

Much of physics has been known and documented for centuries, and perhaps for many thousands of years as speculative theory or common sense feelings of truth. Greek lovers of wisdom divided into inward and outward philosophies. Inward philosophy became psychology. Outward philosophy of nature became science (Latin "to know"). Doctoral degrees in science today are still called doctorates in philosophy, Ph D. The study of physics was at one time the study of all science. After the development of specialized sciences, physics is now the leftover science after geology, biology, chemistry, astronomy, and mathematics have been separated from it.

The Laws of Motion and Aquatics

We begin with Sir Isaac Newton in the 1600's. Newton wrote the *Principia* or *Mathematical Principles of Natural Philosophy* comprising three laws. Newton's first law of motion: A body continues in its state of constant velocity (which may be zero), unless acted upon by an external force. A force is that which can impose a change of velocity on a material body. A vector quantity has size and direction. Force can be quantified as a vector. Without direction, the quantity is scalar. Displacement is a vector that combines size, direction and distance. The convention in aquatic exercise is to call the result negative velocity when upward acceleration is over powered by the force of gravity. Similarly, when a downward push on aquatic exercise equipment is overpowered by the force of it's buoyancy, if it has buoyancy like foam dumbbells, it is also a negative velocity.

Land-based weighted exercise incorporates simple vectors. A weight lifter moves in one direction with a fixed weight for a specified distance that is related to either body structure or the limitations of exercise machinery. However, in aquatic exercise, vectors go to extremes of complexity that are nearly impossible to measure or track. Joint circumductions, rotations, and continual velocity alterations allow each scalar vector to be an

independent variable capable of influencing the force at any point in time during the exercise.

Newton's second law of motion: The acceleration produced by a force acting on a body, is directly proportional to the magnitude of the force and inversely proportional to the mass of the body. A force produces acceleration. The size of the acceleration is a measure of the force. Higher inertia or mass requires a larger force to produce the same acceleration. The inertia of the body is proportional to its mass (the constant of proportionality). In aquatic exercise, the mass of the body is the water itself. The force needed to move against water is influenced by all the isokinetic variables applicable throughout the movement, including angles, surface irregularities, temperature, water currents, body mechanics, drag coefficients, and other variables. From the standpoint of the physics of action and reaction, both the contractile muscle tissue that is moving the aquatic exercise equipment and the resisting water are

the sources of two different forces of equal importance.

Newton's third law of motion: In a system where no external forces are present, every action force is always opposed by an equal and opposite reaction force. For every action, there is an equal and opposite reaction. For a force to exist, it must be exerted on or by something. Whenever one body exerts a force on a second body, the second body exerts a force on the first body. These forces are equal in magnitude and opposite in direction. More accurately, this is a law of interaction. Vector addition does not cancel out the forces because the two separate bodies impose equal and opposite forces on eachother. The water is pushing against the aquatic exercise equipment with a force equal to that applied by the user.

The pressure of a liquid is transmitted perpendicularly to the walls of its container and to the surface of any solid object within the liquid. An object has a greater upward force of pressure from the liquid beneath it than from the liquid above it. Using

Archimedes' principle we can understand buoyancy as the upward force of a liquid against an object in the liquid. The liquid will exert an upward force on the object equal to the weight of the liquid displaced by the solid object. The weight of the solid after submersion is equal to its original weight minus the weight of the displaced water. In water, buoyancy is the counterforce to gravity.

There is a unit of force named after Newton. One **newton (N)** is the force required to give a mass of one kilogram an acceleration of one meter per second squared (N = gram-force x 0.01; 1N = 100 dynes; 1 sthene = 1000 N). Converting between measurement systems, one pound-force equals 0.225 newtons force. Example: 168.1 newtons = 38 pounds. 1 Kg of mass exerts 9.8 newtons of force in Earth's gravity. Weight is proportional to mass but not synonymous. Weight is the force. Weight is mass times acceleration. Mass is the inertia. Mass is force (weight) divided by acceleration. Mass and weight are related by gravity.

Centripetal force is inward towards the earth's center. Centrifugal force is outward away from the earth's center. Both of these forces are active during aquatic exercise. Centripetal force keeps your feet on the pool floor. Centrifugal force is created during the radial motion of hinge and ball & socket bone joints using aquatic exercise equipment (Fig.160).

.

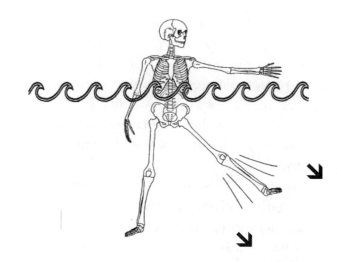

Centrifugal

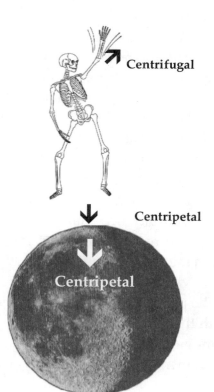

Centrifugal

Centripetal

Centripetal

(Figure 160)
Centripetal/Centrifugal

Centripetal and centrifugal forces shape galaxies of spheres into flattened rotations. Orbits of electrons are spheres. Planets, moons, stars, they are all ellipsoid in shape, elongated spheres. As you move in the water, if you were to track all your potential movements, the image would be a sphere, the perfect shape. Leonardo DaVinci filled a circle with a human figure that had outstretched legs and arms. Putting him in motion would turn the circle into a sphere.

How is force measured in water? I will go over this briefly because the Stokes equation is detailed in its own chapter, Chapter 11, *The Kinetics of Water*. Assume that you are using aquatic resistance equipment. Its shape and contours determine the drag characteristics as a coefficient in an equation. Other components of the equation are the velocity, the viscosity and density of the water, temperature, and the resistive surface area of the exercise equipment.

Using a disc shaped device, the Wasilowski interpretation (see Appendix: Wasilowski, 2000) of the Stokes equation is as follows:

$$F_D = \frac{(0.25)\pi\, d^2 C_D \rho\, V^2}{2}$$

V = Velocity
d = diameter
F_D = Drag force
C_D = drag coefficient
ρ = water density in slugs

What is a "slug" in this equation? A slug is the gravitational unit of mass in the *fps* (foot, pound, second) system to which a pound force can impart an acceleration of one foot per second per second. In this equation, slugs are per cubic foot of water.

Professor George Huang at the University of Kentucky Department of Mechanical Engineering has also supplied an equation to determine force in water but leaves off water density (2002):

$$F_D = \frac{(0.25)\pi\, C_D\, d^2\, V^2}{2}$$

Drag coefficients are charted in Chapter 11.

A gallon of water weighs 8 1/3 lbs (4 liters/3.78kg). One cubic foot of water = 7 ½ gallons and weighs 62.5 lbs (30 liters/28.4kg). When you push water with aquatic exercise equipment that has a relatively small surface area of 144 square inches, a lot more than 62 .5 lbs of water is affected. Every drop of water in the pool is affected by your energy. Because water is incompressible, you make waves in the pool and water can splash out of the pool at the opposite end from just one strong person vigorously exercising with large muscle endurance aquatic exercise equipment. Water in a swirling vortex, like that of a rapid stream or in a whirlpool, has a higher apparent density than stagnant water.

Aquatic Physics and the Senses

What sound comes from the turbulence of water to your ears above water? What are the sounds heard throughout the oceans of the world? Is there a difference between the sounds below and those above the surface? It is an error to think that the water surface is only the level, horizontal surface between the body of water and the atmosphere. The surface of water is wherever water touches something other than itself. There are boundary layers that separate the body of water from surface contact with objects. There are separate surfaces around particles and droplets of different substances in emulsion. There are boundary surfaces between water and insoluble fluids in the water. There are many types of water surfaces. Let's get down into pure, deep water, away from the surfaces and listen. There is a big surprise waiting for you. Sound travels at an average of 758 miles per hour (1220 km/h) through the air but in water sound travels at 3,240 miles per hour (5213km/h). Why?

Intermolecular forces in liquids and solids bring about a much quicker rebound after compression. The more rigid the substance is, the greater the velocity of sound going through it. In steel, sound travels at 11,200 miles per hour (18,020km/h). Supersonic in the air is not necessarily supersonic in water. See Figure #18 for a photograph of the effects of sound on water and Chapter 1, *Healing Waters,* that includes the use of sound in aquatic therapy.

Waves of water in the ocean are transverse to the water itself and confined to the upper surface due to the force of gravity. The wave moves but the water remains in one place. The entire body of water has weight. Within the body of the water, each portion of it is suspended by surrounding portions of water. Viewed within the larger body of water, that 62 ½ lb cubic foot of water has mass but it does not have weight. It weighs nothing in relation to its surroundings. It is suspended just like a person is suspended in neck deep water with their 8 lb cranium being more or less the total weight against

the pool floor (depending on their lean body mass).

There is a visual distortion of objects that are partially submerged in water. This can make a difference in what a therapist sees from above the water and what a patient is doing underwater. Being aware of this phenomenon will help therapists visually compensate for this optical illusion for documentation of more accurate observations. The sense of sight is fooled by water. Standing in waist deep water and reaching your straight arm out at a 45° angle causes the arm to appear bent at the air/water surface when it is actually straight. Can you really trust the accuracy of where you think you see yourself or another partially submerged person nearby? The answer is no. The light bends. The arm is not bent. And you thought that light always traveled in a straight line except when it was reflected. You were wrong. The law of physics we are working with here is the Snell-Descartes law of refraction discovered and unpublished by Dutch physicist Willebrord Snell and independently discovered and published by Rene Descartes, both in the early 1600's. Whenever light passes from one transparent medium into another, the ratio of the sine of the angle of incidence to the sine of the angle of refraction is a constant.

To understand this phenomenon of visual distortion in water, we will define the terms. A sine can be understood by looking at a right triangle. There are three angles, a 90° right angle and two acute angles that are dependant on the length of the two perpendicular sides. From one of the acute angles, go the opposing side. There is a ratio between that side and the hypotenuse of the triangle. That ratio is the sine of the angle.

An index of refraction is the constant when light passes obliquely from a vacuum into transparent matter. The index of refraction of air is 1.00029. Water is 1.33. Glass and diamond are higher. Higher optical density results in a higher index of refraction. When light travels from air to water at an angle, it is going to a substance of higher optical density that bends the light towards the normal. The normal is the line perpendicular to the water at the point of entry. In the reverse direction, from a substance of higher optical density to one of lower optical density, the bend is away from the normal.

There is a critical angle of 48.6°. An angle of incidence greater than that when the line of light is closer to the water surface will entirely reflect the light traveling from air to water. Substances with a greater refractive index have smaller critical angles.

How far can you see in water? In a vacuum, light passes without obstruction. Water is transparent but its transparency has limits. Light is not visible more than 450 feet in water – more water than this is effectively opaque. Light is converted into heat when it enters opaque matter. Lambert's third law (J.H.Lambert 1728-1777): The luminous intensity of light decreases exponentially with distance as it propagates through an absorbing medium.

Enter a therapy pool. You sense the warmth of the water as waves of heat. You sense the stimulation of water compressing epidermal nerves as waves of turbulence and pressure. You sense the olfactory irritation from the antibiotic oxidizing agents and pool chemicals. With the retina in your eyes, you sense the nebulous images of the rippling reflections of light on the water surface as waves of photons and you hear the sounds of anatomical appendages entering and exiting the water as waves of audible frequencies. You feel the contraction of muscles that initiate and control the motion of your body. You sense your own buoyancy as you subconsciously analyze and compare differences in density between the water and your particular body composition, and you sense the pull of gravity mostly on portions of your body that are above the water line.

Sensory perception receives these electrochemical nerve transmissions in the brain and processes them for interpretation and response. A response, dependant on the initial interpretation of the stimuli, can be the desire to increase one or more of these sensory inputs. You might want to experience more muscular effort by increasing energy output in aquatic exercise if the pool is cooler. You could be overwhelmed by a fear of drowning. The stress of this situation could induce a panic attack. You could pronate your body without effort and experience an overall tranquilizing effect by the activation of your parasympathetic nervous system, the ideal state for returning from dysfunction and illness to homeostasis. There are many possible reactions to sensory perceptions while you are in the water. What are these stimulators, the electrochemical nerve impulses, and what is the nature of your interpretations from sensory stimuli? What is matter and what keeps it all together? Looking into the atoms of a water molecule, simplicity rules. It is all organized waves of motion, movement of waves and nothing more. Allow *Nalu* to now take a closer look into this smallest world.

The Microsphere

Down to the elusive electron we go, to that invisible hermit, and to the nutrino, the quarks and their subatomic layers of motion, all moved by the forces of bosons. We will be defining these entities, elementary particles with and without mass, some with the ability to occupy the same space at the same time. Traveling through the smallest world is almost an unbelievable exploration. Max Planck and Albert Einstein led the way.

There is possibly no end to the microsphere just as there are no boundaries to the theoretical macrouniverse. The reciprocal could even be that space is imploding with an illusion of material expansion. These massless force interactions that affect particles with mass are: the infinite reach of gravitation, electromagnetic interaction that establishes the position of electrons and the atomic nucleus, the strong force that keeps quarks together in triplets, and the weak interaction. The weak force is beta radioactivity that governs thermonuclear reactions, the source of that warm ray of sunlight on your back as you walk in the water. Without the weak force there would be no heat from our star and life could not develop.

Knowing how the atoms within water maintain their integrity leads us to the definitions of some of the more common terms used in quantum mechanics and particle physics (Stonybrook State University of New York; Lakehead University, Ontario; Michigan State University Physics Department)

Particles – bosons (energy) and fermions (matter)
Leptons – elementary particle that participates in weak interactions
Hadrons – elementary particle that interacxts strongly with other particles
Lepton bosons – photons, gravitons
Lepton fermions – electrons, muons, nutrinos
Hadron bosons – mesons
Hadron fermions – baryons
Meson – one quark and an antiquark plus a gluon; a hadronic boson

Baryon – three quarks (fermions) held together by gluons (bosons); a hadrionic fermion

Antiparticle – one of a pair of particles of equal mass but with opposite sign like the electron/positron

Quark – fermion constituent of a hadron mediated by gluons; the only particles that can couple with gluons; several types in generations; protons and neutrons are composed of different combinations of quarks

Gluon – eight distinct neutral particles without mass

Photon – a gauge boson without mass that mediates electromagnetic interaction, interacts with any particle that has an electric charge

Gauge boson – particles of energy that carry fundamental interactions

Graviton – boson particle without mass or charge that carries the gravitational force and affects all fermions to infinity

Muon – heavy lepton that decays into an electron, nutrino and an antinutrino

Pion – the lightest meson, made of quarks, interacts with nuclei to transform neutrons into protons and vice versa

Quantum electrodynamics (QED) is the theory that heavier bosons with shorter ranges of interaction mediate the strong exerted forces between fermions. Forces do not exist without bosons. Quarks increase their force with distance so that their flights are the source of their force. Here again, motion controls cohesion. Under the influence of electromagnetic force, any shape can be formed. The mediator boson for electromagnetism is the massless photon, light. Light is an electromagnetic wave. It is motion. The boson mediator for the strong force is eight different gluons. The characteristics of electronic orbitals between atoms assure the attraction that binds them together to form complex molecules.

Photons are emitted when electrons penetrate the fields of other electrons. This diffusion creates the electromagnetic force and this is the source of all chemistry, all changes in molecular structures, of your own anaerobic and aerobic production of energy, all nerve impulses, all feelings, all tissue repairs, and all healing. The accepting, rejecting, expelling, sharing, capturing, repelling, accommodating, hyperpolarizing, destabilizing, attracting, and penetrating nature of electron orbits is the sole source of our memory, instincts, genetics, intellect, and our ability to sequence and plan an exercise routine in the water, either in place or entirely within our imagination The electromagnetic force is the source of language, emotions, and our senses. The infinite variables of the complexity of life can be condensed all the way down to the invisible electron and the massless photon. We are the algebraic sum of the potentials of billions of neurons.

When electrons share orbits between atoms of a molecule, a protein molecule with five million atoms for example, all the electrons in the atomic fringe orbits that are vulnerable to invasion, moving at nearly the velocity of light, fill every other outer orbit in a commonality of motion without collisions at close to 186,280 miles per second. The forces that hold the molecule together and keep the electrons from spiraling into the nucleus are a balance of electrostatic and centripetal forces. The outer shell electrons are diffused everywhere in the field of orbitals as one unified mass. This can easily be compared to the human body and the relation between fascia, muscles and organs. Considering muscles, the myofascia surrounds each muscle, each fiber, each tendon, and merges with the periosteum that surrounds the bones. The fascia is connective tissue, a continuous and uninterrupted mesh of collagen all connected with one purpose, to hold everything together as one intact being, to give integrity to shape, like the molecule being glued together with a common electromagnetic force.

Waves of sound, waves of light, electromagnetic radiation, these relatively recent discoveries are the result of pure science and our curious search for truth emerging long ago when the first humans threw stones into Lake Turkana and observed the rippling waves spreading out in circles away from the splash,

weakening ever so gently to an unnoticeable calmness. For two hundred thousand years our thoughts did swirl in the African Rift Valley. A stone is thrown. The response from the water is art. Two stones are thrown. The waves become complex. Our intellect, once equal to that of a primitive prosimian, adapted to survive until we had enough tools and inventions to free up some time to think about the why and how of the physical world. We began to see the laws of physics in the water and now we see luxon waves of massless momentum traveling at the speed of light (671 million miles per hour; 1.08 billion km/h) between ergospheres and event horizons, from the distance of the farthest galaxies within our telescopic vision (Figure 160B).

When you enter the water, know that the most fundamental forces in the universe are with you. Know that the surface of this planet and all life upon it would not exist without water and waves of motion, the motion that is the entire universe. The diversity and interaction of motion's velocity,

vibration and frequency is the key to the development of a complex world.

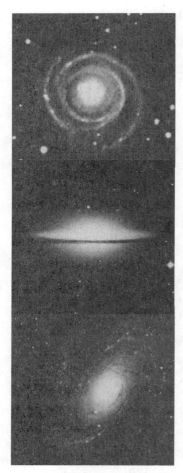

(Figure 160B)
Galaxies are Fluids. Earth is traveling at a half million mph around the center of our Galaxie.

Chapter 11
The Kinetics of Water

Let's get physical…. When physical force is applied to an object and it is moved through water, the water is physically changed. It moves out of the way and around the object creating eddies and turbulence around and following the moving object (Figure 164, p. 311). The amount of force used to move an object like the Aquatoner aquatic exercise equipment can be calculated considering the shape, size, velocity, and distance it is moved through the water.

Water has viscosity. It is a continuous medium. In fluids like water, viscosity is "thickness" or the behavior of water molecules when they move against each other or when their layers shear against each other. Surrounding surfaces like walls and riverbanks influence viscosity. It is also influenced by temperature and by objects that create turbulence within the water. The dynamic and kinematic viscosities of water

decrease with heat and increase with cold. In this book we will explore objects in the water that have shapes useful for creating resistance against the water's viscosity for aquatic exercise. Relative viscosity is the ratio of absolute viscosity to the viscosity of water. Absolute viscosity, which is highly dependant on temperature, is the characteristic of a fluid that causes it to resist flow. It is viscosity times density. Kinematic viscosity is the ratio of relative viscosity to relative density, viscosity divided by density.

Water in a gravitational field such as earth's has pressure. Greater depth has greater pressure. Water has density. Colder water has higher density than warmer water. A whirlpool or any swirling vortex of water has a higher density than water that is not moving. Boundary conditions are yet another variant. There is a molecular attraction between a fluid and the surface of a solid body. Though an object can be moving rapidly through molecules of water, they are at complete rest adjacent to the solid surface because they adhere to the surface. This was

first suspected by French scientist Henry Darcy (1803-1858), who identified the boundary layer as being where molecules of fluid at rest are shearing against the molecules of fluid that are rapidly moving.

When an object is moved through water, the water attempts to get out of the way, so to speak, but it is slowed by its molecules colliding with one another in the process. These collisions of the water molecules increase friction. A shear stress is created between the slower and faster water molecules. Some water molecules will actually interchange with others across the boundary layer.

Water that is not moving has no preferred directions in molecular motion. The molecules are moving randomly, not in unison. Each molecule is isotropic in relation to other water molecules. There is an equal value of physical characteristics along axes in all directions. It makes no difference if water is moving past a stationary object, or if an object is moving through stationary water. Both flows are equivalent. The shapes of objects create the differences in flow characteristics, which are expressed as drag coefficients (Cd). Bodies with significant thickness have higher drag coefficients than essentially two-dimensional bodies. Rough surfaces with projections have higher drag coefficients than smooth surfaces. Flat surfaces against a flow direction have higher drag coefficients than rounded, hydrodynamic shapes. A cupped hand has a higher drag coefficient than a fist or an open hand. Dimensional analysis shows that a drag coefficient is a function of both the geometrical configuration of the immersed body and its velocity (Cheremisinoff, 1983). Reynolds number (Re) is a dimensionless ratio of inertial drag to viscous drag, turbulent flow to laminar (smooth & layered) flow. It is a measure of the nature of flow.

Text continued on page 312.

(Figure 161) Absolute Viscosity vs. Temperature

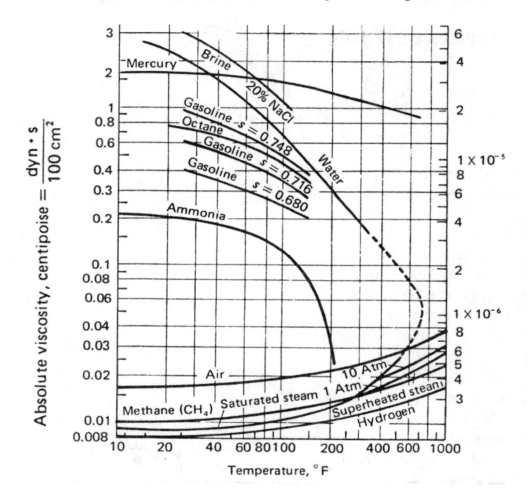

Adapted from R.L. Daugherty and A. C. Ingersoll
(1954) *Fluid Mechanics.* McGraw-Hill

(Figure 162) Drag Coefficients (Cd)

Drag coefficients for two-dimensional bodies						Drag coefficients for three-dimensional bodies					
			C_D							C_D	
Shape	C_D	Shape	Laminar flow	Turbulent flow		Shape	C_D	Shape	Laminar flow	Turbulent flow	
Plate → 2.0		Ellipses:				Disc → 1.17		Sphere: → 0.47		0.27	
		2:1 ⊂ 0.6		0.20							
Half cylinder {→ 1.2 / → 1.7		4:1 0.35		0.10		60° cone → 0.49		Ellipsoidal body of revolution:			
		8:1 0.28		0.10		Cube {→ 1.05 / → 0.80					
Half tube {→ 1.2 / → 2.3		Cylinder: → ○ 1.2		0.30				2:1 → 0.27		0.06	
Square cylinder {→ 2.1 / → 1.6		Rectangular plate → l: $\left(\frac{b}{h}\right)$	1 1.18 / 5 1.2 / 10 1.3 / 20 1.5			Hollow cup {→ 0.38 / → 1.42		4:1 → 0.20		0.06	
								8:1 → 0.25		0.13	
Equilateral triangle {→ 1.6 / → 2.0		b / h ▭				Solid hemisphere {→ 0.38 / → 1.17					

Figures 162 and 163 contain data commonly found in many elementary fluid mechanics textbooks. Examples are: Munson, Young & Okushi (1998) *Fundamentals of Fluid Mechanics.*Wiley; White, F.M.(2003) *Fluid Mechanics.*McGraw Hill.
For sources of this information online visit the following URL's: http://wright.nasa.gov/airplane.shaped.html;
http://www.insideracingtechnology.com/tech102drag.htm;www.smartfish.ch/index.cfm/fusaction/show/path/1-53-55.htm;
www.engineeringtoolbox.com/21_627.html; http://aerodyn.org/drag/tables.html#bluff

(Figure 163)
Reynolds Numbers (Re)
for Various Shapes
(see note on page 309)

Formula for Reynolds number:

$$Re = \frac{DV\rho}{\mu}$$

D = characteristic length , ft.(m)
  Ex: diameter of an object or pipe
ρ = density, slugs/ft³ (Kg/m³)
μ = viscosity, lb.s/ft² (centipoise, cPs)
V = velocity, ft/s (m/sec.)

Reynolds numbers can be automatically calculated online at:
www.processassociates.com/process/dimen/dn_rey.htm

www.efunds.com/formulae/fluids/calc_reynolds.c

Type of Body		Proportional Dimension	Re	Cd
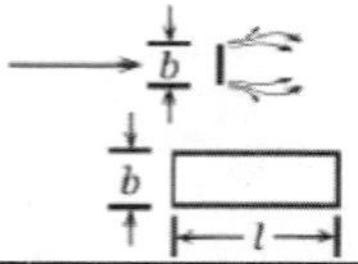	Rectangular plate	$l/b = 1$	$>10^4$	1.18
		$l/b = 5$	$>10^4$	1.20
		$l/b = 10$	$>10^4$	1.30
		$l/b = 20$	$>10^4$	1.50
		$l/b = \infty$	$>10^4$	1.98
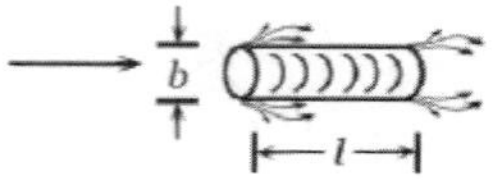	Circular cylinder- axis // to flow	$l/d = 0$ (disk)	$>10^4$	1.17
		$l/d = 0.5$	$>10^4$	1.15
		$l/d = 1$	$>10^4$	0.90
		$l/d = 2$	$>10^4$	0.85
		$l/d = 4$	$>10^4$	0.87
		$l/d = 8$		0.99
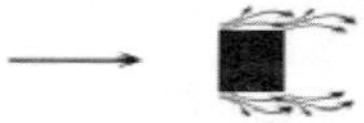	Square rod	∞	$>10^4$	2.00
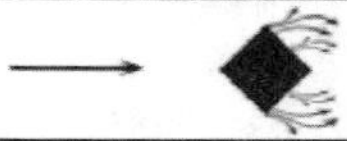	Square rod	∞	$>10^4$	1.50
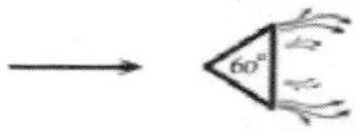	Triangular cylinder	∞	$>10^4$	1.39
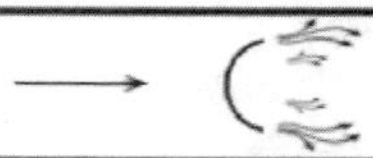	Semi-circular shell	∞	$>10^4$	1.20
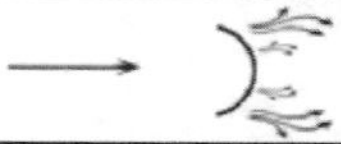	Semi-circular shell	∞	$>10^4$	2.30
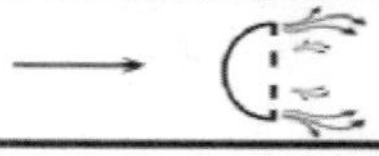	Hemispherical shell		$>10^4$	0.39
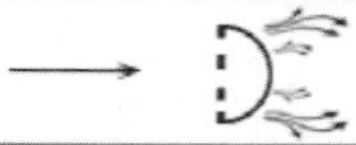	Hemispherical shell		$>10^4$	1.40
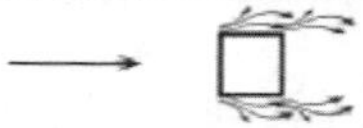	Cube		$>10^4$	1.10
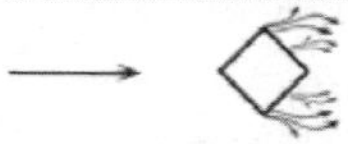	Cube		$>10^4$	0.81
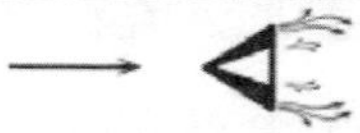	Cube - 60° vortex		$>10^4$	0.49

Re = Reynolds Number   Cd = Drag Coefficient

Nalu: The Art and Science of Aquatic Fitness, Bodywork & Therapy

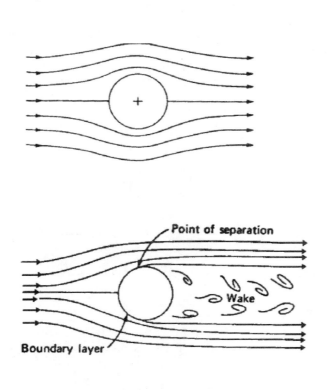

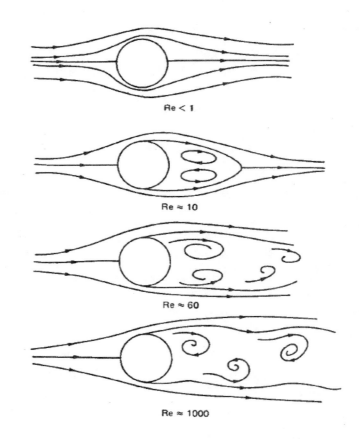

(Figure 164) Water Patterns around a Cylinder Produced by Turbulent Flow

(Figure 165) Effect on Wake around a Cylinder Produced by an Increase in Reynolds Number

Figures 164 and 165 adapted from
Starr, Victor (1968) *Physics of Negative
Viscosity Phenomena*. McGraw Hill

Nalu: The Art and Science of Aquatic Fitness, Bodywork & Therapy

As shown in Figures 164 and 165, extreme variations occur between the effects of the drag coefficient and the Reynolds number with varying velocity. If you move a large disk or sphere very slowly through the water, the drag coefficient is a negligible contributor to resistance and the Reynolds number predominates. If you move the disk or sphere rapidly through the water, the Reynolds number has little effect and the drag coefficient effect is big. In this case, at the molecular level, the inertial forces can be neglected as the viscous forces alone dominate. This is called deformation drag. The water particles are deformed by the movement of the solid disk or by the sphere.

An adverse pressure gradient occurs when an increasing fluid pressure in the flow direction separates the boundary layer from the object moving through the water. Minimizing pressure drag delays the boundary layer separation. This can be done by reducing the object's size, speed or drag coefficient. If the goal is high resistance and viscous forces, we want high drag coefficients and thick boundary layers. Minimizing pressure drag by streamlining delays, prevents or eliminates the separation of the boundary layer. A disk or Aquatoner can be streamlined by tilting it on its side, parallel to the flow direction.

If a boundary layer— the water molecules that are between the surface of the object and the fast flow— becomes turbulent, the still molecules become mixed in the viscous flow and the boundary layer becomes thinner. The separation of the boundary layer from the object's surface is then delayed and the drag is consequently reduced. Turbulence does not reduce the drag coefficient. It reduces drag by causing a thinner boundary layer. A thick boundary creates drag on the outer water molecules. In fact, many applications in hydrodynamics and in aerodynamics are intentional vortex generators for a smoother glide like the top surfaces of airplane wings, the fuzz on tennis balls, the dimples on a golf ball and under autos (Lexus), or the new dimpled polo balls that go farther. The roughened surfaces lower the effect of viscosity by creating just enough turbulence to degrade the heavy dragging boundary layer molecules of the fluid – air or water. (Air is a fluid too, a gaseous fluid.) Fluids are consistent freely moving particles that stay together when moved as a whole, in other words a group of particles that are easily moved under pressure without a separation of the mass.

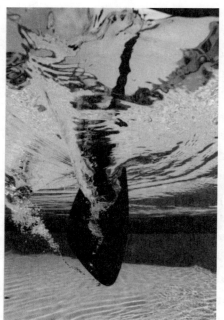

(Figure 166) Double Vortices with Opposite Spin During a Canoe Paddling Stroke

To increase drag, the Aquatoner® (Figure 181) has overlapping paddles with long perimeters that fill a circular area for greater surface in an opened configuration. The Aquatoner with an 18" diameter has 144" of total perimeter length around the three paddles. Those edges are the drag components.

The force needed to move an object with a high drag coefficient in the water increases with the square of its speed. Therefore to increase the exercise speed of an Aquatoner attached to the bottom of your foot, using the powerful quadriceps and gluteus muscles to move the device three feet takes about 120 lbs of force to move it that distance in 2 seconds compared to only 30 lbs to move 4 seconds. The force is quadrupled as the velocity is doubled or time is halved to move the tree feet. So there is a dramatic increase in resistance during the exercise when the speed is increased. For a given distance, if the time is cut from four seconds to two seconds the resistance is increased by a factor of four. A decrease in time from three seconds to one second

multiplies the resistance nine times and moving it in a half second from three seconds increases resistance by thirty-six times.

Stress tensors are a combination of internal stresses like the pressure of the water acting on itself plus the stress from viscous forces.

Water is a Newtonian fluid. A Newtonian fluid is a viscous fluid whose shear stress area is a linear function of the fluid strain rate. A streamline is a path in a steady flow field along which a given fluid particle travels. Turbulence is a flow field that cannot be described with streamlines. In turbulent flow, the inertial stresses dominate over viscous stresses leading to a chaotic type of fluid motion. The eddies and vortices introduce a time-dependent flow field and the turbulent system does not reach a steady state. Viscosity is a fluid property that relates the magnitude of fluid shear to the fluid strain rate or simply to the acceleration in the fluid velocity field. Viscosity is the relationship between the parallel and perpendicular shear

stresses to the fluid flow. This kinematic property in fluid dynamics deals with aspects of motion apart from considerations of mass and force.

Velocity affects force. Faster flow produces higher force against a stationary object. A faster moving object in stagnant water has higher resistance to movement than a slower object. Another variable is current. If water is already in motion this will have an effect on the moving object. Energy is dissipated from the moving object when it encounters an external force from the moving water, a function that is in proportion to the velocity and direction of the moving water against the moving object. In these calculations to follow it will be assumed that the water being encountered by the object is initially still, not moving on it's own.

We will soon be calculating how many pounds of drag force a moving object has in water. The variables are: shape, size, surface, and velocity.

Looking at this overall concept from a distance, it appears to be simple. Don't be confused by the math. It is only a means for communication between people. The details of the calculations are a way of considering all possible variables that influence the outcome.

Fluids resist deformation. Higher applied shear stress increases the rate of shear deformation. Normally in most fluids this relation between stress and rate of strain is linear.

The primary equation of computational fluid mechanics is the Navier-Stokes equation. It relates pressure and external forces acting on a fluid to the response of the fluid flow.

$$F_D = \frac{(0.25)\pi d^2 C_d \rho V^2}{2}$$

(Wasilowsk interpretation, terms defined in Step 3, page 315)

Claude-Louis-Marie Navier derived the Navier-Stokes equation of motion in 1827, and Simeon-Denis Poisson derived it independently in 1831. Their derivations of the stress tensor were based on what amounts to a molecular view of how stresses are exerted by one fluid particle against another. In 1843, Barre de Saint Venant derived the equation, as did George Gabriel Stokes in 1845. Stokes lived a long 84 - year life, long in those days from 1819 to 1903.

There are four fundamental equations that describe laminar flow. These equations are: fluid continuity, equation of motion, constitutive relation, and fluid kinematics. The Navier-Stokes equation is obtained by combining the relation of constitutive and kinematic components into the fluid equation of motion, eliminating the fluid stress and strain rate.

Below is the general equation used to determine forces to move the Aquatoner through water at various frequencies and amplitudes. (Liburdy, 1992). Further discussion of the analytical equations used in the research and the calculation of the energy dissipation rate is located in the Appendix (page 370).

$$F = -k M_0 (dV/dt) \div \tfrac{1}{2} C_d S \, V|V|$$

F = force
k = inertia of added mass
C_d = drag coefficient
M_0 = mass of the fluid displaced by the disk
S = projected area of the disk in the direction of motion
V = velocity of the disk
|V| = absolute value of the disk velocity
dV/dt = time derivative of the velocity (acceleration)

In December 2000 a retired mechanical engineer in Lilburn, Georgia, Bronislaw Wasilowski, simplified pages and pages of Navier-Stokes equations for me so that I could recalculate forces used by physical therapists with the Aquatoner. Not being a physicist I needed simplification. Dr. Bronislaw did his homework and made easy-to-use graphs for determining drag coefficient (see Appendix page 369).

The following is Dr. Wasilowski's procedure for determining force from liquid against the face of a disc moving through water:

Example: What is the drag force in the fps (foot, pound, second) system on a disc having 11" diameter moving in 70°F water at 5 mph?

Step 1

Calculate the Reynolds number with the following equation (Efunda, 2004) or locate it on one of the websites on page 308:

$$Re = \frac{\rho V d}{\gamma}$$

Re = Reynolds number
ρ = water density (see slugs page 301)
V = velocity of disc in water in ft./sec.
d = diameter of disc in feet
γ = the kinematic viscosity of water for a given temperature in sq.ft/sec.

ρ = 1.94 slugs/ft³
V = 7.33 ft/sec.
d = 11" = 0.917ft.
Using the *Physical Character-istics of Water* chart in the Appendix, p.369, at 70°, γ = 0.0000106 (1.06 x 10⁻⁵) sq. ft per second.

$$Re = \frac{7.33 \times 0.917}{1.06 \times 10^{-5}} = 634,000$$

Step 2

Determine Drag Coefficient, C_d, from the Rationalized Relation of Drag Coefficient to Reynolds Number graph (page 369). Cd = 1.1

Step 3

Solve for drag on disc with the Navier-Stokes equation.

$$\mathbf{F_D} = \frac{(0.25)\pi d^2 C_d \,\rho V^2}{2}$$

F_D = drag force
d = 0.917 ft.
C_d = 1.1
ρ = 1.94 slugs/ft³, from the *Physical Characteristics of Water* chart in the Appendix, page 369.

$$F_D = \frac{(0.25)\pi d^2 C_D \rho V^2}{2}$$

$$= \frac{(0.25)(3.14)(0.917)^2(1.1)(1.94)(7.33)^2}{2}$$

$\cong$ **38 lbs**

Rework the procedure in the mks (meter/ kilogram/ second) system:

70°F = 21.1° C
V = 5mph = 2.23 m/sec.
d = 11" = 0.279 meters
γ = 0.977 x 10⁻⁶ (from chart p. 369)

$$Re = \frac{Vd}{\gamma} = \frac{(2.2352)(0.2794)}{0.97 \times 10^{-6}} = 637,000$$

The slight difference is due to interpolation and rounding.

$$F_D = \frac{(0.25)\pi d^2 C_d \rho V^2}{2}$$

C_d = 1.1
ρ = 998 Kg/m³ (from chart p. 369)

$$= \frac{(0.25)\pi(0.279)^2(1.1)(998)(2.23)^2}{2}$$

= 167 newtons
A "newton", named after physicist Sir Isaac Newton(1642-1727), is a unit of measurement in the mks system where 1 kilogram force can impart an acceleration of 1 m/sec./sec. under its influence (see newtons page 300).

167 newtons $\cong$ **38 lbs**

The results are consistent between both systems.

In an effort to verify pages of complicated Stoke's equations as they related to using exercise equipment in water, I discussed my project with other professors in 2000, Dr. Riester at Clemson University, Dr. Huang at the University of Kentucky, and Dr. Moore at Florida International University. Between these professors, the retired Engineer Dr. Wasilowski, and the original work of Dr Liburdy at Clemson, I was able to cross check the calculations using condensed interpretations of the equations of fluid dynamics developed from 1827-1845 by Navier, Poisson, Venant, and Stokes. Using the equations below, a predetermined Aquatoner surface configuration, a measured distance of movement, and the time it took for one specific movement in a uniform direction, all simplified equations produced the same result in pounds of exerted force.

$$F = \frac{C_d \, A \rho \, V^2}{2}$$

$$F = 0.5 \, C_d \, V^2 \rho \, A$$

$$F = \frac{C_d \, A \, (1.93 \times V^2)}{2}$$
(for water @ 80º to 100ºF)

$$F = 0.5 \times 1.3 \times 1.93 \times A \times V^2$$
(When estimating Cd = 1.3 at typical Re's)
(Huong, 2000)

Drag force = half the drag coefficient x the water density x the square of the velocity x the surface area of the front profile.

Conversion Formulae

$°C = (°F-32) \div 1.8$
$°F = (°C \times 1.8) + 32$

mph = x 0.621
km/h = mph x 1.61
mph = ft/s x 0.682
ft/s = mph x 1.47
mph = m/s x 2.24
m/s = mph x 0.453

ft = m x 3.25
m = ft x 0.308

lb = kg x 2.205
kg = lb x 0.454

newton (N) ⇒ lbs force = x 0.225
lbs force ⇒ N = x 4.448
grams force ⇒ N = x 0.01

All conversions can be obtained at www.onlineconversions.com

Chapter 12
Floating into Therapy

Universal Gravity

There is no escape from gravity. It permeates the universe in various concentrations under the influence of mass and distance. Water does not eliminate gravity. Water provides a greater density than air, one that is similar to the density of our physical bodies which are composed mainly of water. We can adjust our density by inhaling or exhaling air, by increasing lean muscle mass that has a higher density than water, or by adding adipose tissue which has a lower density than water. Oil floats. Our environmental and bodily densities can change and our own relationship with the mass of this planet can change but we cannot increase or decrease gravity. It is beyond our control. Gravity is here to stay, on land, in the air, in space, in the water.

A graviton is a packet of gravity in the way a photon is a packet of light. Both forces are described by quanta with integral spin. A photon has one unit of spin. A graviton has two units of spin. Matter is made of quarks and leptons with a half unit of spin. My view is that all these particles in the universe can be completely unified in the form of supersymmetry demonstrated with complex equations containing hundreds of terms in the equations. Supersymmetry can only exist, however, at the moment the universe changes from dormant potential to everything, when energies are instantly enormous.

A single force of explosive genesis begins as vibrations of multi-dimensional hyperspace with trillions of degrees of heat. It is an emitter of an opaque fog of radiation. The vibrations include forces and subatomic particles. After time, cooling, spreading, and dissipating the radiation changes to a lower frequency, and condensation produces subatomic particles that begin to organize into stable atoms of hydrogen. Light particles are then able to travel between them. The forces within the vibrations include:

electromagnetic, including electricity, magnetism, and light; strong nuclear forces that fuel the stars like our sun; weak nuclear forces in radioactive decay; and gravitational force, a very weak yet plentiful force in the universe that holds planets in orbit and keeps a galaxy or clusters of galaxies together during continued cooling. There is continued development of atomic elements using increasingly diverse groups of subatomic particles.

According to Cambridge Mathematics Professor Sephen W. Hawking (1990) extremely small black holes are numerous, two or three per cubic light year. Gravity always wins in the universe. Matter gravitates into black holes. They are the size of a proton yet weigh a billion tons. Exploding stars yield black holes. The center cores of some galaxies are gigantic black holes. With energy going into the production of radiation and particle emission, the gravitational field of some of the smallest black holes with life expectancies of a brief ten billion years weakens and they explode into high-energy gamma rays. Then they are not black holes. I believe they become the beginnings of their own universes. Potentially, this happens to the large black holes too but the time needed is considerably greater than the present age of our contemporary universe. See Chapter 9, *Kealawai (The Path of Water)*, for more on this subject.

Buoyancy

The most accurate scale to calculate lean body mass or body density is hydrostatic. A person is weighed on a scale underwater. He or she exhales all air out of the lungs and carefully totally submerges for the seconds it takes to measure the weight. For accuracy, the water must be stagnant.

The submerged person in the procedure above still has weight. Gravity is not eliminated in water. Gravity is always there pulling towards the Earth's core. The moon is also continually pulling, creating high and low tides in our oceans. If a person in a pool wears a foam flotation belt, gravity is still there, unchanged. What is added is an

opposing force that is greater than the gravitational force, buoyancy. If there were no gravity, the person would float into space.

If you have two magnets of equal strength with the same poles facing each other and they are equidistant from a steel ball bearing, the ball bearing will not move. But if one of the magnets has a slightly stronger force, the ball bearing will begin to move slowly towards the stronger magnet with increasing velocity. That doesn't mean that the smaller magnet's force has vanished. If it had, the ball bearing would have moved very swiftly from the start. Instead the original forces are unchanged. So too is gravity in a body of water.

Standing on buoyancy devices in the water can assist the development of balance. Adding flotation to the body core is a good method to allow the legs to move freely without floor contact, or to suspend the body in a supine position when the flotation is added under the neck and knees. Partial buoyancy lessens weight bearing on the joints. If a person

without added buoyancy goes into deeper and deeper water while walking on the pool floor, they effectively weigh less and less up until complete submergence; after that their effective weight will remain the same regardless of depth.

If one person has more adipose tissue and less lean muscle mass than another person, they will have more buoyancy since the density of the adipose tissue is less than water, and the density of lean muscle mass is higher than water. Stability of the feet on the pool floor is an inverse proportion to a person's natural buoyancy. The stability can be adjusted by being deeper or shallower, by wearing flotation or by adding weights.

Unless a person is exercising in water to passively isolate range of motion for a limb with the assistance of flotation, or to re-learn balance, buoyancy devices should be restricted to the torso and worn around the center of the body. Buoyancy out on an appendage restricts natural movement. It interferes with the forces applied by the person exercising. Confining buoyancy to the core area allows more natural movements uncontrolled by the influences of anything other than a persons' own musculature, connective tissue, and body mechanics.

Hydrotherapy

In the archaic New World, Sioux hunters and Navajo farmers stumbled upon pure thermal mineral waters erupting and most probably couldn't resist a foot soak. Ah, what relief hydrotherapy offered the hunter, causing reflex actions to many organs and other parts of the body. When the Indian came upon cold springs there was another foot soak. The sensation was different. It was stimulating and the reflex action was much longer lasting. Without a written language it remained an undocumented feeling, passed on to others only in conversation, as a carving, petroglyph, or other form of expression. What we today call reflexology, shiatsu, myofascial release, structural integration, Thai stretches, Rolfing, Trager , cranio-

sacral therapy, Swedish tapotement, Reiki, Feldenkrais Method, Alexander Technique, neuromuscular therapy, polarity, these and many other therapeutic modalities were given and recieved in and next to the hot springs with unknown or local identifying nomenclature. There is nothing new in massage and aquatic therapy.

At the opposite side of the globe, Egyptians constructed bath chambers for health and rituals thousands of years ago. Then, very ancient Greeks created luxurious hot public baths. The Greeks developed the therapeutic use of water between 3400 and 3700 years ago (Barron, 1995). Some of the bath ruins are still standing on Crete. About 400BC Hippocrates and Celsius recorded their studies on their development of the therapeutic use of water for healing many diseases. Hippocrates knew and reported that the human body has a powerful capacity for self-healing (Buchman, 2002). The information about his aquatic work was preserved in monasteries and in Arabic libraries, documenting the use of cold baths

combined with friction massage to treat fevers, inflammations, gout, rheumatism and other acute and chronic disease.

In the remainder of this section I will summarize many current hydrotherapies as described by Buchman (2002), Barron (1995), and in courses I attended at Western Illinois University and at the Atlanta School of Massage. Cold water applications are at temperatures of 40-55° F (4.4-12.8°C). Hot water applications are at temperatures of 100°-113° F (38-45°C).

*F*ighting a forest fire in Alaska was a dirty job. Some of the battles lasted for over a month. Imagine a month of dirt and sweat without a bath. After one such experience, two Indians from Ft. Yukon and I came upon a large, clear, pond outside the fire perimeter. We knew what we had to do. Within seconds we were all undressed and jumping into the water. The water was on top of permafrost 365 days a year so I would say it was borderline ice. In less than a minute I was flying out of the water so fast my heart was ready to stop. It was more than refreshing and there were leeches from the bottom were clinging to my feet. Hypothermia is a dangerous, near-death experience. I would never join a "Polar Bear" club for an annual deep-dip into water below 40° F.

What I learned was that it takes a while for body heat alone to warm cold muscles and connective tissue to their normal temperature. If added heat is applied the change in tissue temperature is much faster. As a massage therapst I have used this contrast concept successfully where it was needed on clients many times to move tissue temperatures to their comfortable extremes.

><((((O>   ><((((O>   ><((((O>

A short cold running water footbath is a treatment for insomnia, chronic fatigue syndrome, and depression. A prolonged cold footbath treats sprains and inflamed bunions. A short warm footbath treats circulation problems and is a preparation for cold footbaths. A hot footbath relieves foot

and leg cramps, menstrual cramps, neuralgic pains, and like cold it treats insomnia. Hot is a preparation for cold.

Alternating hot and cold applications as a contrast treatment on painful or injured parts of the body are remarkably successful when the hot water precedes cold, when the cold water treatment is ¼ the duration of the hot, and when the treatment ends with cold. Contrasting back and forth from cold to hot increases blood flow 100% when all extremities are treated and 70% when the lower extremities only are treated (Buchman, 2002). One minute cold followed by four minutes hot in a continuous sequence for as long as a half hour makes an ideal contrast between repeated vasoconstriction and vasodilation. Vasoconstriction is rapid while vasodlation is slower. The objective is to widen the relative blood flow rate between the two so the change in flow becomes greater. Heat may be used locally to pull blood from a distant area, increasing its flow in the direction of the heat application. This is called derivation. When cold

application is used to reduce accumulation of blood in a local area and increase it in another area, it is called depletion. The act of using cold to move blood away from an area towards internal organs is called retrostasis. A good example of combining derivation with retrostasis is a hydrotherapeutic method of treating a high blood pressure headache. Blood is diverted from the head towards the feet by soaking the feet in a hot bath while applying moist cold to the head. The blood quantity is then relocated away from the head and distributed to the internal body core. The headache disappears.

Hydrotherapy manipulates circulation to achieve homeostasis through thermal applications. The response of the person being treated to thermal waters causes healing. Water conducts heat quickly to or from the body and changes the characteristics of blood flow. Blood flows toward heat and away from cold. Optimum treatment employs both derivation and retrostasis. Derivation and retrostasis can be used simultaneously and collaterally where arterial trunks split into deep and superficial arteries. A single application of hot water prepares for a more powerful single treatment of cold water with revulsive effects. The arterial trunk reflex occurs when heat dilates an arterial trunk and as a consequence also dilates distal arterial branches of the trunk.

Reflex points are more successfully stimulated when thermal applications are concentrated and focused in a small area and when either the cold or heat application is greater in terms of temperature and duration. An expectoration reflex results from heat to the chest. After a meal the digestive reflex and increased gastric secretion follow abdominal heat application if the temperature is mild. Spinal cord reflexes are also successful using reflex points on the skin (Buchman, 2002).

Cold constricts blood vessels. Heat dilates them. Ischemia can be caused by the functional constriction of a blood vessel or by obstruction. In either case, cold can be dangerous if there is ischemia because cold is constricting and restricts blood flow. Heat makes it flow faster. Heat increases hemorrage and cold slows it down. Cold increases blood viscosity while heat thins the blood. Carbon dioxide accumulates in the blood when flow is restricted. Oxygen reaches more tissue when flow is increased. Cold slows pain and touch neurons and heat speeds up nerve function. In most cases, except when swelling is initiated by prostaglandins, cold reduces edema. Heat aggravates inflammation. Cold slows healing by decreasing the metabolic rate. Heat speeds healing by increasing the metabolic rate. Cold is more deeply felt than heat. Cold increases the rate of breathing because of the accumulated carbon dioxide. Heat slows breathing because blood flow is more efficient and oxygen is more plentiful. A simplified explanation is that cold application reduces fatigue and stimulates the body while heat causes relaxation. Cold stimulates the movement of bowels, but heat slows the movement. Cold reduces sensations of the skin. Heat elevates the sense of touch. Cold slows reflex and heat promotes a faster reflex. If too much heat or too much cold is applied for a prolonged time, both can damage tissues. Muscle spasms respond positively to heat which reduces metabolites in the muscle, not to cold. Trauma that produces inflammation and consequent pain responds positively to initial cold treatment, not heat. Arthritis, with one exception, responds favorably to heat, not cold. Acute rheumatoid arthritis also responds favorably to cold. Mild heat and mild cold are sedative while extreme heat and extreme cold stimulate the autonomic nervous system.

Moving, swirling, direct hot water promotes the relief of chronic pain more than stagnant water (Buchman, 2002). If not in the superior environment of a natural hot spring, a man-made whirlpool will do.

Herbs, minerals, and nutrients can be added to baths to promote health. Added sulphur reduces to sulphurated hydrogen and is a powerful antiseptic for the skin.

Added ascorbic acid (vitamin C) heals hemorrhoids.

A tonic friction bath is taken in cold stimulating water using friction massage with a loofa sponge, mitten, brush, or salt crystals. The increased circulation promotes internal self-healing. This is known today and it was known by Hypocrates 2400 years ago. It is most useful for weak and bedridden people.

Hot water can be dangerous. It systemically elevates blood pressure because there is a shift in lymph fluid from tissues to the blood vessels, increasing blood volume. Heart rate and pulse rate increase and remain high for a while after leaving the water. Acutely injured tissue can be further damaged with heat if it is applied less than 72 hours after an injury. Arteriosclerosis is a contraindication for hot baths because weak vessel walls would be exposed to increased blood flow. More than occasional use of hot baths is also contraindicated for individuals with impaired urine flow because the heat normally increases urine production.

Applying hot water to the skin results in vasodilation and increased blood flow. Remember that "hot" refers to a temperature range of 100 - 113° F maximum (38-45°C). Increased nutrient transport to the skin and the superficial muscles leads to healing and the removal of accumulated pain-causing metabolites. Joint capsules and tendons become more stretchable from heat. This increases range of motion where collagen tissues have been shortened by scar tissue from injury. Range of motion can increase by as much as 20% after hot water immersion of the area at 113° F (45°C). (Barron, 1995).

A lot is going on in the spinal cord, too. There are nerve fibers in parallel paths through the length of the spinal cord. Some carry messages about pain sensations that originate from peripheral nerve organs called nociceptors. Others control skeletal muscle contraction or internal organs. Others still – the Golgi tendon organs called proprioceptors – monitor body positions. There are touch receptors on the skin that send messages to the brain. Temperature differences are sensed through their own nerve tracts. These neurons are all parallel to each other and in very close proximity. When two different kinds of nerve impulses are traveling at the same time, one impulse can be dominant. In the case of hot water immersion, neurons that carry the messages of elevated temperature dominate the pain pathways. The result is analgesia. Muscle spasms subside. Joint pain temporarily fades away and internal organs that are in pain become calm.

Rehabilitation

It's time to put this all together for one of the most important uses of your knowledge, aquatic rehabilitation.

We will begin in 1984, on a long bus journey from the West Coast to the East Coast with nothing more than a bicycle, a backpack, a trunk of tools, and an idea. George Orwell's 1984 predictions hadn't happened so there was freedom to be an entrepreneur. With the idea to start manufacturing the Aquatoner, I descended from the alpine mountain-tops of Idyllwild, California, and brought the project to some of the oldest mountains in the world, found on North Carolina's Cherokee Indian Reservation in southern Appalachia. There I was encouraged by Chief Robert S. Youngdeer to develop an aquatic exercise program for the tribe. With the generous help of Jim Cooper, owner of the reservation's Holiday Inn with its large pool, I settled into a cabin. From there I would bike up and down the hills to and from the pool. Carving the first Aquatoners out of wood was time consuming, but an inventory accumulated and there was a motivated group of people wanting to participate in classes. First came Jim Cooper's elderly mother with osteoarthritis. Then came people from Jim's church with rheumatoid arthritis, cardio-respiratory deficiencies and other needs. Then came other business owners needing various kinds of exercise. The word was getting around Cherokee that something good was happening at the Holiday Inn pool. Everyone paid for their aquatic exercise sessions and began to purchase Aquatoners.

The Cherokee Health Delivery System contracted the Aquatoning Program to serve clients from the tribal sheltered workshop, some of whom were the mentally and physically challenged. They came by bus every day. There was a pool full of people from 6AM until late afternoon. Adding to the group were people from the surrounding communities in the Smokey Mountains: Sylva, Bryson City, Andrews, and Whittier. Each had disabilities with adaptive needs.

An older couple brought in their thirty-five year old daughter who had been in a wheelchair most of fifteen years, unable to take one step because of advanced multiple sclerosis. It was a long drive for them to get to the pool. They had tried many physical therapists in Western North Carolina but Jennifer didn't feel they did anything for her, so there she was being lifted to the water from her wheelchair, first time in a pool. She was nervous at first and wanted to please me but couldn't do much of anything except lean against the pool wall in shoulder deep water while I caught her first on one side and then the other as she lost balance.

Casual conversation made her more comfortable so that she was then able to be still and not tip over. Her parents brought her every day, seven days a week, luckily at a time when few other participants were in the pool, so I could give her more or less undivided attention. By that time the sheltered workshop group had finished their day's session and departed in their bus. After a while, many of the people that started had their own equipment and knew what they were doing so all I had to do was offer encouragement at the right time, monitor their progress, and demonstrate new exercises when they were ready for them.

After a week of getting accustomed to being in the deeper water, leaning against the pool wall, being on her feet, and weighing next to nothing, Jennifer began to move. At first it started as a leg lift. When I saw she could lift her foot off of the pool floor an inch I knew we had made a start. Although she would never recover from the damage to the insulating sheaths that once surrounded her nerves, atrophy had been a greater enemy than the MS. My question was: How much of her disability was due to MS and how much was from the disuse atrophy and extensive muscle weakness that prevented her from overcoming the gravitational weight of her own legs? It was a beginning. The Iliopsoas muscles, extremely weak, were still functioning and able to start to flex the femur when the water buoyed the weight of her legs. That was where we started.

We developed an exercise routine for her whole body. Part of the time I would have to hold her upright. The movements were brief, weak, and had limited range of motion, but Jenny was determined to get the most out of it and looked forward eagerly to her time in the pool every day. In two months she was using the Aquatoner in it's smallest (lowest resistance) configuration for all the exercises.

Then we began adding resistance. I attached the Aquatoner to the bottom of one foot around the metatarsal arch and she struggled to lift her leg, then we repeated this on the other leg. As the months went by she could lift her legs higher and higher. One day I put Aquatoners on both feet at the same time, and lifted her into a horizontal position to do a bicycle type motion with her legs. It was a disaster. There was no coordination between the legs. She persisted the following days and coordination gradually improved over a period of weeks. Now we were onto something, both legs going in circles with increasing Aquatoner resistance. We measured all exercises with time, 1-2 minutes to achieve a perceived near maximal effort, not a certain number of repetitions. It was truly a routine for muscle endurance, not pure strength or aerobics.

Full body exercise continued with an emphasis on the bicycle exercise. After the first year of this I asked Jennifer to walk towards me, still in shoulder deep water, holding my hands and facing me. She would fall from side to side, dragging her MS-

afflicted legs toward me. I could feel much unsteadiness in her hands. She was embarrassed about the whole thing, considering that other people were around. But they kept her motivated. She did well and used every ounce of her effort to become stronger. During that second year, in the ten minutes of water walking after each workout, I began to guide her to shallower water little by little, day by day, allowing gravity to creep into the routine almost unnoticeably. After nearly two years of aquatic exercise and assisted water walking, there was a day when things automatically happened. As Jennifer walked forward we both suddenly and gently let go of the other's hands and there she was momentarily on her own, independent and mobile. But then balance and coordination took a giant step backwards - she had been totally dependent on holding my hands as she walked and so she stumbled. However it was worth the stumble because in subsequent sessions she began to make rapid improvement, walking in very shallow waist deep water with 60% of her body weight on the pool floor, totally on her own, back and forth, from one side of the pool to the other while I was at a considerable distance. Jennifer's smile from that moment on was worth the many months of work. She was walking on her own. Yes it was in water, and no she never could do the same thing on land, but she smiled and life was fun. It was self-mobility and independence for Jennifer.

Eight-six-year old arthritic client Myrtle Cooper, Jim Cooper's mother, was another success story for aquatic therapy. She progressed from a slow moving walker, to a cane, to dancing at her family's Christmas Party all within six months. A Hoyer hoist with a soft sling seat was installed at the poolside for her to get in and out of the water. She would sit in that hoist and do the two-Aquatoner bicycle exercise, splashing and laughing. Her progress was more rapid than Jenny's but just as much fun. It took a while to coordinate the reciprocal movements of arms and legs, swinging the arms, because, using a walker for all those years, her body had forgotten how to walk naturally. We too would walk after each workout but we would walk on land.

Two Cherokee Indians from the sheltered workshop had particularly successful experiences in the Aquatoning program. One man had a disfigured, atrophied left arm from cerebral palsy. Using an Aquatoner attached to the forearm, he worked on his deltoid muscles over a period of eighteen months until the left shoulder became sufficiently normal to give him a symmetrical appearance. The other man was deaf, had lost a leg just below the knee to diabetes, and couldn't walk without prosthesis. He attached an Aquatoner to his remaining thigh to develop his hip flexors, extensors, adductors, and abductors and learned to walk better with his prosthesis.

Aquatic rehabilitation has a very bright side. The above examples are a testament to the rewards. As a therapist, never give up on a patient or client. Willpower is stronger than our infirmities.

Before Cherokee, back in Idyllwild, I put together a long bar with triple paddles on the ends (Fig.181). All I could do with this "Aquatoning Bar" was use it for conventional exercises like a barbell in the weight room or like a canoe paddle. It was great for pulling and pushing, lifting a ton of water straight up out of the pool, and generally making waves to impress onlookers. Bringing the bar idea to Cherokee in 1984 led to a more comprehensive discovery of it's therapeutic potentials by allowing some of the stroke patients to utilize the device for carefully controlled self-destabilization and re-stabilization, an effective method to relearn balance and proprioception.

><((((O>   ><((((O>   ><(((O>

While some aquatic activities are more effective with assistance, there are times when a client's self-discovery and independent feel of progress are most beneficial. Positive changes are more permanent when the client decisions is allowed to fully participate in decisions such as how hard to push, how large to set the paddle configuration, how far to comfortably reach an appendage in any direction, or what needs to be repeated. If they feel that they are making some of those important decisions, they are truly participating in the therapy and results come quicker.

Whether working aquatically for improved range of motion, core stability, coordination of authentic movement, increased strength, power, cardiac stamina, increased circulation, connective tissue stretching, or muscle endurance, the endurance factor should have priority amidst all of the above for well-rounded physical rehabilitation. The most effective approach to serve clients is interdisciplinary.

Certain disorders contraindicate high-intensity, vigorous exercise. High velocity, for example, is not prescribed for osteoarthritis patients in physical therapy. While low to moderate activity is beneficial and safe for patients with autonomic or peripheral neuropathy, high intensity exercise can cause foot problems due to vascular insufficiency that may

accompany peripheral neuropathy, and inadequate thermoregulatory capacity can cause hypotension and hypertension patients with autonomic neuropathy (Colberg and Swain, 2000). Exercise itself reduces the development of hypertension and stroke (Kiely, 1994).

The reduced blood viscosity during deep-water immersion described in Chapter 3 lowers the proportion of blood protein. During unloaded aquatic movement, the contrast of the lower viscosity with higher protein concentrations in the synovial fluid of cartilaginous abrasions promotes filtration, regeneration, and healing (Lieb, 2003).

During one hour of neck-deep aquatic therapy, the spinal column lengthens approximately 2 cm due partially to fluid engorgement of the intervertebral discs (Lieb, 2003) because blood supply is optimized and the anti-gravity muscles relax. This helps release pressure on nerve roots and vertebral mobility is improved. Departing the pool safely requires preparation because of this

hypermobility and hypotonicity. Prior to coming back to full gravitational influence on the spine, prepare the postural musculature by contracting and tensing all the major muscles. Avoid spinal twisting and rapid turning or bending movements for a while. Depart the water slowly to avoid dizziness, and drink ample amounts of water with added electrolytes if possible. A cold shower on the legs improves the tone of the muscles in their veins. It is helpful for those with varicose veins to elevate the legs for a while after exiting the pool.

Improved joint articulation is the primary reason why aquatic strength and endurance conditioning is prescribed for patients at orthopedic and physical therapy clinics. The therapy typically involves the low back, the knee, or the rotator cuff. This book works with examples rather than every part of the entire body. It is assumed that you are prepared with comprehensive anatomy books to extend this learning process to all parts of the body. In the section on joint articulations, you will find the example I have chosen is the rotator cuff and shoulder. The rotator cuff is not one muscle. It is sometimes confused with the anterior, lateral, or posterior deltoid or with the biceps tendon long head where it passes through the intertubercular bicipital groove at the proximal humerus. aBicipital tendinitis is a common location of tendonous frictional overuse microtearing. The rotator cuff may also be confused with the triceps brachii at its origin.

There are functional assessments used to identify and differentiate rotator cuff injury, chronic strain damage, tendon impingements, tendinitis, bursitis, subluxations, dislocations, adhesive capsulitis and other regional syndromes. Each condition has its own diagnostic testing and treatment. There are the Speed's Test, the Drop Arm Test, the Hawkins-Kennedy Impingement Test, the Empty Can Test, and the Apley Scratch Test among others. Physical therapists will be familiar with the appropriate assessments and treatments.

Rotator cuff injuries are most common to the muscles that insert above and below the spine of the scapula. The injuries result from repeated eccentric loading of the humerus during such typical activities as serving in tennis. pitching, lifting barbells overhead or swinging a hammer overhead. The purpose of the rotator cuff is to hold the humerus in the glenoid fossa of the scapula. Aquatic resistance conditioning is at the top of the treatment list for all of the conditions mentioned in the previous paragraph.

Physical therapists measure range of motion (ROM) in degrees of an angle by using a goniometer. In my view, this can be measured more conveniently in a pool from using radians (Figure 167). A radian(or rad) is the central angle of a circle whose subtended arc is equal to the radius of the circle. Full circumference is about 6.3 rads (2π). A normal healthy full range of motion for hip or shoulder abduction and adduction in water seems to be over 1 rad. In some aquatic situations it is not convenient to use a goniometer to measure ROM.

Using the symbols in Figure 167, the formula for calculating ROM angle in radians is: $M = a/r$, where M = ROM angle, r = the radius, and a = the lengthy of the arc made at the tip of the radius.

Converting to degrees of an angle is the product of rads x 57.3°, the constant for 1 rad.

Example 1: The distance from the shoulder joint (superior glenoid fossa) to the elbow (olecranon process) on a patient is 14". The motion is shoulder abduction. The patient can move the elbow through an arc of only 9". In this example r = 14"; a = 9", M = a/r = 9/14; ROM = 0.64 radians.

Example 2: Calculate hip ROM in cm where r = 51cm, a = 76cm, M =a/r = 51/76; ROM = 0.67 radians.

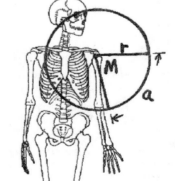

**(Figure 167)
Radians**

Igor Burdenko and The Burdenko Institute

Igor In an interview for *Nalu* I asked 64-year old Dr. Igor N. Burdenko about his early years in Russia. Out of all the information online about this extraordinary individual, there is nothing to be found about his childhood. How did he become the person known throughout the world as the one to coalesce sports medicine with aquatics?

"My parents told me that I started swimming before I started walking. What I liked most as a child were all outdoor sports. I participated in a lot of soccer, speed skating and cross-country running." You can see that Dr. Burdenko has a solid foundation in endurance.

Young Igor grew up in the rugged Ural Mountains during World War II. He was an only child for his first twelve years, then he had a baby brother. "I did not have any toys," said Dr. Burdenko as he traveled far back into his memory. "My toys were rocks and sticks. They are perfect for exercise. I still design many programs using materials from nature for exercise. I experience rocks and sticks differently than the way most people do." This is from a childhood without conventional toys. What he did have was far more valuable. It was the opportunity to develop an interest in his natural environment in the Ural Mountains and to find practical uses for objects in the forest around him. With an intuitive mind, young Igor created exercise devices out of variously shaped tree branches and different sizes of rocks. This was his entertainment.

"Life is complicated enough. I like simple things. I never had a bicycle until six years ago."

At the N. K. Krupskaya State Pedagogical University in Moscow, Dr. Burdenko received his Ph.D. in Sports Medicine and his M.S. in Physical Education. He is the founder and chairman of the Burdenko Water and Sports Therapy Institute. He has worked as a rehabilitation and training consultant, is on the board of directors of the National Youth Sports Safety Foundation for the Prevention of Athletic Injuries and is a member of the Aquatic Exercise Association Research Committee.

Dr. Burdenko has authored or co-authored four books and over one hundred articles on training, conditioning, health and fitness. He presents seminars and lectures throughout the world and consults on the design and start-up of therapeutic facilities. Lecturing extensively as he does, it is hard to believe that this excellent communicator feels that his greatest failure in life was not learning formal English in school as a child. "My wife, Irina, was a university professor of English and I still did not make the effort to improve. I didn't make enough effort to learn the language. When I first came to the US it set me back for quite a while."

Founded in 1984, The Burdenko Institute has been dedicated to healing programs that combine traditional and alternative therapies.

The Institute was also established to provide health professionals with a means of certifying their knowledge of the Burdenko Method: a unique, innovative system for rapid conditioning and injury prevention.

Balance training, range of motion exercises, biomechanical training, strengthening and gait training are available through his rehabilitation process. Dr. Burdenko is an advocate of water as a unique environment in which the effects of gravity are minimized and the effects of buoyancy take over, allowing for non-weight bearing and partially weight bearing exercises. "This allows individuals to use the water to assist or resist their movements at a pace they can tolerate."

The Burdenko Method focuses on the **qualities of movement** and is a lifestyle approach to health and fitness. Described as a pyramid beginning with rehabilitation, restoring the center of balance is the foundation at the base, to establish freedom to move the extremities without pain. The second level of the pyramid is the quality of optimal coordination, combining multi-directional movement with postural alignment. The third level is flexibility and pelvic stability with enhanced maneuverability. At the the top are endurance with total body alignment,

(Figure 168)

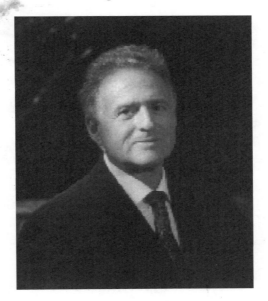

Igor N. Burdenko, Ph.D.

speed with proximal stability, and functional or sport-specific strength. The conditioning program progresses through three levels and the training program is geared for competitive, world-class athletes.

Dr. Burdenko says, "Exercises in the vertical position promote body awareness, postural control and movement patterns which have carryover to activities of daily living. An added benefit is that water therapy involves the use of the entire body, not just the injured part, thereby enhancing overall conditioning." On land and in the water, individuals at the Burdenko Institute are instructed in a progression of exercises that safely address their specific limitations and goals. The Burdenko Institute is in the Boston metropolitan area. For more information about certification in the Burdenko Method and about products used in these techniques go to http://www.burdenko.com.

Dr.Burdenko's writings:
Ultimate Power of Resistance, An American-Russian Approach to Fitness and Health. Igor Publishing, 1992,1998.
Overcoming Paralysis. Avery, 1999.

The Burdenko Exercise Guide, Part I, levels I-III .Igor Publishing, 2001.
The Burdenko Exercise Guide, Part II, levels IV-VI. *Igor Publishing, 2002.*
2 chapters attributed to **Artistry on Ice** with *Principal authors Nancy Kerrigan and Mary Spencer. Human Kinetic,. 2003.*
National Water Fitness Newsletter. *Articles throughout 1995. National Water Fitness Association.*

A client, Holly Chaplin, a resident of Key West, recently came to me for aquatic exercise sessions after undergoing therapy with Igor Burdenko at the Burdenko Institute. She had been in a high-speed head-on auto accident five months previously resulting in multiple leg and foot fractures. This is her story:

"I received extensive bilateral injuries to my legs in a car accident in the Florida Keys where the head-on collision trapped both feet in folded metal. I was airlifted from Florida to Massachusetts General Hospital Orthopedic Trauma Center in Boston for extensive surgeries. I was in the hospital for 1 ½ months feeling nausea and pain much of the time. PT exercises like quad sets were painful particularly in my hips and back because my right knee would only bend less than half way. Two months after surgery when the infection danger was over the last pins were removed from my left foot.
I signed up for aquatic therapy at the Burdenko Institute in Bedford, Massachusetts. My understanding was the Instutute's conditioning program of water and land exercises increases joint motion and muscle strength based on six essential skills: balance, coordination, flexibility, endurance, speed, and strength."

Dr. Burdenko shook his head while viewing my X-rays. He said the way this puzzle of bones was put together in alignment with numerous plates, pins and screw was a miracle. He asked about my objectives for rehab. I replied quietly, I want to run, I want to play tennis again! He looked pleased - a very different reaction than my operating physicians who told me I'd probably never run again. I instantly loved this man Burdenko."

The doctor guided me through some stretching and balancing on land on a half-round of foam beneath my spine. Our session was nearly over and I asked if I could get into the water. Wearing a water vest for flotation, I was wheeled down the pool ramp. The water rose around me. I slipped off the chair and maneuvered into the deep water. Tears streamed down my face. I felt supported, light, pain free for the first time in two months. I was off my butt floating happily in the 88-degree water. Igor asked me to cross walk, making my steps definite. This hurt and felt lopsided but I kept up the intention of lifting up from the pelvis and keeping my legs and feet beneath me. I walked in the deep water using force and control, moving forward then backward."

I knew this was just the beginning of my rehab but felt incredible achievement, moving with effort, energy, and success. That night I slept deeply for the first time in months. My dreams were peaceful. I'd found water."

Holly Chaplin is now simulating tennis moves in the pool, running in the water with a buoyancy vest, and exercising vigorously while working on balancing techniques. Thanks to Dr Burdenko, Holly is able to walk and is reaching her goals. It is helpful for clinical therapists to hear a patient's perspective on their rehabilitation. Christopher Reeve is also using aquatic therapy and we wish and anticipate success for him and for all people using water in their rehabilitation.

><((((O>   ><((((O>   ><((((O>

Arthritis Precautions

Arthritis hurts millions of people. Examinations are sometimes inadequate with results that are confusing to the patient. Medical treatment is not always successful. Prevention and relief leaves few options. Aquatic exercise is one of the few comfortable physical treatment options.

In osteoarthritis, there is degeneration of articular cartilage where bones meet other bones. It is the most prevalent joint disease in the United States, afflicting over 43 million Americans – a 20% increase in just the last decade. Rheumatoid arthritis is characterized by bone and cartilage damage from inflammation believed to be caused by a faulty immune system. Osteopenia, a low bone mass risk factor for osteoporosis, affects 54% of all postmenopausal women in the world (Kanis, 1994). The Arthritis Foundation in Atlanta, Georgia has a YMCA Aquatic Program that recommends daily joint exercise for all types of arthritis. The exercise should be resistive, slow but dynamic, without torsional stress, and through a full range of motion in warm water over 83° F (28.3°C).

Passive motion in warm water with a therapist certified by the Worldwide Aquatic Bodywork Association is also beneficial. To learn more about different types of bodywork in the pool that can relieve the discomforts of arthritis, see Chapter 2, *Aquatic Bodywork* by the founder of Healing Dance, Alexander Georgeakopoulos.

Be advised that for older aquatic muscle endurance class participants with arthritis in the wrist, holding exercise implements in their hands using a high resistance may not be safe. There is professional equipment that can be fastened to an arm for the upper body exercises to avoid a possibly harmful situation for those at risk of damaging their hands or wrist (Bedgood, 1988).

For further information about continuing education pool activities for arthritis, and easy-to-use products, contact the Arthritis Foundation at: 800-283-7800
www.arthritis.org
Arthritis Foundation
PO Box 7669
Atlanta, GA 30357-0669 USA

For subscriptions to *Arthritis Today:*
Customer Service Center
PO Box 4284
Pittsfield, MA 01202-4284 USA

For information about research grants and awards:
Research Department
Arthritis Foundation
1330 W. Peachtree St.
Suite 100
Atlanta, GA 30709 USA
404-872-7100

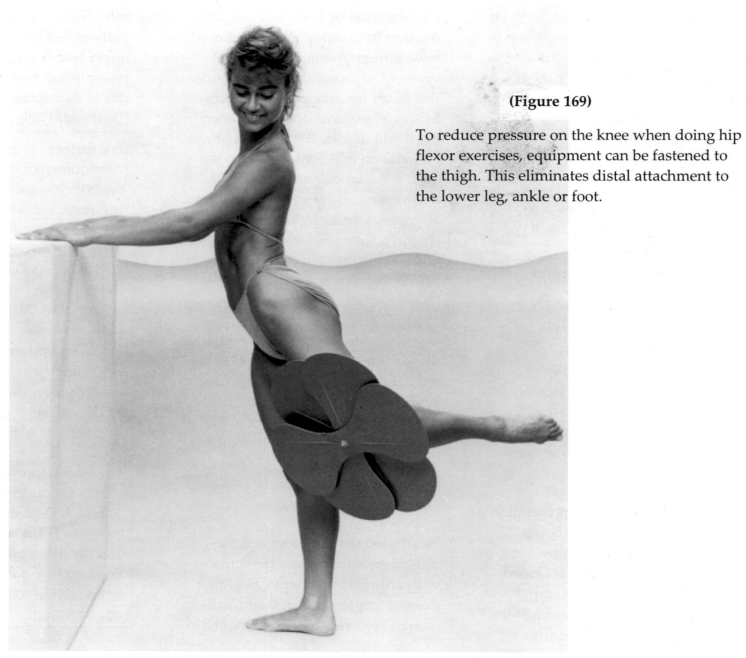

(Figure 169)

To reduce pressure on the knee when doing hip flexor exercises, equipment can be fastened to the thigh. This eliminates distal attachment to the lower leg, ankle or foot.

Nalu:The Art and Science of Aquatic Fitness, Bodywork & Therapy

Chapter 13 Paddling

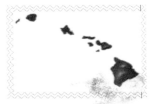

The Islands of Hawaii

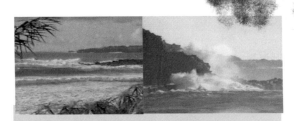

*I*t was the peak season

for outrigger canoe racing in Hawaii in 1981 when contestants in the double hull Liliuokalani International Long Distance Canoe Race were lining up for the start offshore from Keauhou Bay. Each entry was made up of two forty foot long koa log canoes connected by a common outrigger and manned by twelve paddlers.

Our canoe was the last to line up. Pierre Kimetete, our Tahitian coach, was a giant. He rode on the outrigger

as we paddled to the starting position while we tried to figure out a method of coordinating the strokes. We were quite unorganized at first until the timing was more synchronized between all twelve of us. We had to quickly determine which crewmembers would be paddling on the right or left side, and how the call commands would be used to change sides, all this as we paddled to the starting position for the big race. One thing we could count on as a crew was that we were all in top physical condition and anxious for the race to begin.

The paddlers in our Kouikeouli Canoe Club (Figure 175) were locals from the Big Island on the Kona coast, experienced from a lifetime of racing outrigger canoes, except for myself. I was the "houli," the newcomer from the mainland, quiet, humble, a fast learner, and determined obsessively to give it my best effort in every race. I sat at #2 in the hull on the right side in this race which was against canoe clubs mostly from other Hawaiian Islands as well as California, Australia and Tahiti.

As our twelve-man double hull canoe made of 840 pounds of koa wood propelled by 2000 pounds of muscle and twenty pounds of paddles approached the starting lineup , I began to join in with the calls of the stroker who sat at #1 in the left canoe. Out of the blue, during the second two calls out of the three the stroker used each time the crew changed paddling sides (every ten or twenty strokes), I intuitively joined in the call like it was an echo or a chant. The idea spread within seconds. Without any conversation between the crew we all knew that this was going to be a different race. The chanting unified us immediately. Pierre didn't know what to make of this. He dove off like a giant seal towards the escort boat. Being last to the starting line, we placed ourselves farthest from shore.

It was an "ironman" race (Figure171). There would be no relief paddlers on the escort boat. The gun sounded and the mighty first pull was pure power. After the first change, the other side was pure power. The sets continued at a rapid pace. After a couple of minutes we had used much of our stored glycogen and our breathing became deeper. Perceived maximal effort continued as the race became a powerful aerobic event.

Normally the #1 seat in front would call the changes. He was the stroker. The call would be one sound during the last two or three strokes in a set, something like "hey-hut," or "hee-hee-hey," The others would follow his timing and stroke while the #6 would steer and be the captain that would call out occasionally to a paddler who was off timing. The captain would encourage the crew.

W e had ten miles to go to get to Kailua Bay. Early on, I glanced towards all the other canoes that were spread out to our right, all in front of us. That was a shocker to be in back of the entire competition. How did we get into this situation?

We had some fast learning to do to get coordinated. As a crew, we had never practiced in a double hull

before. It was always six paddlers per canoe in the regattas and other long distance races. We were a strong club. There are two photos of winning crews in this chapter. Among the men, besides myself always wearing a torn white towel on my head for luck in the races, are two paddlers from Tahiti and one each from Hawaii, Canada and California. The women in the club were all from the Big Island. We were all lightweight, strong, and extremely fast. There were over 130 members in the Kouikeouli canoe club. Sometimes our crews would practice with one or two large truck tires over the front of the canoe to add tremendous resistance. Paddling is tremendous aquatic exercise. The coach would be standing out in the shallow water in the bay and as we passed, Pierre would decide to throw a tire over the long, slender front of the beautifully carved koa log canoe or over one of our fiberglass canoes and force us to work harder. We had power and endurance but every newly arranged crew had to relearn timing as a team. That was the problem and the chanting had to solve it or we would remain dead last.

All twelve of us contributed every ounce of effort and we approached each canoe in the race with our powerful chanting and intense focus until we passed them all, pulled clearly into the lead and won the race by a long distance (Figure 172B). That was the power of unity.

(Figure 170A)

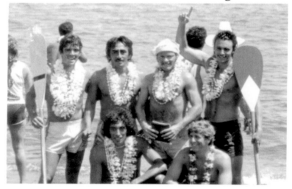

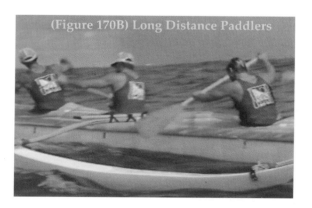

(Figure 170B) Long Distance Paddlers

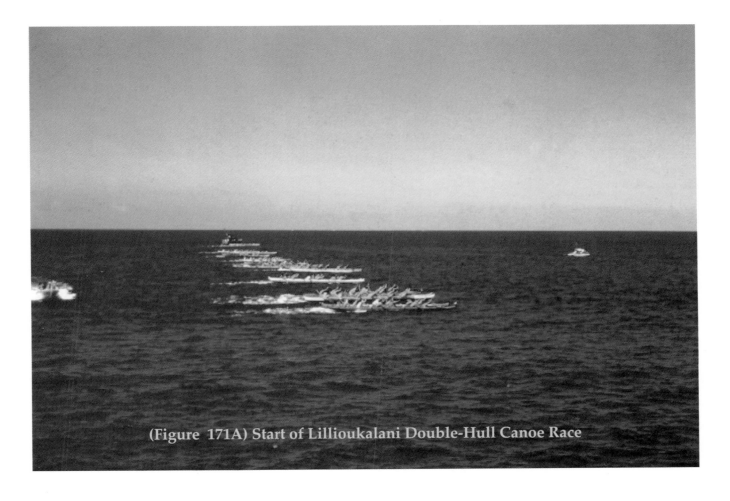

(Figure 171A) Start of Lillioukalani Double-Hull Canoe Race

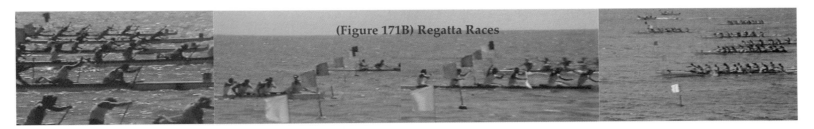

(Figure 171B) Regatta Races

Nalu: The Art and Science of Aquatic Fitness, Bodywork & Therapy

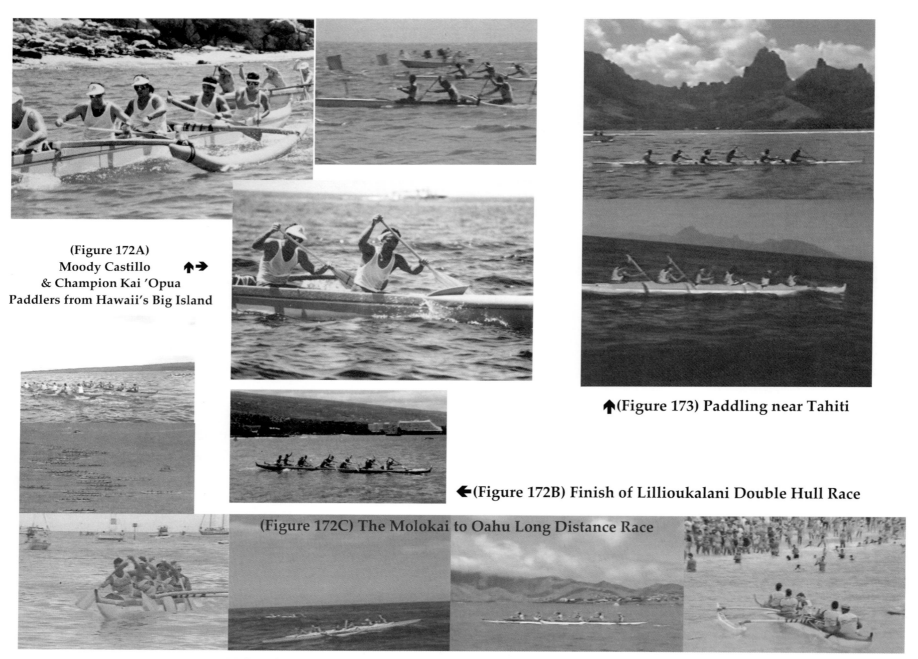

(Figure 172A)
Moody Castillo ↑➡
& Champion Kai 'Opua
Paddlers from Hawaii's Big Island

↑(Figure 173) Paddling near Tahiti

←(Figure 172B) Finish of Lillioukalani Double Hull Race

(Figure 172C) The Molokai to Oahu Long Distance Race

(Figure 174) Paddling Strokes

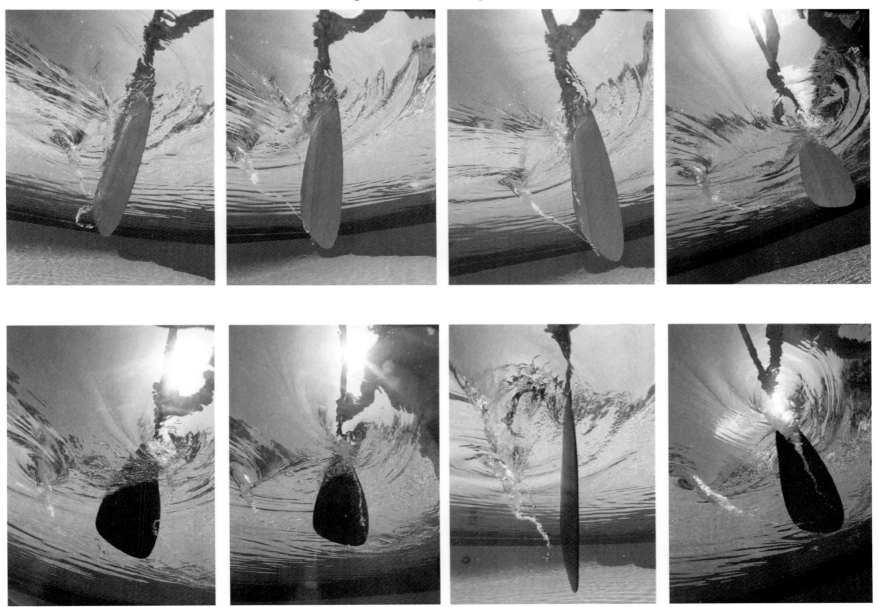

Nalu: The Art and Science of Aquatic Fitness, Bodywork & Therapy

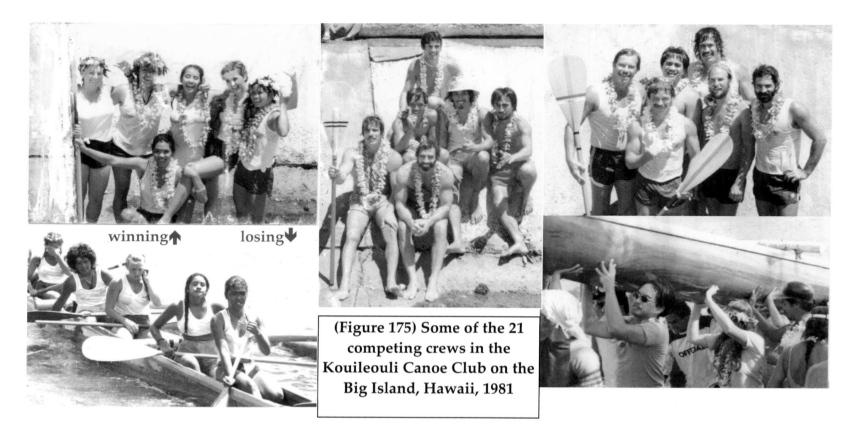

winning⬆   losing⬇

(Figure 175) Some of the 21 competing crews in the Kouileouli Canoe Club on the Big Island, Hawaii, 1981

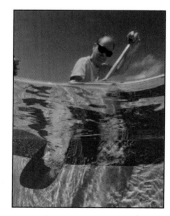

(Figure 176) The Author Practicing a Paddling Stroke

Nalu: The Art and Science of Aquatic Fitness, Bodywork & Therapy

Chapter 14
Water Boxing with Cassius Clay

In a Miami pool in 1960-61, nineteen-year-old Cassius Marcellus Clay dreamed of becoming the world heavyweight-boxing champion. Wearing a gold medal fresh from the Olympics, Clay knew he needed water to reach his dream. There was mighty competition in the professional sport and young Cassius was still an amateur.

In to the pool he went. With trainer Angelo Dundee, Cassius boxed in water for a year. In a 1961 issue of Life Magazine, after professional bout #8, Clay says, "They say I'm the fastest heavyweight in the ring today. That comes from punching under water." He explains, "You try to box hard. Then when you punch the same way out of the water you got speed." Clay also optimized his footwork underwater. "Speed's the main reason for it." said Clay, soon to call himself Muhammad Ali.

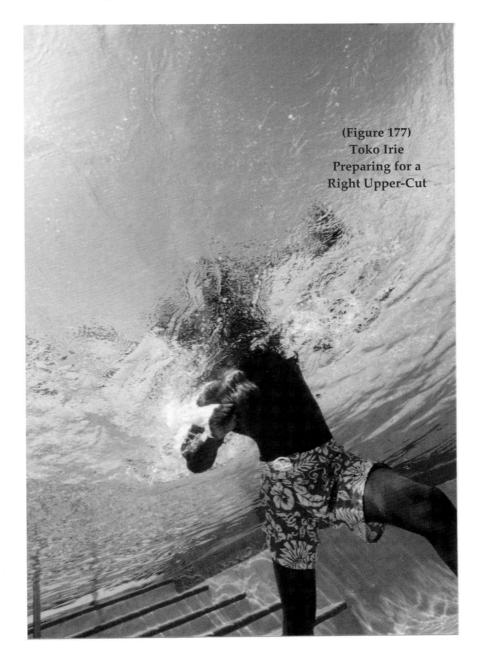

(Figure 177)
Toko Irie
Preparing for a
Right Upper-Cut

Nalu: The Art and Science of Aquatic Fitness, Bodywork & Therapy

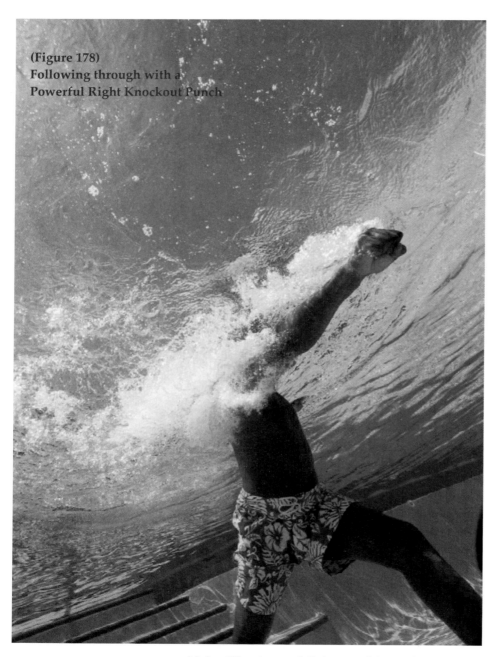

(Figure 178)
Following through with a
Powerful Right Knockout Punch

*A*li *floated in the ring*

with the strongest legs in the history of boxing. His trademark "Ali Shuffle" was literally born in the water. While doing an elevated and distracting speed-dance with fancy footwork he delivered a powerful punch to his opponent. The speed and grace of Muhammad Ali were unprecedented, developed as the young Cassius Clay boxing in water like Toko Irie from Grenada in these photographs (Fig.177-180). Ali was, in fact, the greatest fighter of all time, with a record of only five losses out of 61 professional bouts. He won thirty-seven of them with a knock out.

Today in Ali's personal office hangs a large print from the water boxing photos by Flip Schulke. They were included in Life Magazine in 1961 and in the Special Anniversary Issue, LIFE 50 Years, Volume 9, No.12, page 273-274 published in 1986. The photos are available at Black Star Productions, New York, 212-679-3288.

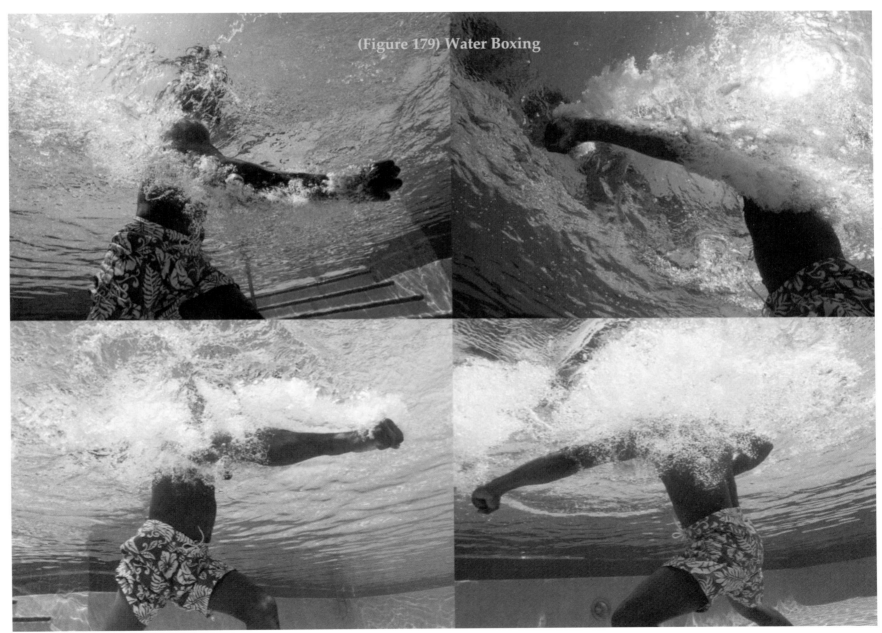

(Figure 179) Water Boxing

Nalu: The Art and Science of Aquatic Fitness, Bodywork & Therapy

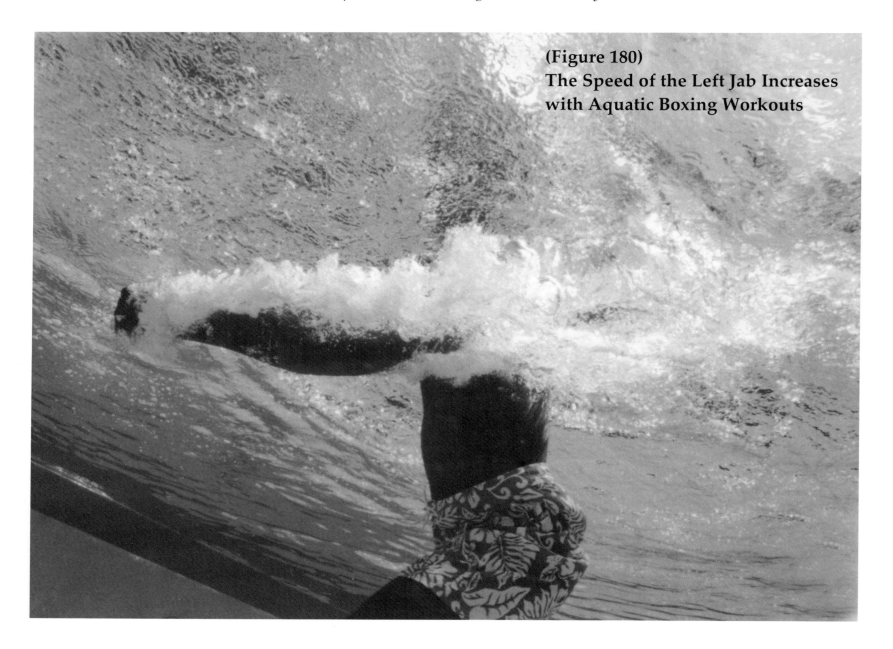

(Figure 180)
The Speed of the Left Jab Increases
with Aquatic Boxing Workouts

Chapter 15 Products, Books and Resources

This chapter is a sampling of excellent products from AquaTherapeutics, Aquatrend, Swimex, Hydrotone, Bioenergetics, HydroFit, Eureka Manufacturing, Aquatic Access, RehabMed, Rio Spas and others.

The Aquatoner

This triple paddle system has a adjustable resistive area over a wide range of 96-250 sq.in. The Aquatoner includes both a handle and a secure attachment for the foot, leg, arm, or disabled hand. The working surfaces are durable polymer or copolyester and the central hardware is stainless steel. A pair of Aquatoners comes with a lifetime warranty.

Text continued on page 349.

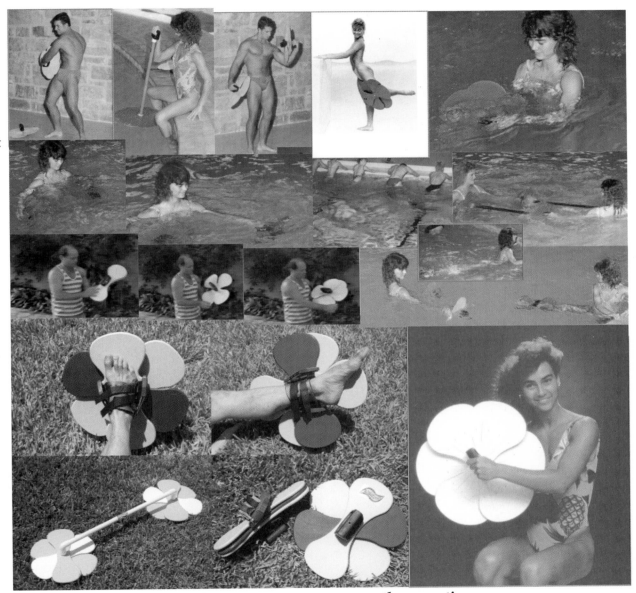

(Figure 181) Aquatoner: www.aquatherapeutics.com

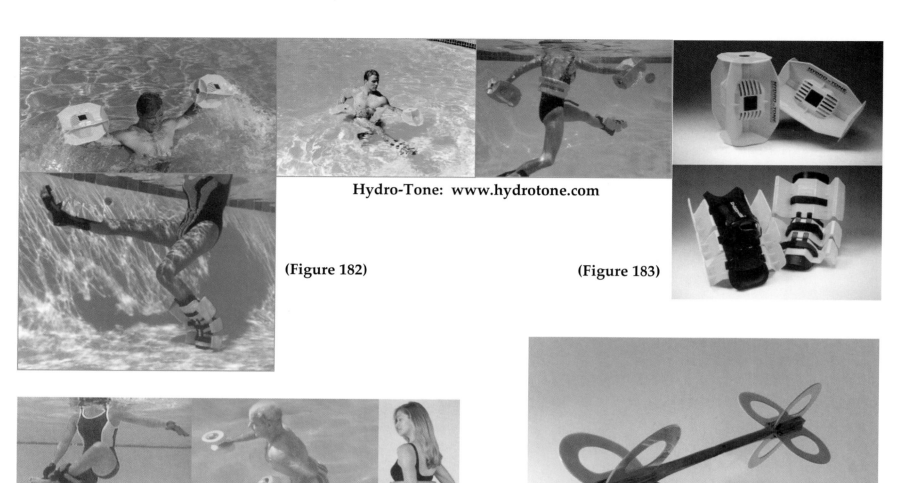

Hydro-Tone: www.hydrotone.com

(Figure 182)

(Figure 183)

(Figure 185) Shapeshifter: www.wavemocean.com

(Figure 184) Hydro Fit: www.hydrofit.com

Nalu: The Art and Science of Aquatic Fitness, Bodywork & Therapy

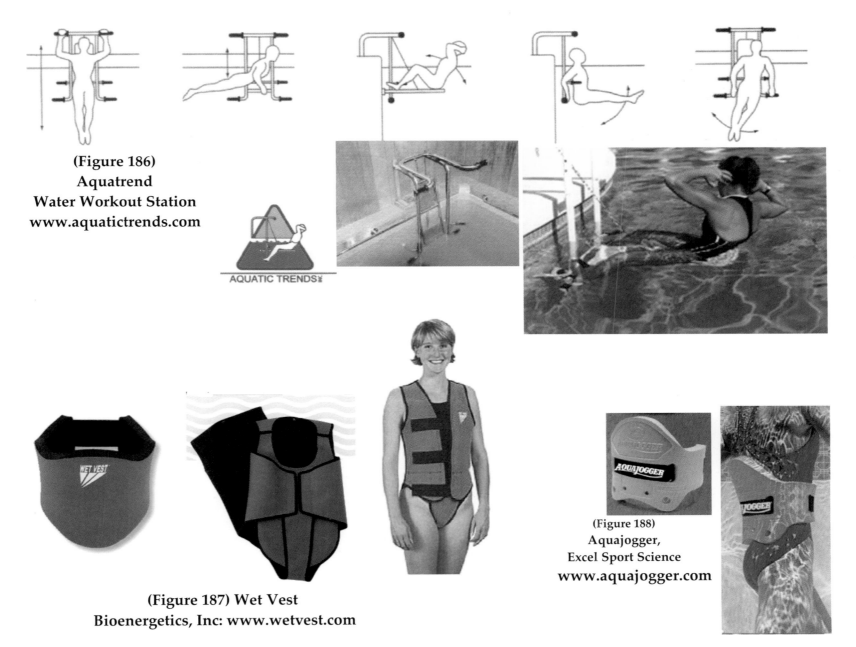

**(Figure 186)
Aquatrend
Water Workout Station
www.aquatictrends.com**

AQUATIC TRENDS™

**(Figure 188)
Aquajogger,
Excel Sport Science
www.aquajogger.com**

**(Figure 187) Wet Vest
Bioenergetics, Inc: www.wetvest.com**

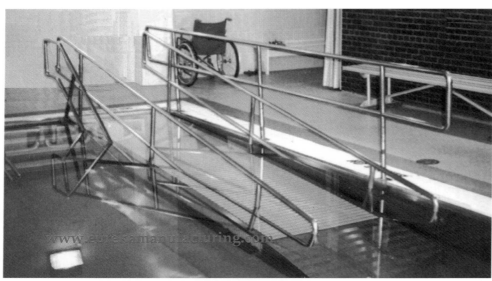

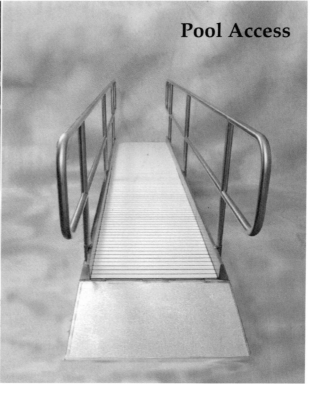

Pool Access

photos courtesy of Eureka Manufacturing Company

(Figure 189) Access Ramp:
www.eurekamanufacturing.com

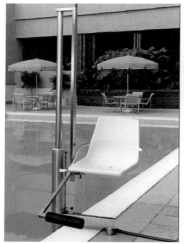

(Figure 190)
Pool Lift: www.ka.net

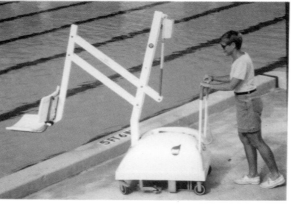

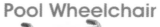

(Figure 191) Portable Aquatic Lift:
www.rehamedlifts.com

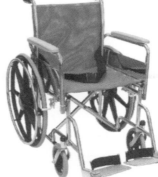

Pool Wheelchair

Creative Living Medical, Inc.
Rehabilitation Pool Wheelchair
888-622-6522

Nalu: The Art and Science of Aquatic Fitness, Bodywork & Therapy

Stationary Cardio Equipment

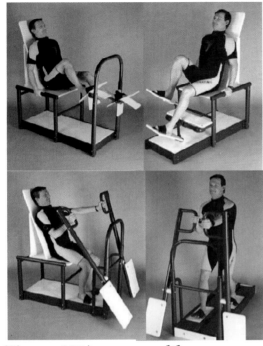

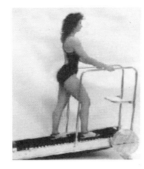

(Figure 194) Aqua Stride Aquatic Treadmill: www.aquastyle .com

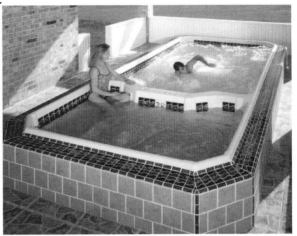

(Figure 193) Aquatic Treadmill: www.aquabilt.com

(Figure 195) Rio Swim Spas and Physiotherapy Pools: www. rioswimspas.com

(Figure 192) www.pooltherapy.com

(Figure 196) SwimExPools — Paddlewheel Propulsion: www.swimex.com

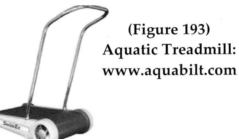

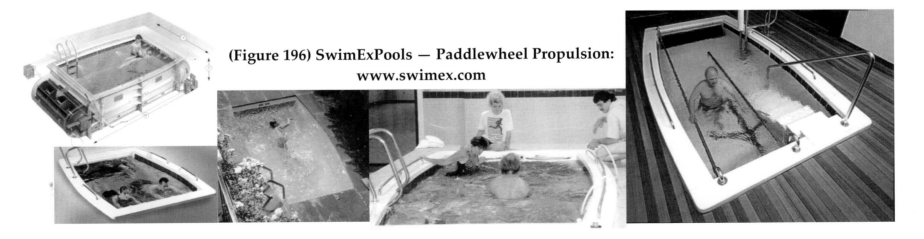

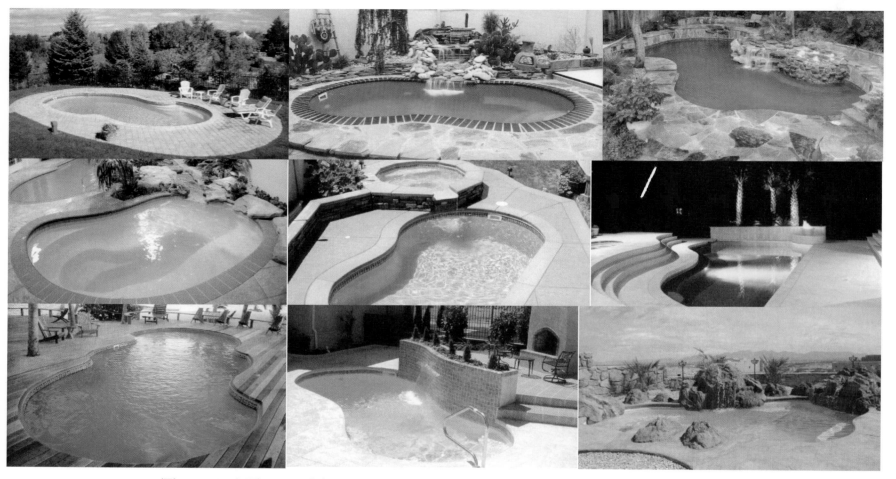

(Figure 197) The trend for in-ground pool custom installations today is for smaller pools with curved perimeters in natural settings that include boulders, quarry rock and waterfalls. These luxurious residential environments above, perfect settings for aquatic fitness, bodywork & therapy are located in Texas, California, New Mexico, Oklahoma, and Ontario. Prices range from $32,000 to $224,000.

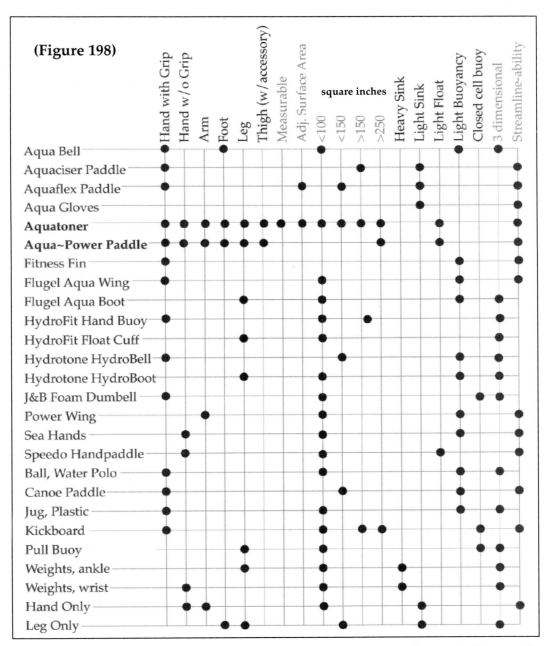

(Figure 198)

Comparison of Water Exercise Equipment

The chart (Figure 198) was first developed by the author in 1986 and revised in 1990. It compares basic equipment and traditional devices of that era and has become a standard method of equipment analysis for aquatic exercise and therapy today. The analytical concept of Bedgood's chart is published by Elsevier Science in the latest edition of the popular *Comprehensive Aquatic Therapy* (Becker, 2003).

The resistance surfaces were measured in a range from less than 100 inch² to more than 250 inch² viewed head-on. On the chart "streamlining" is a laminar flow–isolation technique that returns equipment to the starting position with minimal resistance, turbulence, vorticity and drag. The term "measurable" means there is a surface area scale on the equipment. Closed-cell buoyancy is a strong flotation characteristic. Light float is very close to the specific gravity of water. Attachment is for each individual device, not a combination of products in a system. Equipment prices were not included due to annual fluctuations. There are many more products on the market today.

Nalu: The Art and Science of Aquatic Fitness, Bodywork & Therapy

Books and Resources about Aquatic Bodywork and Aquatic Exercise/Therapy

1983

Bedgood, Douglas. *Aquatoning: A Renaissance in Fitness.* Kona Fitness.

Dulcy, Fayee H. (ed). *Aquatics, a Revived Approach to Pediatric Management.* Hayworth Press.

Fjord, Pauline. *Pool Exercises.* Self Published.

1984

Devarona, Donna, and Tarish, B. *Donna Devarona's Hydro-Aerobics.* Macmillan.

1985

Jetter, Judy, and Kadloc, Nancy. *The Arthritis Book for Water Exercis.* Holt, Rinehart and Winston.

Katz, Jane. *The W.E.T. Workout.* Facts On File.

Krasevec, Joseph. *Hydrorobics.* Human Kinetics.

1986

Bedgood, Douglas. *Exercising with the Aquatoner.* Kona Fitness.

Canadian Police College. *Aquafit: Water Exercise Program.* Independent Publishing Group.

Huey, L., and Knudsen, R.R. *The Waterpower Workout.* Dutton/Plume.

1987

YMCA of the USA. *Aquatics for Special Populations.* Human Kinetics.

1988

Baum, Glenda. *Aquarobics: The Training Manual.* Bailliere Tindell.

Giles, Miriam S. *Aquacises: Restoring and Maintaining Mobility with Water Exercises.* Mills & Sanderson.

McWaters, Glenn J. *Deep Water Exercise for Health and Fitness,* Publitec Editions.

1989

Buhler, Bill, et al. *The Water Workout Recovery Program: Safe and Painless Exercises for Treating Back Pain, Muscle Tears, Tendinitis, Sports Injuries, and More.* NTC/Contemporary Publishing.

Hughes, Helga. *The Complete Prenatal WaterWorkout Book.* Avery Penguin Putnam

Krasevec, Joseph, and Grimes, Diane. *Hydrorobics: A Water Exercise Program for Individuals of All Ages and Fitness Levels.* Human Kinetics.

YMCA of the USA. *Y's Way to Water Exercise Instructors Manual.* Human Kinetics.

1991

Dull, Harold. *Bodywork Tantra on Land and in Water..* Harbin Springs Publishing, Middletown, CA.

Pahlow, Ursula. *The Power of Water: Waterobics and Water Fitness Exercises for All Ages.* Sagamore Publishing.

1992

Bates, A. and Hanson, N. *Aquatic Exercise Therapy.* Online Graphics.

Baum. Glenda. *Aquarobics: Working Out in Water – The Natural Fitness Program.* Trafalgar Square.

Knoph, Karl G., et al. *Water Workouts.* Hunter Textbooks.

Sova, Ruth. *Aquatic Activities Handbook.* Jones & Bartlett.

Sova, Ruth. *Aquatic Exercise.* Jones & Bartlett.

1993

Dull, Howard. *Watsu, Freeing the Body in Water.* Harbor Springs Publishing.

Elder, Terri. *Aquatic Fitness Everyone.* Hunter Textbooks.

Gaines, Marybeth Pappas. *Fantastic Water Workouts.* Human Kinetics.

Huey, Linda, and Forster, Robert. *The Complete Waterpower Workout Book.* Random House.

Rettig, Sam, and French, Duccie. *Sam's Wit: Water Interval Training for Fabulous People of Every Kind.* DFC Seminars.

1995

Katz, Jane.*Water Fitness During Your Pregnancy.* Human Kinetics.

Sova, Ruth. *Water Fitness After 40.* DSL, Ltd.

White, Martha, and Winston, Leland. **Water Exercise:** *78 Safe and Effective Exercises for Fitness and Therapy.* Human Kinetics.

1996

Bates, Andrea and Hanson, Norm. *Aquatic Exercise Therapy.* W.B.Saunders.

Georgeakapoulos, Alexander. *Aquatic Writings.* La Mesa, Ca. Published at http://aquaticwritings.tripod.com.

Katz, Jane. *The All-American Aquatic Handbook: Your Passport to Lifetime Fitness.* Allyn & Bacon.

Katz, Jane. *The Aquatic Handbook for Lifetime Fitness.* Benjamin/Cummings.

Koury, Joanne M. *Aquatic Therapy Programming: Guidelines for Orthopedic Rehabilitation.* Human Kinetics.

Routi, Richard G., Morris, David M., Cole, Andrew J. (editors). *Aquatic Rehabilitation.* Lippincott,Williams & Wilkins.

Sova, Ruth. *Ai Chi – Flowing Aquatic Energy.* DSL, Ltd.

1997

Becker, Bruce,and Cole, Andrew. *Comprehensive Aquatic Therapy.* Elsevier Science.

Cass, Leanne. *Fitness Aquatics (Fitness Spectrum Series).* Human Kinetics.

Kravitz, Len, and Mayo, Jerry J. *The Physiological Effects of Aquatic Exercise.* Aquatic Exercise Association.

Tarpinian, Steve, and Awbrey, Brian J. *Water Workouts: A Guide to Fitness, Training, and Performance Enhancement in the Water.* The Lyons Press.

1998

Lepore, Monica, et al. *Adapted Aquatics Programming: A Professional Guide.* Human Kinetics.

1999

Burdenko, Igor, and Biehler, Scott.*Overcoming Paralysis.* Avery.

Caston, Carole M. Sokolow, et al. *Aqua Aerobics Today! (West's Physical Activities).* Wadsworth Publishing.

Kiss, Agnes. *New Techniques in Aquatic Therapy.* Rivercross Pub.

Larson, Juliana. *Water Dance: Water Fitness for Mind, Body and Soul.* Paper Chase.

Sova, Ruth. ***Essential Principles of Aquatic Therapy and Rehabilitation.*** DSL, Ltd.

Sova, Ruth. ***Ai Chi – Balance, Harmony and Healing.*** DSL, Ltd.

YMCA of the USA. ***YMCA Water Fitness for Health.*** Human Kinetics.

2000

McCormick, Irene Lewis. ***Aquatic Exercise.*** American Council on Exercise.

Sova, Ruth. ***Aquatic Exercise 2nd Edition.*** DSL Ltd.

Sova, Ruth. ***The Complete Reference Guide for Aquatic Fitness Professionals.*** DSL, Ltd.

2001

Coleman, Jill. ***Water Yoga: Water-Assisted Poses for Posture, Flexibility and Well Being.*** Eglantine Press.

Sova, Ruth. ***BackHab – the Water Way to Mobility and Pain-Free Living.*** DSL, Ltd.

Twynham, Julie. ***Waterart Fundamentals Manual*** 2nd ed. Body Check, Inc.

2002

Lindle, June (ed.) ***AEA Aquatic Personal Training Manual.*** Aquatic ExerciseAssociation.

Ogden, David. ***The Unpredictable Command Technique.*** DSL, Ltd.

Rosenstein, Ann A. ***Water Exercises for Parkinson's: Maintaining Balance, Strength, Endurance, and Flexibility.*** Idyll Arbor.

Twynham, Julie. ***Waterart Personal Trainer Specialist Manual*** 2nd ed. Body Check, Inc.

2003

Becker, Bruce, and Cole, Andrew. ***Comprehensive Aquatic Therapy.*** Elsevier Science.

2004

Bedgood, D., Courtney, B. and Georgeakapoulos, A. ***Nalu – The Art and Science of Aquatic Fitness, Bodywork, and Therapy.*** A.E.I.Press.

Continuum Movement Resources

Emilie Conrad
Continuum Movement
1629 18th Street, Studio 7
Santa Monica, CA 90404
(310) 453-4402
www.ContinuumMovement.com

Susan Harper
Continuum Montage
1653 18th Street, #3A
Santa Monica, CA 90404
(310) 449-6653
www.ContinuumMontage.com

Atlantis Rising

For more information on the project *Atlantis Rising*, visit: www.atlantisrising.net. The website provides information about participating in the support and development of the project, as well as how to propose or take part in research. To submit research or descriptions of ongoing work and to be included in the book, *Aquatic Resonant Healing*, please respond to the "call for papers" on the website. Papers on energetic healing involving water, sound, the use of aquatic shamanic practices, and mind-body altered states and related topics are relevant.

Aquatic Exercise Videos

www.atri.org
www.waterart.org
www.aquamagazine.com
www.aquaweb.org
www.distinctivehomevideos.com
www.fitnessmall.com
www.fitnessmart.com
www.hydrofit.org
www.recreonics.com/swim
www.recsupply.com
www.mindspring.com
www.saracity.com
www.sprintaquatics.com
AKWA Shop. Tel. 941-486-8600.
The National Arthritis Foundation Tel. 404-872-7100

Aquatic Bodywork Websites

www.aquaticwritings.tripod.com
   Healing Dance, Alexander Georgeakopoulos

www.jahara.com
   Jahara Technique

www.waba.edu
   Worldwide Aquatic Bodywork Association
   Watsu
   Water Dance
   Healing Dance
   Jahara Technique

www.watsu.com
   Watsu

www.wavemocean.com
   Wave M'ocean
   Resonant Healing
   Sound Healing

To learn about Wave M'ocean workshops, resonant healing or to purchase the Shapeshifter™, visit www.wavemocean.com.

Chapter 16
Reducing Stress with Water Fitness and Aquatic Bodywork

The Hormones

Exercising in water provides the secondary effect of effleurage, lymphatic facilitation, and compression. Muscular compression increases with water depth. Moving in a vertical position in a pool, you will experience more compressive massage from the water on leg muscles and effleurage on all areas submerged. The subchapter on *Massage* directs you to research studies at the University of Miami School of Medicine Touch Research Institute. They conclude that regular massage reduces stress hormones.

Exercise itself produces endorphins that create a feeling of well-being. Opium and morphine block the transmission of pain. They are opioids. LSD and mescaline are also opioids. Endorphins, produced naturally by the brain and pituitary gland, increase during exercise. Like morphine, endorphins are polypeptide opioids containing many amino acids.

The best physical activities to reduce stress are non-competitive and quiet, such as walking, jogging, cycling, rowing, swimming, and aquatic exercise. Aquatic resistance exercise is both invigorating and psychologically relaxing at the same time. In the broad realm of physical fitness, aquatic exercise is non-competitive, at the opposite end of the spectrum from the "How much can you bench press?" mentality.

Stretching in warm water is very relaxing. Other anti-stress methods besides aquatic exercise with its natural massage are: yoga, acupressure, moderate exercise out of water, breathing techniques, body scanning, progressive neuromuscular relaxation, meditation, imagery, having a healthy purpose in life, having pleasant relationships with others, and fulfilling your potentials. Reducing stress involves the parasympathetic nervous system. Operation of the parasympathetic nervous system produces relaxation and conserves energy. The sympathetic nervous system expends energy. Excessive stress is a constant drain on energy; it causes muscular bracing tension, chronic fatigue and many backaches and headaches. However, there is also eustress, a positive and beneficial phenomenon that improves personal growth and performance (Greenberg, 1999). Eustress may involve some of the same challenges as stress, but in selections and quantities and at times that increase rather than decrease well-being. Pulse raising confrontation may be an enjoyable tennis match. Anxiety over the unknown may resolve into the exhileration and pleasure of a new aquatic fitness routine, or even a new child.

Diets that deplete the B vitamin complex or raise blood pressure increase the susceptibility to stress.

Sugar depletes B vitamins while salt increases blood pressure by retaining body fluids and increasing blood volume.

Loud, erratic noise produces disturbance and stress. Stressful noise contrasts with the calming sound of waves and rippling water. The two ingredients of chronic stress are stressors and stress reactions. The stressors of life produce fight-or-flight responses that over many years promote early aging and weaken the immune system. To help live a long, healthy life, limit harmful types of stress and their effects and counteract them with exercise. (Selye,1956).

What are stress hormones, where do they come from, and what is the effect of stress on the body? Incoming stressors detected by signals to the limbic system are aroused through the reticular activating system and thalamus, and the resulting signals are sent to the hypothalamus and pituitary gland. Both the endocrine system and the autonomic nervous system become involved.

The anterior hypothalamus, through activation by the pituitary gland, releases thyrotropic hormone releasing factor that instructs the thyroid gland to excrete thyroxin. Thyroxin (tetraiodothyronine) as a participant in a stress reaction increases gluconeogenesis, respiration, basal metabolism, free fatty acids, heart rate, and blood pressure.

Activated by an autonomic nerve impulse to the adrenal medulla from the posterior hypothalamus, the adrenal glands produce the stress hormones referred to as catecolamines. The catecolamines, epinephrine – adrenalin (Figure 199) and norepinephrine, increase oxygen uptake, accelerate heart rate and pumping force, dilate bronchial tubes and coronary arteries, and speed up metabolism. Epinephrine can save a life at a critical moment.

The other activating pathway to the adrenal cortex also begins at the anterior hypothalamus where corticotropin releasing factor (CRF) stimulates the pituitary gland to produce ACTH, adrenocorticotropic hormone (Makara, 1980). ACTH, sometimes called "corticotropin," in turn stimulates adrenal cortex secretion of the corticoid hormones aldosterone and hydrocortisone. ACTH is a polypeptide containing 39 amino acids.

Cortisol (Figure199) allows the body to cope with immediate stress by controlling blood sugar and affecting mineral balance. But chronically elevated levels of cortisol are harmful. Some of the harmful affects are listed later in this chapter. There is a natural steroid hormone produced in the body that buffers excess cortisol. It is dehydroepiandrosterone (DHEA) (Figure 199), the most abundant steroid in the body that helps cope with stress. Much research in the past ten years has demonstrated that DHEA supplementation neutralizes the affects of high cortisol levels (Morales, 1994). DHEA levels diminish significantly during aging. Low levels have been linked to several chronic diseases.

Compare the molecular configuration of DHEA to those of cortisol, estradiol (estrogen), aldosterone, testosterone, progesterone and cholesterol. There are very few differences in their molecular structures (Figure 199). The small variations make a dramatic difference in their properties.

Cortisol fuels the fight-or-flight response to urgent stress by initiating glucogenesis, the mobilization of blood sugar from amino acids in the liver. Cortisol mobilizes fatty acids and triglycerides in the liver for rapid fuel and suppresses insulin, keeping blood glucose levels high for the immediately stressing emergency. By decreasing thymus and lymph node release of lymphocytes, cortisol also reduces immune response. Aldosterone together with cortisol increase blood pressure for rapid nutrient transport and muscle oxygenation, while aldosterone by itself increases sodium retention, thus increasing blood volume.

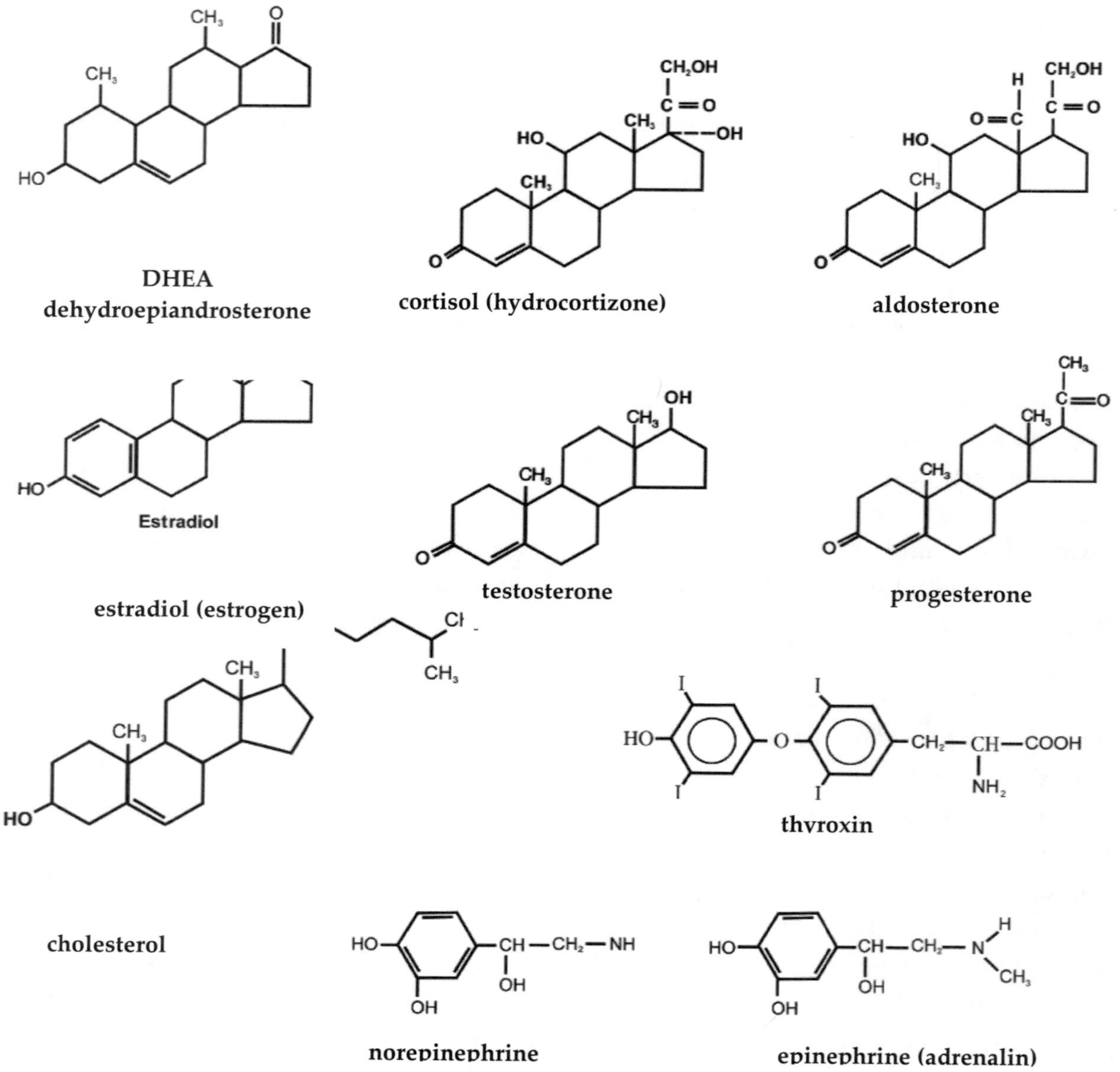

DHEA
dehydroepiandrosterone

cortisol (hydrocortizone)

aldosterone

Estradiol

estradiol (estrogen)

testosterone

progesterone

cholesterol

thyroxin

norepinephrine

epinephrine (adrenalin)

(Figure 199) Hormones

Nalu: The Art and Science of Aquatic Fitness, Bodywork & Therapy

(Figure 200) The Brain

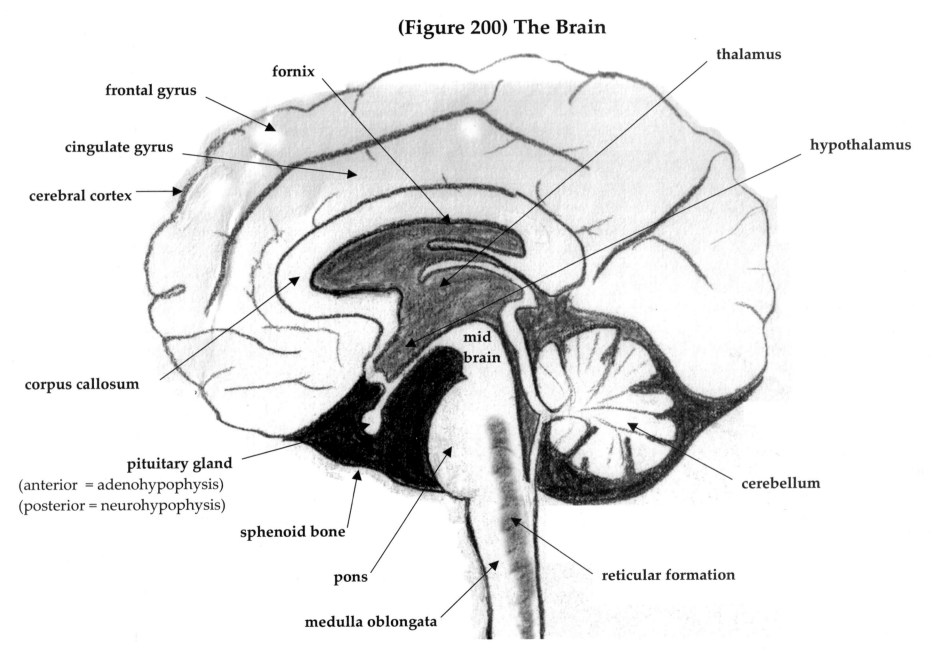

frontal gyrus

fornix

thalamus

cingulate gyrus

hypothalamus

cerebral cortex

corpus callosum

mid brain

pituitary gland
(anterior = adenohypophysis)
(posterior = neurohypophysis)

cerebellum

sphenoid bone

pons

reticular formation

medulla oblongata

Nalu: The Art and Science of Aquatic Fitness, Bodywork & Therapy

Besides consolidating short-term memories (the left for verbal and the right for non-verbal memories), the hippocampus in the limbic system of the brain is the interceptor of emotional and sensory stress and sends alarms to the brain alerting it to stressful situations. It is a large portion of the limbic system and rings the brain stem like a ridge left and right of the hypothalamus and pons area. When stress is prolonged and repeated, there is permanent damage to hippocampus receptors that detect the glucocorticoids (cortisol and aldosterone) released by the adrenal cortex (Greenberg, 1999). This damage reduces the efficiency of future stress detection.

The limbic system is concerned with aspects of emotion, behavior, and reactions that accompany emotions. Anatomically (Figure 200) it includes the hippocampus and pons area), cingulate gyrus of the cerebral cortex, parts of the frontal cortex adjacent to the lateral sulcus, part of the temporal cortex, thalamic and hypothalamic nuclei, the cerebral fornix, parts of the basal ganglia, and amygdaloid bodies between the hippocampus and the pituitary gland. The limbic system is the visceral brain.

In summary, stress hormones are produced in the endocrine glands as directed and controlled by the brain. Emotions originate in the limbic system from stimuli that pass through the reticular activating system and on to the thalamus. The thalamus distributes signals to the hypothalamus. The stressor is then experienced by the hypothalamus that in turn activates the endocrine and autonomic nervous systems to produce hormones for a stress reaction.

There are ideal and less than ideal scheduling sequences for daytime activities, calming meditation, sleep, etc. Morning, afternoon, evening or night, if the timing is not in tune with the individual, stress can result. For many people, the best schedule is for the most demanding high-energy activity, both physically or mentally challenging, to be in the morning, mild exercise in the afternoon, meditative relaxation in the evening or first thing in the morning, and sleep at night. This daily biological clock is the circadian rhythm. Alterations in the usual sequence can be disturbing and trigger a stress response.

Melatonin and serotonin regulate the sleep circadian rhythms by measuring and responding to light and darkness. The chemical name for melatonin is 5-methoxy-N-acetyl tryptamine (Figure 201). It is manufactured in the pineal gland at the top center of the brain. It is inhibited by photosensitivity to bright light via neural pathways from the retina of the eye which send messages to the hypothalamus to instruct the pineal gland to produce or inhibit the melatonin. If you exercise in brightness, you will not get sleepy. Serotonin initiates sleep, reduces carbohydrate cravings, and has the chemical name 5-hydroxy-tryptamine (Figure 202). It is synthesized from tryptophan in protein and is a central neurotransmitter in the brain. In mammals, the melatonin-serotonin control center and master circadian pacemaker is the suprachiasmatic nucleus of the hypothalamus.

(Figure 201) melatonin

(Figure 202) serotonin

(Figure 203) dopamine

Aqua Music & Choreography

Music is art, both creative and interpretive. Music affects emotions and the recall of memories. These moods can be guided with sound.

Music with a dominant, repetitive, rapid tempo is ideal for cardio pool classes and individualized anaerobic muscle endurance workouts. The energetic intensity of the music parallels the intensity of the activity in a turbulent thunder of waves

splashing out of the pool at the opposite end.

Gentle and quiet background music is more suitable for therapy and rehabilitation. See Barbara Courtney's *Sound Awareness Portal* in Chapter 1, *Healing Waters,* for her excellent presentation on resonant and vibrational sound healing in water.

Aquatic bodywork can respond to music of a different kind. Classical music offers an extensive assortment of appropriate music and there are many selections of New Age music like that heard on XM103 Broadband. These are conducive to the flow of aquatic bodywork sessions, but external silence can also open wide musical doors in the mind of the participants. We all use, need and have different drums, flutes, and violins throughout life. One person needs calmness. Another wants to become lively. Others crave stability and the even keel. These needs change during the course of one day and over a lifetime. When several people are in a pool at the same time experiencing aquatic bodywork, each

does best with their own written score and their own "instruments."

There is no need for a distracting boom box that diverts focus away from natural rythms and responses. We can refer to the person or the group of participants as solo or the duet, trio, quartet, octet and the orchestra. The entire body of each person is in an individual concert of their own.

For the practitioner desiring to choreograph a session on paper (Figure 204) there is a shorthand similar to music symbol notations that can be used for pool activity. Instead of the music symbols for pianissimo, fortissimo, storzando, crescendo, trill, staccato, vibrato, swell, decrescendo, forte etc., the symbols for aquatic exercise and bodywork choreography are notations for motion. You can customize your own set of choreographic symbols. The chart that follows is an example of simple notations that can be utilized to save time in session planning and preparation.

(Figure 204)
Choreographic Notations for Aquatic Exercise & Bodywork

intuitive motion	∞		**turn cw**	↻
begin	◖		**turn ccw**	↺
solo	⊙		**turn together**	↻↺
pause	⊙		**rapid reiteration**	≡
submerge	▼		**soft**	ρ
emerge	▲		**very soft**	ρρ
change posture	⌣		**repeat**	≪
relocate	↻		**bilateral/symmetrical**	≈
isolation	∮		**start over**	⤳
entire body	∯		**unpredictably sudden**	✳
maximum effort	∰		breathe deep	ℬ
gradual speed increase	△		**focus**	↗
gradual speed decrease	▽		**finish**	⊕

Massage Therapy

Massage therapy reduces stress hormones (Field, 1992, 1996). When it comes to soft tissue manipulation, nothing is superior to strong, sensitive human hands. A comprehensive, personal aquatic exercise session is best followed with ninety minutes of massage therapy on land such as integrated deep-tissue massage or aquatic bodywork in warm water after a cool down period.

Aquatic bodywork decreases stress. Gentle flowing movement of water itself is a form of calming hydro-massage that diminishes mental and physical stress and tension. Watsu and Jahara are aquatic bodywork techniques that incorporate Shiatsu massage as the primary modality. Two other forms of aquatic bodywork, WaterDance and Healing Dance, both contain Watsu or water Shiatsu. These four bodywork styles require a therapist and contact between the therapist and the client. To learn more about them, go to Chapter 2, *Aquatic Bodywork* by Alexander Georgeakopoulos.

Nalu: The Art and Science of Aquatic Fitness, Bodywork & Therapy

The fifth and newest method of aquatic bodywork is Wave M'ocean. Wave M'ocean is distinct from other forms of aquatic bodywork. It is aquatic mind-bodywork. Wave M'ocean has a profound effect on the mental state of the individual because it introduces several contexts of altered perception. Six portals of awareness are experienced in the water with the intention of creating one's own healing process. Another difference is that here is no physical contact with the therapist. Instead, the individual is encouraged to follow her or his own unfolding movement. The six portals of awareness contained in Wave M'ocean are detailed in Chapter 1, *Healing Waters* by Barbara Courtney.

According to published studies by the Touch Research Institute at the University of Miami School of Medicine, massage reduces excess cortisol. Without adequate recovery time, intensive training and rapid physical exertion in the pool against the powerful viscosity of water, with high resistance equipment, actually produce more cortisol out of the necessity to increase metabolism for energy. Cortisol is a product resulting from many sources of exterior stressors. Cortisol is important in the metabolism of food and some nutrients and as stated in the subchapter, *The Hormones*, cortisol helps the body cope with and adapt to immediate physical stress.

Emotional and mental stress can become chronic for some people. In chronic excess, production of too much cortisol over a long period of time has a number of detrimental effects (Little, 1973).

Excess cortisol -

❶ **hinders protein production**
❷ **is accompanied by an increase in adipose tissue**
❸ **causes a rise in free fatty acids, cholesterol, phospholipids and triglycerides**
❹ **reduces the mobility of connective tissue cell membranes, and hence reduces vascular and connective tissue cell proliferation**
❺ **suppresses calcium and vitamin D absorption**
❻ **reduces the permeability of capillaries, and so affects the cardiovascular functions, electrolyte and water balance, and renal function**
❼ **induces lysis of lymphocytes, reducing mitosis and causing a loss of cytoplasm**
❽ **prevents macrophages from maturing and inhibits their activity**
❾ **hinders cell division of fibroblasts and induces their disintegration of the cells**
❿ **is associated with calcium deficiency.**

In addition, chronically high cortisol levels suppress the immune system leading to many illnesses, and they reduce muscle strength because of the hormone's inflammatory effect.

There are medications that lower cortisol but there is a much better way which avoids the chance of adverse side effects: a long, deep-tissue massage. Massage does much more than lower hormones from physical or emotional stress. It helps to maintain, support, or return to overall homeostasis. It moves waste products out of and oxygen into muscles, separates adhesions, and strengthens the immune system. Massage also reduces diastolic blood pressure, headaches, cephalalgia, soreness, pain, tension, hyperactivity, and anxiety. Soft tissue manipulation alleviates muscle spasms, symptoms of fatigue, post-traumatic stress, anger and depression. It improves sleep patterns and normalizes glucose levels in diabetics. In addition, massage increases serotonin levels, circulation for oxygenation of injured tissues, nutrient transport for healing, mental acuity, job performance and occupational production.

The most relevant clinical studies on the above benefits of massage therapy have been completed or are ongoing at the University of Miami Medical School Touch Research Institute and at the Canadian Touch Research Center in Montreal (TRI, 2004). Generally, massage therapy performed by strong human hands with sensitivity and healing intent are beyond value. The best professional massage is expensive but is a worthwhile investment in a higher quality of life.

How often and when? For recovery the best time is after a workout, after rehydration, and before a meal, ideally after every workout, realistically as often as affordable. Once a week is excellent. Better than nothing is once a month. A massage session of less than one hour is enough to treat specific isolated problem areas but for the best overall therapeutic effect, 75 or 90 minutes works wonders with the right massage therapist. Before a major workout or sports event, a brief sports massage prior to starting time is practical if techniques include vigorous cross-fiber transverse friction to stimulate circulation and elevate muscle temperature. This would not be an appropriate time to do any deep, focused healing work. Pre-event is brief and fast. Post-event is long, deep, and slow.

There is a popular misconception about lactic acid among coaches and personal trainers which says that it builds up during exercise and causes delayed onset muscle soreness, and that massage eliminates it from the muscles. This is incorrect (Vanderbilt 2001). According to Whitney Lowe, author of *Functional Assessment in Massage Therapy* and Owen Anderson PhD, exercise physiologist and editor of *Running Research News*, lactic acid levels return to homeostasis quickly. Lactate has already been converted to pyruvate or glucose by the time any massage has started. Lactic acid does not cause muscle soreness from intensive exercise. Lactic acid provides energy, consumes carbohydrates in the diet and produces glucose and liver glycogen.

According to Anderson and other researchers, muscle soreness comes from muscle tissue damage and free radical attack on muscle membranes, not from lactic acid. When the pH levels of muscle and blood fall below 7 during intense exercise as a result of hydrogen ions dissociating from lactic acid, any dizziness or pain is temporary and the pH returns to normal soon after exercise stops.

Regarding pain and massage:

Keith Grant, head of the Sports and Deep Tissue Massage Department at McKinnon Institute concludes from published research on soft tissue manipulation that massage saturates the body with new sensory input and stimulates the mechanoreceptors that inhibit (pain receptors. The nervous system then allows muscles to relax (Grant, 2003).

Rehabilitative massage reduces pain from muscle adhesions and injuries that adhere other tissues like those at a joint capsule (Lowe, 1995). Many injuries to connective tissues are helped by massage such as loose areolar connective tissue in myofascia and the dense regular connective tissues of tendons and ligaments.

In recent surveys by the American Hospital Association and the American Massage Therapy Association, 91% of one poll said massage therapy reduced pain (AMTA, 2003). In another poll, half of the senior clients received massage for pain relief. A third poll by the AHA surveyed 1007 hospitals with over 70% of the hospitals reporting the regular use of massage therapy for pain management and pain relief.

Contraindications to massage are learned in training. They include acute trauma, acute pain, skin infections, or any abnormality that could increase risk to health from massage such as arthritic joints if the massage is improperly performed, or a person on drugs (licit ir illicit) that could mask sensitivity to injurious pressure. Certain parts of the body have shallow innervations or the potential for plaque deposits in shallow arteries and should be avoided. An example isthe bifurcation of the carotid artery.

What to do after Rolfing, structural integration massage, neuromuscular therapy, or a long therapeutic deep tissue massage: rehydrate, relax, enjoy, and prolong the altered state by avoiding anxiety or any abrupt disturbance like unusually loud noises, bright lights, traffic and congestion, crowds, emotional situations, physical exertion, or anything uncomfortable that could interfere with your tranquil, meditative state. This is the ideal time and condition for healing and repair to occur.

There are manual self deep-tissue muscle massagers that are effective and inexpensive for use between hands-on sessions. An example is the MD4 back massager whose 2003 cost is US$20.00. Temporarily mounted to a vertical surface with two suction cups, it allows self controlled, hands free use on your own body. The configuration of the massage heads allows different techniques to be used. The force of the user leaning on it is concentrated on two small, narrow areas, typically on either side of the spine, with outstanding results. Compared to the electric massagers, vibrators, balls, rollers, the need for another person to use the equipment on you, or items to roll around on the floor with all or none of the user's body weight, or devices too broad to focus pressure for isolated transverse friction, the MD4 would be at the top of the list for manual massagers.

How to find a massage therapist. You work out hard during your exercise sessions in the pool. Now it is your turn for recovery, time for a massage. You want the best. Ask your friends which massage therapists they use. It is a very individual decision. Everyone has different thresholds of response to massage. So it is necessary to shop for your needs.

First determine their qualifications. Are the therapists certified nationally and licensed properly? Where did they go to massage school, how long ago, how large is their clientele, and are there any complaints on record? What are the modalities or kinds of massage they specialize in? Do any local personal trainers utilize their services, and what is their reputation among other healthcare professionals such as chiropractors and orthopedic physicians?

Reduce your list to a handful, and try out three or four of the top massage therapists on your list with a brief trial of a fifteen or thirty minute massage to check out their location, manner, professionalism, feel, knowledge, and comfort level. Then go for the real thing, evaluate the

results for several days to feel how long they last, and choose the winner. That will be your best massage therapist.

The best place to get your massage is poolside, depending on climate, or at your home where you don't have to drive somewhere after the massage. Outcalls are a little more expensive than office visits but worth the convenience as long as you turn off telephones, close doors, put the dog outside, and generally reduce the chances for interruptions to the flow of the massage.

2004 prices range from US$50 an hour at a gym or from a beginner to over US$120 for the best independent contractor in town, or higher at a luxury resort with all the amenities. A top quality therapist will ask about US$85 for an hour long out-call massage and give you more time without cost to work on problem areas when scheduling time permits. Treat them well. They are invaluable to you. Spa massages are sometimes tightly scheduled, rushed sessions with therapists that are often

beginners. A chiropractor with a massage therapist will offer expensive medical massage for a short session on an isolated area and will want to follow the massage with a chiropractic adjustment. An orthopedic physician will prescribe muscle relaxants or cortisone injections more often than not and a massage may not be available at their office. A massage at a gym will be a sports massage, fast action, not what you need after a workout. Find your own personal massage therapist by comparing qualifications, talking to clients, and by the trial method described earlier.

Copies of massage research studies can be obtained by going to http://www.miami.edu/touch-research/home.html. Here you can look for a research topic of interest, record the identification data, and obtain a copy by calling the University of Miami Medical Library in Miami, Florida at 305-243-6749. There is a minimal copying/mailing charge per article.

Information on classes and certification programs throughout the world regarding Watsu, Jahara, WaterDance, and Healing Dance can be obtained at the Worldwide Aquatic Bodywork Association headquarters. WABA, PO Box 889, Middletown, Ca. 95461 USA , tel (707)987-3801, email: info@waba.edu; http://www,waba.edu.

For information on Wave M'ocean Workshops, go to the following website. www.wavemocean.com; Email: lightrain@greennet.net.

Aquatic Bodywork and Waves from the Brain

The gracefulness of an arm flowing through the water in an uninterrupted figure eight pattern is art. Psychologically, the serenity of this smooth creative movement is a perception of individual interpretation, a simple tranquility with profound subconscious effect.

The origins and the effect of these stimuli can be explicated with science and mathematics just as the urban landscapes of Paris in paintings can be seen as individual pigments shaping impressions from the mind of Monet to the canvas. The events involving the motion of the arm through the water begin with a desire, a choice, a need, or a determined "will" that initiates action. The chapter on the Kinetics of Water will be the basis for what is physically experienced.

Enjoy the unplanned, spontaneous moment with your mind drifting off into the sensations of suspended, creative movement. To make this simple movement in the water more effective, change the shape of the hand during the motion of the arm. Go from a flat, opened hand against the water with fingers spread, to a cupped hand by gradually closing the fingers with a delay between each digit flexion culminating in a closed fist. Reverse the sequence to an opened hand. Tilt your hand to feel maximal and minimal drag. All these moves take place without stopping. Slowly change the angle at the elbow. Rotate the arm to alternately supinate and pronate at different places throughout the figure eight pattern. Enlarge and reduce the size of the shape. Feel the difference between laminar and turbulent velocity, but return to laminar.

In water the variations have become endless, resembling the free form of modern dance rather than the structured discipline of ballet. This is not a battle. It is an embrace.

During changes in the three dimensional geometry of aquatic exercise multiple drag coefficients in the hydrodynamic equation are in constant alteration. Tendon insertion points on the bones influence leverage. Depending on the shape of the hand, drag coefficients can more than triple from a convex hollow cup shape at 0.38 to a concave hollow cup shape at 1.42. The changing length between the axillary fulcrum and the distal fingertips due to the bending of the arm at the elbow can alter the sensation of force by up to 50%. At the other extreme, with sensitivity a change in resistive force can be detected by the closing of one finger.

Different electrochemical locations in the brain perceive the overall experience as oscillations of voltages producing synchronized waves of electric current (Gray, 1994). These wave frequencies are measured in cycles per second or Hz. Hz is simply an abbreviation honoring German physicist Heinrich R Hertz (1857-1894). Scientists categorize and identify separate levels from low frequency/high amplitude to high frequency/low amplitude. The highest frequency levels indicate increased brain activity and arousal during a strongly engaged mind while lower levels reflect non-arousal and a slowing down of activity. Frequency ranges are identified by Greek letters.

0.1-4 Hz .... Delta
4 -7 Hz .... Theta
7-13 Hz .... Alpha
14-30 Hz.........................Beta
30-100 Hz .... Gamma

These brain wave frequencies are approximate. There are minor differences between research results and there are some overlapping characteristics. With meditation training, the brain can learn to maintain frequencies at will. Humor itself effects brain waves (http://web.sfn.org/content/Publica tions/BrainWaves/)

To put these low frequency brain waves into perspective we will look at two other electromagnetic waves, radar and light. Radar works at various frequencies in a range of about 400,000,0000 to 1 trillion Hz. Visible light ranges from about 430 trillion Hz for red light to 750 trillion Hz for violet.

Ordinarily we experience beta brain waves in our daily activities when we are consciously alert, mentally engaged, stressed, or emotionally tense. They are the brain's normal response. Delta brain waves, the slowest, are the deep sleep waves and the cycles per second come close to zero. Delta brain waves are associated with healing, triggering the release of Human Growth Hormone and regeneration (Genet, 1995). There is a fine line between 0.1 and 0.0 Hz. At zero is brain death.

The theta state is characterized by reduced consciousness, drowsiness, daydreaming with vivid imagery, and long periods of mental relaxation. Marathon runners float in the rain of theta brain waves. Theta is a positive time when clear ideas occur and flow freely. Theta is the twilight between delta and alpha states with an opportunity to increase memory and learning capabilities.

The fast gamma band or gamma rhythms overlap beta brain waves and are associated with the neural networks of higher mental activities. Gamma rhythms bind and unite perceptions and the conglomerate of sensory components into a single cognitive experience (Barinaga, 1989).

If there is an absence of high adrenalin from such environments as competitive sports, alpha brain waves have an opportunity to emerge. Alpha waves are "turned on" during water immersion and flowing aquatic movements just as they are during massage therapy, meditation, or deep breathing while standing on a sunny mountaintop. Alpha waves indicate attentive mental relaxation, quiet alertness, clarity, and heightened awareness. Calming, alpha brain waves provide the ideal condition for learning, memory formation, beta-endorphin production, and the release of the powerful natural painkillers dopamine, norepinephrine, and serotonin. Impaired synthesis and depletion of these neurotransmitters are related to depression. Cortisol levels from stress and anxiety decrease during the production of alpha range brain wave frequencies.

In the alpha state there is less neural degeneration from lack of use. Alpha-brain waves help to establish new neuronal connections and the potentials for diverse skills.

The low frequencies from the classical music of Mozart and Hayden accelerate learning by slowing the heartbeat and respiration, which in turn lowers the brain wave frequency by the pulsing rhythmic entrainment process. The waves slow in sympathetic resonance.

At any given moment we are experiencing a changing mix of frequencies within the spectrum of brain waves. The interrelationship of these continuously circulating waves of electromagnetic energy gives us mental individuality. The uncommon ability to control brain waves allows those who have trained themselves to maintain desired frequencies (Kamiya, 1968). With this gift they experience optimal accomplishments, knowing the brain waves that are associated with their goals.

Understandably, the movement in the water that we started out with is the perfect antecedent to any task requiring spatial visualization or the need to learn new information. Tranquil movement in the water helps to lower the brain waves to alpha, the state of mental being that opens the doors to non-cognitive levels of intelligence and awareness of our self-altering abilities.

(Figure 204) Brainwaves

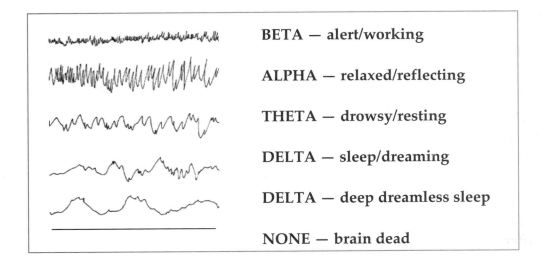

BETA — alert/working

ALPHA — relaxed/reflecting

THETA — drowsy/resting

DELTA — sleep/dreaming

DELTA — deep dreamless sleep

NONE — brain dead

Envoi

Together we have
journeyed far on Nalu,
the wave, and learned
from the healing waters.
Aquatic fitness,
bodywork and therapy
were born in the amniotic
fluid of the womb. The
art and science behind
Nalu will intoxicate many
of you to do more of this
research and motivate
you to reach deep within
your creative minds as it
has for the authors. To
those in the professions,
may you be buoyantly
uplifted throughout your
lifetimes. To you the
enthusiastic pool owners
in your back yards, may
Nalu improve your life's
quality and joy.

Thou gracious starry maid,
  By Heaven blest,
Pour from thy urn of jade
  Eternal rest.

Manley P. Hall
The Space-Born
(1930)

Nalu: The Art and Science of Aquatic Fitness, Bodywork & Therapy

Appendix

Physical Characteristics of Water for a Given Temperature

Refer to kinematic viscosity in the Wasilowski equation in Chapter 11, p. 315

Temperature	Density	Specific weight	Dynamic viscosity	Kinematic viscosity	Vapor pressure
	kg/m³	N/m³	N·s/m²	m²/s	N/m² abs.
0°C	1000	9810	1.79×10^{-3}	1.79×10^{-6}	611
5°C	1000	9810	1.51×10^{-3}	1.51×10^{-6}	872
10°C	1000	9810	1.31×10^{-3}	1.31×10^{-6}	1230
15°C	999	9800	1.14×10^{-3}	1.14×10^{-6}	1700
20°C	998	9790	1.00×10^{-3}	1.00×10^{-6}	2340
25°C	997	9781	8.91×10^{-4}	8.94×10^{-7}	3170
30°C	996	9771	7.97×10^{-4}	8.00×10^{-7}	4250
35°C	994	9751	7.20×10^{-4}	7.24×10^{-7}	5630
40°C	992	9732	6.53×10^{-4}	6.58×10^{-7}	7380
50°C	988	9693	5.47×10^{-4}	5.53×10^{-7}	12,300
60°C	983	9643	4.66×10^{-4}	4.74×10^{-7}	20,000
70°C	978	9594	4.04×10^{-4}	4.13×10^{-7}	31,200
80°C	972	9535	3.54×10^{-4}	3.64×10^{-7}	47,400
90°C	965	9467	3.15×10^{-4}	3.26×10^{-7}	70,100
100°C	958	9398	2.82×10^{-4}	2.94×10^{-7}	101,300
	slugs/ft³	lbf/ft³	lbf-s/ft²	ft²/s	psia
40°F	1.94	62.43	3.23×10^{-5}	1.66×10^{-5}	0.122
50°F	1.94	62.40	2.73×10^{-5}	1.41×10^{-5}	0.178
60°F	1.94	62.37	2.36×10^{-5}	1.22×10^{-5}	0.256
70°F	1.94	62.30	2.05×10^{-5}	1.06×10^{-5}	0.363
80°F	1.93	62.22	1.80×10^{-5}	0.930×10^{-5}	0.506
100°F	1.93	62.00	1.42×10^{-5}	0.739×10^{-5}	0.949
120°F	1.92	61.72	1.17×10^{-5}	0.609×10^{-5}	1.69
140°F	1.91	61.38	0.981×10^{-5}	0.514×10^{-5}	2.89
160°F	1.90	61.00	0.838×10^{-5}	0.442×10^{-5}	4.74
180°F	1.88	60.58	0.726×10^{-5}	0.385×10^{-5}	7.51
200°F	1.87	60.12	0.637×10^{-5}	0.341×10^{-5}	11.53
212°F	1.86	59.83	0.593×10^{-5}	0.319×10^{-5}	14.70

*Notes: (1) Bulk modulus *E.* of water is approximately 2.2 G P, (3.2 × 10⁵ psi); (2) Water–air surface tension is approximately 7.3 × 10⁻² N/m (5 × 10⁻³ lbf/ft) from 10°C to 50°C.

SOURCE: Reprinted with permission from R. E. Bolz and G. L. Tuve, *Handbook of Tables for Applied Engineering Science*, CRC Press, Inc., Cleveland, 1973. Copyright 1973 by The Chemical Rubber Co., CRC Press, Inc.

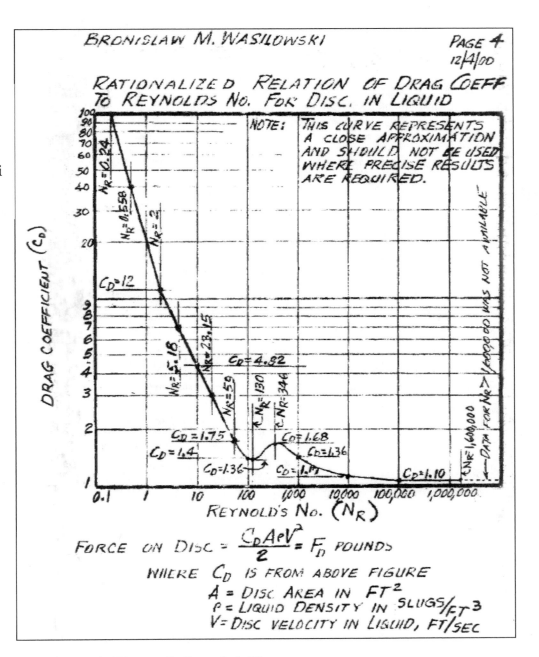

Nalu: The Art and Science of Aquatic Fitness, Bodywork & Therapy

College of Engineering
DEPARTMENT OF MECHANICAL ENGINEERING

May 7, 1992

EVALUATION OF THE AQUATONER PERFORMANCE

by
James A. Liburdy
Professor

INTRODUCTION

The performance of the Aquatoner as an aquatic exercise device was carried out using experimental and analytical methods. The experiments were used to verify the analysis which in turn was used to develop a complete description of the performance. The device is designed to provide a flexible exercise program where the effective area can be changed to provide variable water resistance. The primary goal of this evaluation was to (i) determine the force required to move the Aquatoner in water and (ii) determine the total energy expended in moving the Aquatoner. Both items (i) and (ii) were evaluated over the range of Aquatoner seyttings representing different effective areas and for a range of amplitudes and frequencies which are representative of a range of typical users. The amplitude is a measure of the distance of extension of thye Aquatoner. The frequency is the inverse of the time required to complete one complete cycle on movement of the Aquatoner.

Listed in Table 1 are the various configurations the Aquatoner can be placed in which change the effective area. Also indicated are the associated area percent of the maximum surface area obtained when the Aquatoner is fully open. Also listed is the actual surface area in square inches and square centimeters for the various settings and the effective diameter which is the diameter of a round disk with the same corresponding area as the effective area. Listed in Table 2 are the amplitudes studied and the associated amplitude ratios with each of the paddle positions. If it is desired, other conditions of amplitude and frequency can be analyzed by using the computer code that was written for the present analysis.

TABLE 1

GROOVED MARKING NUMBER				PERCENT OF MAXIMUM SURFACE	RESISTIVE SURFACE AREA 18", 46cm diameter	
TOP- MIDDLE PADDLE PADDLE		MIDDLE-BOTTOM PADDLE PADDLE			SQ.INCHES	SQ cm
1 - 1		1 - 1		40%	97	626
1 - 2		1 - 1		50%	121	780
1 - 2		1 - 2		60%	146	942
1 - 3		1 - 2		70%	170	1096
1 - 3		1 - 3		80%	194	1251
1 - 1	cross	1 - 0		84%	207	1335
1 - 4		1 - 3		90%	219	1413
1 - 4		1 - 4		100%	243	1567

TABLE 2

EFFECTIVE DIAMETER (cm)	AMPLITUDE RATIO (a/d)	
	a= 60 cm.	a= 90 cm
28.23	2.1254	3.1881
31.51	1.9042	2.8562
34.63	1.7326	2.5989
37.36	1.6060	2.4090
39.91	1.5034	2.2551
41.23	1.4543	2.1829
42.42	1.4144	2.1216
44.67	1.3432	2.0148

EXPERIMENTAL ARRANGEMENT

The experimental program was designed to test a few of the conditions to validate the analysis. A large tank filled with water was used as the test medium. A support structure was designed and built to hold the aquatoner in place and to accelerate the aquatoner through the water at a predetermined rate. The aquatoner was attached to the base of the moveable support brace. A known loading was supplied to the support brace which rode along the top track system. Data were obtained consisting of the acceleration of the aquatoner by means of a piezoresistive accelerometer mounted to the brace of the aquatoner where it was mounted to the support brace. The output of the accelerometer was recorded using a strip chart recorder after being amplified. The acceleration data were combined with the known mass of the device to determine the force on the aquatoner as a function of time during the acceleration. The force required to move the support brace independent of the aquatoner was subtracted from the total force. This support brace force component was measured by accelerating it without the aquatoner attached.

ANALYSIS

An analysis was made of the oscillation of a disk with varying area to determine the total force required to move the disk in oscillatory motion in water. The general equation for the force can be written as:

$$F = kM_0 (dV/dt) \div 1/2\, C_d\, S\ V/V/$$

with the following definitions:

   k - inertia of added mass
   C_d - drag coefficient
   M_0 - mass of the fluid displaced by the disk
   S - projected area of the disk in the direction of motion

V - velocity of the disk
/V/ - absolute value of the disk velocity
dV/dt - time derivative of the velocity

In this analysis the disk is assumed to oscillate sinusoidally such that the time dependent velocity vector is:

$$V = -a\, \omega \sin(\omega t)$$

where a is the amplitude of the oscillation and ω is the frequency of oscillation.

Substitution of the velocity expression into the force equation results in the following:

$$F = k\frac{\pi}{6}d^3 \rho a \omega^2 \cos(\omega t) + C_d \frac{1}{2}(a\omega)^3 \sin(\omega t)|\sin(\omega t)|\pi\frac{d^2}{4}$$

There have been several experiments reported in the literature which have determined the value of the added mass coefficient. Kanwal (1) determined the following relationship:

$(d^2 w/v)c < (d^2 w/v)$:

$$k = 2/\pi + 4.42(d^2 w/n)^{-0.43}, \qquad 0.083 < a/d$$

$(d^2 w/v)c > (d^2 w/\ )$:

$$k = 1.10(a/d)^{0.12}, \qquad 0.083 < a/d < 0.2$$
$$k = 1.64(a/d)^{0.37}, \qquad 0.2 < a/d$$

where (d^2w/v) represents a flow Reynolds number. $(d^2w/v)c$ is a critical flow Reynolds number which is determined by the amplitude ratio, a/d using the relationship:

$$(d^2w/v)_c = 27.0 \ (a/d)^{-1.7}$$

There are several studies which have determined the value of the drag coefficient from both experimental and theoretical methods as a function of amplitude ratio and Reynolds number. Minamizawa et al. (2) present correlations from experimental data as:

for $(d^2w/v) < (d^2w/v)c$ and $0.083 < a/d$

$$C_d = 8.52(\log(d^2w/v)) - 2.1(a/d)^{-0.93}$$

for $(d^2w/v) > (d^2w/v)c$ and $0.222 < a/d < 0.308$ and
         $(d^2w/v) > 200$ and $0.308 < a/d$

$$C_d = 2.37 \ (a/d)^{-0.57}$$

The above expressions were used to determine the force, F, exerted by the disk to move through water for the range of amplitude ratios shown in Table 2. Each case was run for three frequencies, 0.5, 1.0 and 2.0 cycles per second (cps).

In addition to the determination of the force the energy dissipation rate, E, caused by exerting the necessary force was also calculated. This was determined from the definition:

$$E = (F) \ (V).$$

The above expression for the energy dissipation rate was then numerically integrated over the time during one cycle to determine the total energy used per cycle.

RESULTS

The results were obtained for a range of amplitude ratios and frequencies. The drag coefficient and added mass coefficient was calculated using the above relationships which were verified from a series of experiments, and were found to be within 15% over the full range of paddle positions. Based on an overall uncertainty analysis the results are expected to be within +/- 20% and most and nominally within +/- 15%. The results presented were calculated using a computer code developed for this analysis. Results for other operating conditions can be readily obtained.

The time variation of the force is shown in Figures 1 through 6 where each figure is divided into parts (a) and (b) to accommodate the full range of amplitude ratios, a/d. All of the plots have the same basic form, the maximum force occurs for the lowest amplitude ratio for a given frequency. The variation over time occurs due to both the variation in drag and inertia which are a direct result of the time variation of velocity and acceleration, respectively. Maximum acceleration occurs when the disk changes direction and at this point the velocity is zero resulting in maximum inertial force and minimum drag force. Maximum velocity occurs when the displacement is zero (its neutral position) and at this point the acceleration is a minimum, this condition results in minimum inertial force and maximum drag force.

For the same amplitude, Figures 1-3 and Figures 4-6, and for the same paddle settings giving the same effective area, as the frequency increases the forces increases dramatically. For instance comparing Figures 1 and 3 show that for a/d = 2.0148 the maximum force increases from approximately 290 N to 4700 N (or 65 lb to 1057 lb). For the same frequency and amplitude ratio, for example Figure 1, when the paddle setting changes from its minimum are (a/d = 3.1181) to its maximum area (a/d = 2.0148) the maximum force increases from approximately 90 N to 290 N. (or 20 lb to 65 lb).

The maximum force to move the disk increases as the oscillation amplitude increases. For instance, compare the 60 and 90 cm amplitudes in Figures 1 and 4, for 0.5 cps frequency. To compare identical paddle positions look at the effective diameter of 37.36 in Table 2 which corresponds to a/d of 1.6060 and 2.4090 for the 60 cm and 90 cm amplitudes respectively. The maximum force, from Figure 4, for the higher amplitude is approximately 175 N (or 39 lb) and for the lower amplitude, Figure 1, is approximately 90 N (or 20 lb). This represents almost a doubling of the maximum force when the amplitude increasing 50% from 60 to 90 cm. This ratio is fairly consistent for other frequencies. Comparing Figures 2 and 5 for the 1 cps frequency and using the same effective diameter of 37.36 shows a rise from 1500 N to 2950 N (or 337 lb to 663 lb) again approximately a doubling of the maximum force.

The energy dissipation rate, in watts, is shown in Figures 7 through 12 for the range of conditions shown in Figures 1 through 6. In all of the plots the peak dissipation rate occurs when the drag force is a maximum. The smaller peak occurs when the inertia force is a maximum. This result indicates that if future design modifications are contemplated it would be of most benefit to increase the drag component of the device rather than the inertia component.

The energy dissipation rate was used to calculate the total energy dissipated in one cycle, in joules (1 joule is 0.000239 calories, based on kg). This is shown in Figure 13 versus effective diameter which corresponds to different paddle settings. The results are presented for the 90 cm amplitude and three different oscillating frequencies. There is a steady nearly linear rise of energy use versus effective diameter but the slope is dramatically influenced by the operating frequency. High frequency operation, from 0.5 to 2.0 cps will increase the energy use by approximately a factor of 23 from 2,000 to 46,000 at the largest effective diameter. While at the lower effective diameter the increase over the same change in operating frequency is approximately 13 times, from 1,000 to 13,000.

CONCLUSIONS

An analysis was carried out to determine the force, energy dissipation and total energy consumed per cycle of operating the aquatoner in a oscillatory manner in water. The results were based on the experimental verification of the drag coefficient and added mass coefficient of the accelerated aquatoner. The results show the effect of paddle position, operating frequency and operating amplitude or extension. It is evident that a wide range of operating forces and energy use rates can be achieved with this device.

REFERENCES

1. Minamizawa, M. and Endoh, K., , J. Chemical Engineering of Japan, 17, n. 2, 1984, pp 186.

2. Kanwal, R.P., J. Fluid Mechanics, 19, 1964, p. 631.

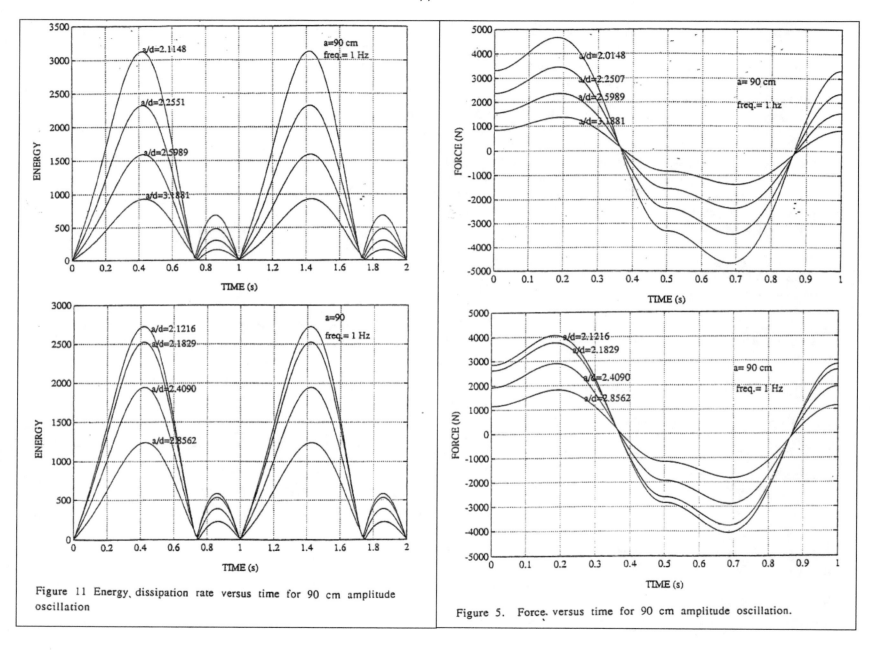

Figure 11 Energy, dissipation rate versus time for 90 cm amplitude oscillation

Figure 5. Force, versus time for 90 cm amplitude oscillation.

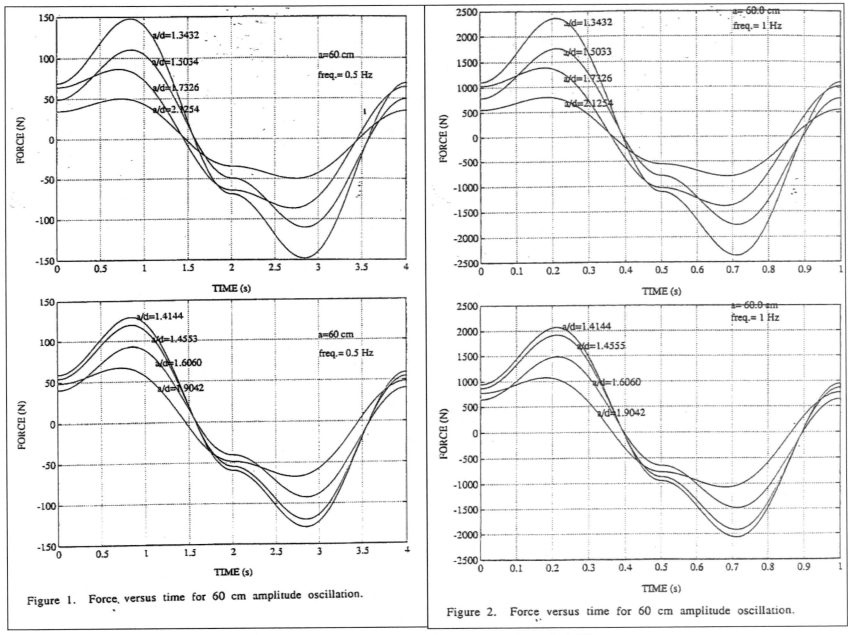

Figure 1. Force versus time for 60 cm amplitude oscillation.

Figure 2. Force versus time for 60 cm amplitude oscillation.

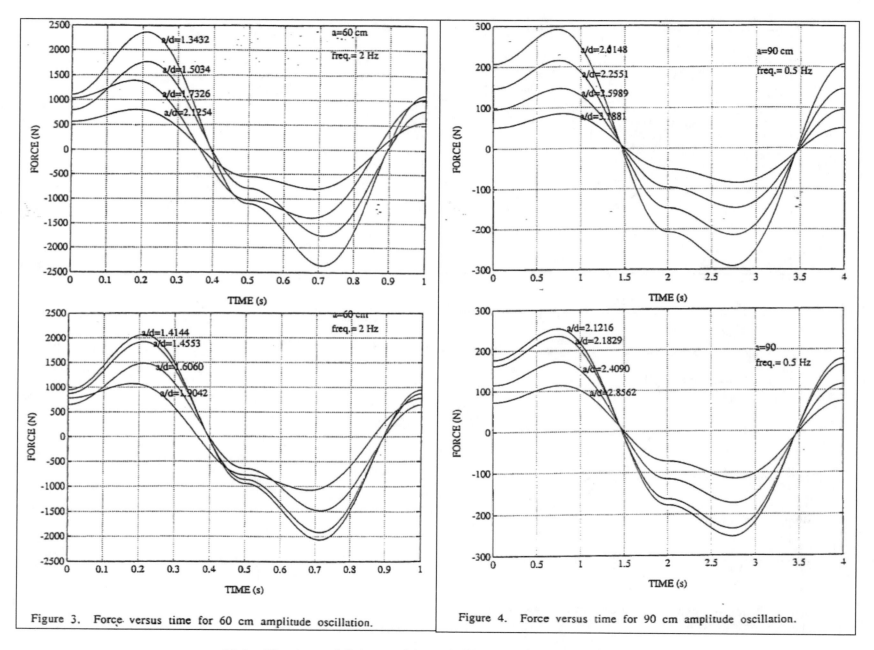

Figure 3.   Force versus time for 60 cm amplitude oscillation.

Figure 4.   Force versus time for 90 cm amplitude oscillation.

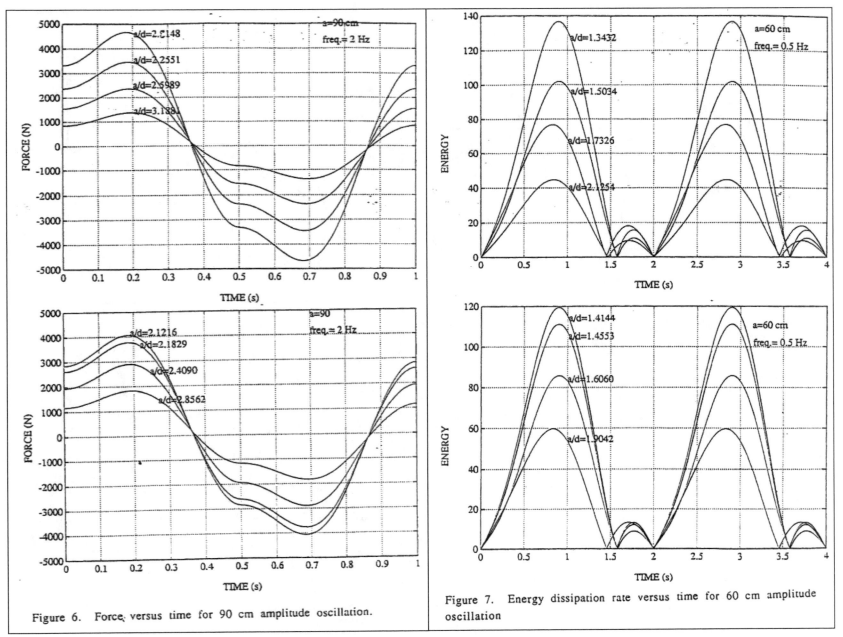

Figure 6. Force versus time for 90 cm amplitude oscillation.

Figure 7. Energy dissipation rate versus time for 60 cm amplitude oscillation

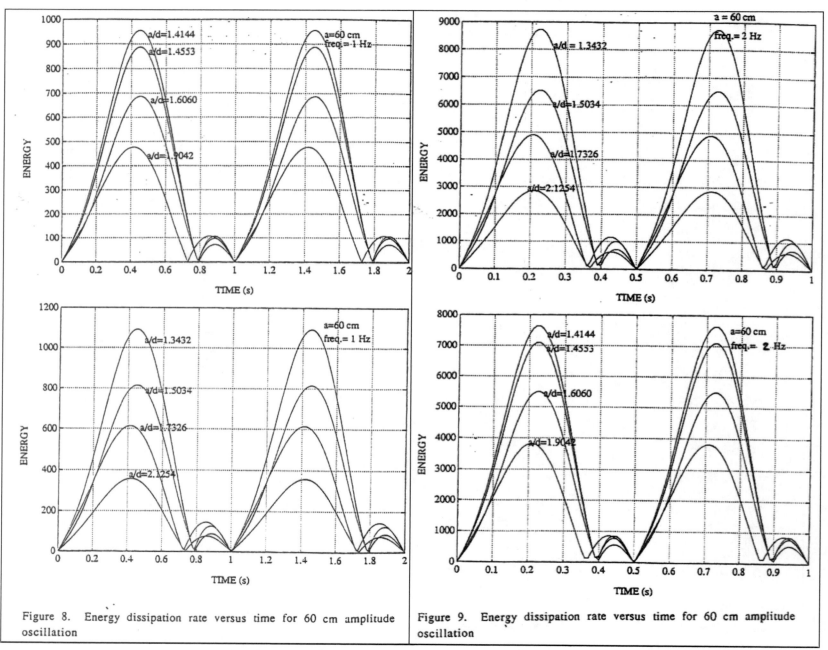

Figure 8. Energy dissipation rate versus time for 60 cm amplitude oscillation

Figure 9. Energy dissipation rate versus time for 60 cm amplitude oscillation

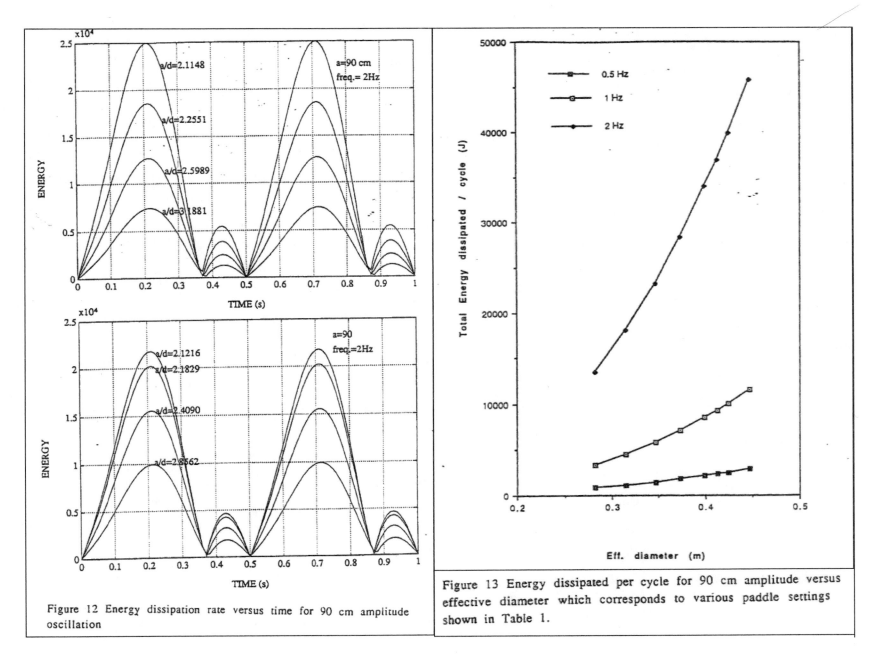

Figure 12 Energy dissipation rate versus time for 90 cm amplitude oscillation

Figure 13 Energy dissipated per cycle for 90 cm amplitude versus effective diameter which corresponds to various paddle settings shown in Table 1.

Nalu: The Art and Science of Aquatic Fitness, Bodywork & Therapy

References & Credits

ACSM (1998) The American College of Sports Medicine recommended quantity and quality of exercise for developing and maintaining cardiorespiratory and muscular fitness and flexibility in healthy adults. *Medicine and Science in Sports and Exercise.* 30(6):975-991.

Aitken, G.S. (1986) Syndromes of lumbopelvic dysfunction. *Modern Manual Therapy of the Vertebral Column.* G.P.Grieve (ed). Churchill Livingston.

Alberts, Bruce et.al.(2002) *Molecular Biology of the Cell.* 4th ed. Garland Pub.

Alaimo, K. et al. (1994) Dietary intake of vitamins, minerals, and fiber of persons ages 2 months and over in the US. Third National Health and Nutrition Examination Survey, Phase 1. *Advertising Data.*258:1-28.

Altman, Nathaniel (2000) *Healing Springs, The Ultimate Guide to Taking the Waters.*Healing Arts Press.

AMTA (2003) *Massage Therapy Increasingly Sought for Pain Relief.* Press Release 10/15/03 www.amtamassage.org.

ADA, American Diabetes Association(2000) Clinical Practice Recommendations 2000: diabetes mellitus and exercise. *Diabetic Care.*23(1):S50-S54.

Anderson, J.W. et al. (1994) Health benefits and practical aspects of high fiber diets. *American Journal of Clinical Nutrition.* 59:5S0, 1242S.

Anderson, R.A. (1986) Chromium metabolism and its role in disease processes in man. *Clinical Physiology and Biochemistry.*4:31.

Alexander, R.M., and Bennet-Clark (1977) Storage of elastic strain energy in muscle and other tissues. *Nature.*265:114-117.

Anderson, F.C. and M.G.Pandy(1993) Storage and utilization of elastic strain energy during jumping. *Journal of Biomechanics.* Dec;26(12):1413-1427.

Anderson, I.C. and C. Ericksson (1970) Piezoelectric properties of dry and wet bone. *Nature.*227: 491-492.

Anderson, P.A. and Sprecher, H.W. (1987) Omega-3 fatty acids in nutrition and health. *Dietetic Currents.* 14(2):7.

Applegate, E. A.(1991) *Power Foods, High Performance Foods For High Performance People.* Rodale Press.

Arborelius, M. et al. (1972) Hemodynamic changes in man during immersion with the head above water. *Aerospace Medicine.* 43:592-598.

Aris, Rutherford(1990) *Vectors, Tensors, and the Basic Equations of Fluid Mechanics.* Dover.

Aronson, W. et al. (2001) Diet, exercise slow prostate cancer as much as 30%. *Journal of Urology.* Sep.2001.

Arroll, B., and R. Beaglehole (1992) Does physical activity lower blood pressure: a critical review of the clinical trials. *Journal of Epidemiology.* 45(5):439-447.

Ashcroft, Frances M.(2000) *Life at the Extremes.* University of California Press.

Atkinson,P.J. (1965) Changes in resorption spaces in femoral cortical bone with age. *Journal of Pathology and Bacteriology.* 89:173-178.

Avellini, B.A. et al.(1983) Cardio-respiratory physical training in water and on land. *European Journal of Applied Physiology and Occupational Physiology.* 50:255-263.

Ball, Philip(2000) *Life's Matrix.* Farrar, Straus, & Giroux.

Barinaga, Marcia. (1989) The mind revealed. *Science.*vol.249.

Barron, P. (1995) *Hydrotherapy Theory and Technique.*Oviedo Physical Medicine and Rehabilitation, Inc.

Barton, R.N.E.(2003) *Paleolithic Archeology* GIBCEMED and.Oxford Brookes University. Gibraltar Museum Site Research Team www.gib.gi/museum/p58.htm

Bassett, C. and R.O. Becker. (1962) Generation of electric potentials by bone in response to mechanical stress. *Science.*137, 1063-1064.

Batchelor, G.K.(2000) *An Introduction to Fluid Mechanics.* Cambridge University Press.

Bates, Andrea and Norm Hanson (1996) *Aquatic Exercise Therapy.*W.B.Saunders Co. Philadelphia.

Batmanghelidj, Fereydoon(1995) *Your Body Cries for Water.* Global Health.

Beck, B.R. and M.R.Shoemaker(2000) Osteoporosis: Understanding key risk factors and therapeutic options. *The Physician and Sportsmedicine.* 28:2.

Becker, Robert O. and Gary Selden.(1985) *The Body Electric.* William Morrow & Co.

Bedgood, D.(1983) *Aquatoning, A Renaissance in Fitness.* Kona Fitness, Inc.

Bernard, T.N. and J.D.Cassidy.(1991) The sacroiliac joint syndrome. *The Adult Spine: Principles and Practice.* .J.W.Frymoyer(Ed). Pp2111-2112. Raven Press

Biewener, A.A. and T.J.Roberts(2000) Muscle and tendon contributions to force, work, and elastic energy savings: a comparative perspective. *Exercise and Sports Science Review.* Jul;28(3):99-107.

Biewener, A.A. and C. R. Taylor (1986) Bone strain: a determinant of gait and speed?. *Journal of Experimental Biology.*123: 383-400.

Bilezikian, John P. Ed.(1996) *Principles of Bone Biology.* Academic Press.

Billig, H. and Loewendahl, E. (1949) *Mobilization of the Human Body.* Stanford University Press; Oxford University Press.

Blair, S.N., et al. (1989) Physical fitness and all-cause mortality: a prospective study of healthy men and women. *Journal of the American Medical Association.* 262:2395-2401.

Blake, G.M. and I. Fogelman(1996) Principles of Bone Densitometry. *Principles of Bone Biology* (J.P.Bilezikian, Ed.). Academic Press.

Bonner, John Tyler(1952) *Morphogenesis. Princeton* University Press.

Bronner, F. (1994) Calcium and osteoporosis. *American Journal of Clinical Nutrition.* 60(6):831.

Bortz, W.M.(1982) Disuse and Aging. *JAMA.* 248(10):1203-1208.

Bosbough, John(1985) *Stephen Hawking's Universe.* William Morrow & Co.

Bridges, P.S. (1989) Spondylolysis and its relationship to degenerative joint disease in the prehistoric southeastern United States. *American Journal of Physical Anthropology.* July, 79(3):321-329.

Bridges, P.S. (1991) Degenerative joint disease in hunter-gatherers and agriculturalists from the Southeastern United States. *American Journal of Physical Anthropology.* August, 85(4):379-391.

Bridges, P.S. (1994) Vertebral arthritis and physical activities in the prehistoric southeastern United States. *American Journal of Physical Anthropology.*93(1):83-93, January.

Brookes, Murray and W.J. Renell(1998) *Blood Supply of Bone: Scientific Aspects.* Springer Verlag.

Buchman, Dian D.(2002) *The Complete Book of Water Healing.* Contemporary Books.

Buckwalter, J.A. et al.(1995) Bone Biology Part I: structure, blood supply, cells, matrix, and mineralization.*Journal of Bone Joint Surgery.*77-A, 1256-1275.

Bulgen, D.Y.et al.(1984) Frozen shoulder:a prospective clinical study with an evaluation of three treatment regimens. *Ann Rheumatic Dis.* 43(3):353-360.

Byatt, Andrew, et al.(2002) *The Blue Planet.* D.K.Publishing.

Calkin, M.W. Ed.(1948) *The Metaphysical System of Hobbs.* Open Court Publishing.

Campbell, Don (1990) *Healing Powers of Tone and Chant.* Quest Books.

Carter, D.R. and W>C>Hayes (1976) Bone compressive strength: the influence of Density and Strain Rate. *Science. Dec 10; 194(4270):1174-1176.*

Cavanaugh, D.J. and C.E.Cann (1988) Brisk walking does not stop bone loss in postmenopausal women. *Bone.* 9(4):201-204.

Cech, Donna and Suzanne Martin(2002) *Functional Movement.* W.B.Saunders.

Chard, M.D. et al.(1991) Shoulder disorders in the elderly: a community survey. *Arthritis and Rheumatism.* 34(6):766-769.

Cheng, David K.(1989) *Field and Wave Electromagnetics.* 2ned. Addison. Wesley Pub.

Cheremisinoff, Nicholas P. and Gupca, R. Eds.(1983) *Handbook of Fluids in Motion.*Butterworth-Heinemann.

Chernoff, R. (1994) Thirst and fluid requirements. .*Nutrition Review.*52. *Archives of Internal Medicine.* 152(3):655.

Chodorow, Joan (1997) *Encountering Jung on Active Imagination.* Princeton University Press.

Clemens, T.L. and J. O'Riordan(1995) Vitamin D. *Principles and Practice of Endocrinology and Metabolism.* 2nd ed. (Becker, K.I. Ed.).pp 483-490. J.B.Lippincott.

Christensen, N.J. and Galbo, H. (1983) Sympathetic nervous activity during exercise. *Annual Review of Physiology.* 45:139-153.

Clementz, G.L.(1990) The spectrum of vitamin B12 deficiency. *American Family Physician.* 41(1):150.

Cohen, Neil S.(1989) *The Principles of Proper Food Combining.* Legion of Light.

Colberg, S.R. and D.P. Swain(2000) Exercise and diabetes control. *The Physician and Sportsmedicin.,* 28(4).

Conrad, Emilie (1997) Continuum Movement Training Class. Santa Monica, CA.

Cook, J.L. et al.(1997) A cross-sectional study of 100 athletes with jumper's knee managed conservatively and surgically. *British Journal of Sports Medicine.*31(4):332-336.

Cook, J.L. and K.M.Kahn et al.(2000) Patellar tendon ultrasound in asymptomatic elite junior basketball players: a 12-month longitudinal study in 52 tendons. *Journal of Ultrasound Medicine.* Press.

Cooper, C. et al. (1988) Physical activity, muscle strength, and calcium intake in fracture of the proximal femur in Britain. *British Medical Journal.* 297:1443.

Cooper, C.(1997) The crippling consequences of fractures and their impact on quality of life. *American Journal of Medicine.* 103(2A):12S-19S.

Cordell, Linda S. Ed. (1989) *The Dynamics of Southwest Prehistory.* Smithsonian Institution Press.

Cosman, F. and R. Lindsay(1998) Is parathyroid hormone a therapeutic option for osteoporosis? A review of the clinical evidence. *Calcified Tissue International.*62(6):475-480.

Convertino, V.A. et al.(1996) American College of Sports Medicine position stand on exercise and fluid replacement. *Medical Science in Sports and Exercise.* 28(1):I-vii.

Coyle, E.F. and S.F.Montain. (1992) Benefits of fluid replacement with carbohydrate during exercise. *Medicine and Science in Sports and Exercise.* 24:33S.

Cromie, W.J.(2000) Exercise reduces cancer risk. *The Harvard University Gazette.*May 11.

Curry, J.(1984) *The Mechanical Adaptations of Bones.*Princeton University Press.

Curry, J.(2002) *Bones: Structure and Mechanics.*Princeton University Press.

Dalen, N. and Olsson. K.E. (1974) Bone mineral content and physical activity. *Acta Orhop. Scand.* 45:170-174.

Daugherty, R.L. and Ingersoll (1954) *Fluid Mechanics.* McGraw-Hill.

Davis, J.M., et al. (1990) Fluid availability of sports drinks differing in carbohydrate type and concentration. *American Journal of Clinical Nutrition.*51:1054.

Day, Sean (2003) *Esquire Magazine.* quote in August issue p.70.

Delmas, P.D.(1993) Biochemical markers of bone turnover. *Journal of Bone Mineralization.*8, S549-S554.

DiPietro, L, and J. Dziura(2000) Exercise: a prescription to delay the effects of aging. *The Physician and Sportsmedicine.* 28:10.

Denes, Thomas A. and Diana D. DeMedina (1997) *The Waterproof Coach.*Ancient Marine Aquatics.

Dilsen, G. et al. (1989) The role of physical exercise in prevention and management of osteoporosis. *Clinical Rheumatology.* S2:70-75.

Domen, R.E. (1981) Paleopathological evidence of rheumatoid arthritis. *Journal of the American Medical Association JAMA.* 246(17):1899, Oct.

Dreyfuss. P. et al. (1996) The value of medical history and physical examination in diagnosing sacroiliac joint pain. *Spine.* 21(22):2594-2602.

Dull, Harold (1993) *Watsu, Freeing the Body in Water,*Harbin Springs Publishing, Middletown, CA.

Eastell,R. et al.(1991) Interelationship among vitamin D metabolism, true calcium absorption, parathyroid function and age in women. *Journal of Bone Mineralization.* 6:125-132.

Efunda (2004) www.efunda.com. Engineering Fundamentals Online Publisher

Einborn, Thomas A. (1996) Biomechanics of Bone, *Principles of Bone Biology,* (J.P.Bilezikian, Ed.).Academic Press.

Ellenbecker, T.S.(1995) Rehabilitation of shoulder and elbow injuries in tennis players. *Clinical Sports Medicine.* 14(1):87-110.

Elmore, William C. and Mark A. Heald.(1985) *Physics of Waves.* Dover.

Emoto, Masaru (2002) *Messages from Water.* Hado Kyoikusha, Tokyo.

Engstrom, G. et al. (1999) Hypertensive men who exercise regularly have lower rate of cardiovascular mortality. *Journal of Hypertension.*17(6):737-742.

Epstein, M.(1992) Renal effects of head out immersion in humans: a 15-year update. *Physiology Review.*72:563.

Eriksen, E.F.(1986) Normal and pathological remodeling of human trabecular bone. *Endocrinology.*7, 379-408.

Erickson, L.(2002) *The Tendinosis Injury.* Published at www.tendinosis.org/injury.html.

Eriksson, J. et al.(1998) Aerobic endurance exercise or circuit-type resistance training for individuals with impaired glucose tolerance? *Hormone Metabolism Research.*30(1):37041.

Ettema, G.L.(2001) Muscle efficiency: the controversial role of elasticity and mechanical energy conversion in stretch-shortening cycles. *European Journal of Applied Physiology.* Sep;85(5):457-465.

Ettema, G.J. (1996) Mechanical efficiency and efficiency of storage and release of series elastic energy in skeletal muscle during stretch-shorten cycles. *Journal of Experimental Biology.* Sep;(Pt.9):1983-1997.

Fabiani, D. et al.(1996) Rheumatological aspects of mineral water. *Clinics in Dermatology* 14:573.

Field, T. et al. (1996) Massage therapy reduces anxiety. *International Journal of Neuroscience.*86:197-205.

Field, T. et al. (1992) Massage therapy reduces anxiety in child and adolescent psychiatric patients. *Journal of the American Academy of Child and Adolescent Psychiatry.* 31:125.

Fish, F.E. and B.R.Stein.(1990) Functional correlates of differences in bone density among terrestrial and aquatic genera in the family Mustelidae (Mammalia). *Zoomorphology.* 110:339-345.

FNB, Food and Nutrition Council, National Research Council. (1994) *Recommended Dietary Allowance, 11ᵗʰ ed.* National Academy Press.

Fortin, J.D. et al. (1994) Sacroiliac joint: pain referral maps. *Spine.* 19(13):1475-1482.

Fortin, J.D. et al. (1999) Three pathways between the sacroiliac joint and neural structures. *American Journal of Neuroradiology.* 20(8):1429-1434.

Fox, S.M., et al.(1971) Physical activity and the prevention of coronary heart disease. *Annals of Clinical Research.* 3(6)404-432.

Frost, H.M.(1964) *The Laws of Bone Structure.* Charles C. Thomas Co.

Frost, N.E. (1965) The growth of fatigue cracks. *Proceedings of the First International Conference on Fracture.* 3:1433-1459.

Fucada, E., and I. Yasuda. (1957) On the Piezoelectric Effect of Bone. *Journal of the Physical Society of Japan.* 12: 10.

Fullmer, C.S. (1992) Intestinal calcium absorption. *Journal of Nutrition.* 122:644.

Gage, J.P.et al.(1995) Collagen type in dysfunctional temporomandibular joint discs. *Journal of Prosthetic Dentistry.* 74(5):517-520.

Georgeakopoulos, Alexander (1996, 1998) *Aquatic Writings.* La Mesa, Ca. Published at http://aquaticwritings.com.

Gallegos, Eligio Stephen (1985) *The Personal Totem Pole Process.* Moon Bear Press.

Germain, Blandine (1993) *Anatomy of Movement.* Eastland Press.

Genet. J.C.(1995) The brain wave frequencies of health. *Health/Science, New Mexican.* 04/07/95 issue.

Gohil, K. et al. (1986) Vitamin E deficiency and vitamin C supplements: exercise and mitochondrial oxidation. *Journal of Applied Physiology.* 60(6):1986-1991.

Goldberg, Donald et.al.(2002) *The Best Supplements for your Health.* Kensington Pub.

Goldstein, Herbert et al.(2002) *Classical Mechanics.* Prentice Hall.

Gondhalekar, P.(2001) *The Grip of Gravity.* Cambridge University Press.

Goodman, A., D. Dufour and Gretel Pelto , Eds.(1999) *Nutritional Anthropology: Biocultural Perspectives on Food and Nutrition,* McGraw Hill.

Grant, Keith (2003)McKinonmassage.com/articles. Oakland, CA

Gray, C.M.(1994) Synchronous oscillations in neuronal systems. *Neuroscience.* 1:11-38.

Greenberg, Jerrold S.(1999) *Comprehensive Stress Management.* 6ᵗʰ edition. McGraw Hill.

Guyton, A.C. (1996) *Textbook of Medical Physiology, 9th ed.* W.B. Saunders.

Haddleston, A.L. et al. (1980) Bone mass in lifetime tennis players. *JAMA.* 244: 1107-1109.

Hall, J., Bisson, D. and P. O'Hare (1990) The physiology of immersion. *Physiotherapy.* 76:517-521.

Hall, Manly P.(1930) *Space-Born.* Skelton Publishing Co.

Haapenen, N. et al.(1997) Association of leisure time physical activity with the risk of coronary heart disease, hypertension and diabetes in middle-aged men and women. *International Journal of Epidemiology.* 26(4):739-747.

Hagberg, J.M. (1995) Physical activity, physical fitness, and blood pressure: *NIH Consensus Development Conference: Physical Activity and Cardiovascular Health.* pp.69-71.

Hamer, T. and A. Morton.(1990) Water running: training effects and specificity of aerobic, anaerobic and muscle parameters following an eight-week interval training program. *Australian Journal of Scientific Medicine.* 22:13-22.

Hansen, J.P. and I.R. McDonald (1990) *Theory of Simple Liquids,* .2ⁿᵈed. Academic Press

Harner, Michael (1990) *The Way of the Shaman*. Harper, San Francisco.

Harris, S.S. and B. Dawson-Hughes (1994) Caffeine and bone loss in healthy postmenopausal women. *American Journal of Clinical Nutrition*.60:573.

Haskell, W.L. and W. T. Phillips (1995) Exercise training, fitness, health, and longevity. In *Perspectives in Exercise Science and Sports Medicine: Exercise in older adults*. D.R.Lamb, et al., (Eds.)vol.8. pp11-52.

Hawking, Stephen(1988, 1990) *A Brief History Of Time*. Bantam Books.

Harrison, D.E. et al. (1997) The sacroiliac joint: a review of anatomy and biomechanics with clinical implications. *Journal of Manipulative Physiology and Therapy*. 20(9):607-617.

Heinonen, A. et al. (1995) Bone mineral density in female athletes representing sports with different loading characteristics of the skeleton. *Bone*. 17: 197-203.

Hertler, et al. (1992) Water running and the maintenance of maximum oxygen consumption and leg strength in women. *Medicine and Science in Sports and Exercise*. 24:S23.

Herzog, W. et al. (1999) Electromyographic responses of back and limb muscles associated with spinal manipulative therapy. *Spine*. 24(2):146-153.

Hillman, R.A. and T.M. Skerry (1995) Inhibition of bone resorption and stimulation of formation by mechanical loading. *Journal of Bone Mineralization*.10: 683-689.

Hoeger, W.K. et al. (1992) Comparison of maximal VO2, HR and RPE between treadmill running and water aerobics. *Medicine and Science in Sports and Exercise*. 24:S96.

Hoeger, W.K. et al. (1992) A comparison of selected training responses to water aerobics and low impact aerobic dance. *National Aquatics Journal*.Winter 13-16.

Hoffman, N.B. (1991) Dehydration in the elderly: insidious and manageable. *Geriatrics*. 46:35.

Hoffer, A.A. et al.(1991) Effects of water immersion on cardiac output of lean and fat male subjects at rest and during exercise. *Aviation and Space Environmental Medicine*.62:125.

Hopper, J. and E.S. Seeman(1994) The bone density of female twins discordant for tobacco use. *New England Journal of Medicine*.330:387.

Huong, George (2000) personal communication Re: Computational Fluid Dynamics. Faculty, Univ. of Kentucky, Lexington.

Huxley, H.E. and M. Kress(1985) Crossbridge behavior during muscle contraction. *Journal of Muscle Research and Cell Motility*. 6(2):153-161.

INTERSALT(1988) Intersalt Cooperative Research Group: An international study of electrolyte excretion and blood pressure. *British Medical Journal*.279:319.

Ireland, D et al.(2001) Multiple changes in gene expression in chronic human Achilles tendinopathy. *Matrix Biology*.(3):159-169.

Ivy, J. et al.(1988) Muscle glycogen synthesis after exercise: effect of time of carbohydrate ingestion. *Journal of Applied Physiology*. 64(4):1480-1485.

Jackson, M.J.(1987) Muscle damage during exercise: possible role of free radicals and protective effect of vitamin E. *Proceedings of the Nutrition Society*. 46(1):77-80.

Jahara, Mario (1997) Jahara Technique; Jahara Concepts. www.jahara.com

Jasmuheen (2000) Living on Light. *Monthly Aspectarian*. August issue.

Jenny, Hans (2001) *Cymatics*. MACROmedia.

Jequire, E. (1994) Carbohydrates as a source of energy. *American Journal of Clinical Nutrition*. 59;3S,682S.

Johnson, R.L. (1973) The lung as an organ of oxygen transport. *Basics of Respiratory Disease*. 2:1-60.

Johnson,Leland G.(1983) *Biology*. Wm.C.Brown Co.

Johnston, I.A.(1991) Muscle action during locomotion: a comparative perspective. *Journal of Experimental Biology*. 160:167-185.

Jordan, Paul (1999) *Neanderthal Man and the Story of Human Origins*. Sutton.

Juhan, Deane (1987) *Job's Body: A Handbook for Bodywork*. Station Hill Press.

Kamiya, Joseph (1968) Conscious control of brain waves. *Psychology Today*. 1:57-60.

Kampert, J.B. et al.(1996) Physical activity, physical fitness, and all-cause and cancer mortality: a prospective study of men and women. *Annals of Epidemiology*. 6(5):452-457.

Kanehisa, J. and J.N. Heersche(1988) Osteoclastic Bone Resorption. *Bone*. 9: 73-79.

Kanis, J.A. et al.(1994) The diagnosis of osteoporosis, *Journal of Bone Mineralization*. 9(8):1137-1141.

Kannus, P. (2000) Structure of the tendon connective tissue. *Scandinavian Journal of Medicine & Science in Sports*. 10(6)p.312-320.

Kapandji, I.A. (1974) *The Physiology of Joints, Vol.2, Vol.3*, Churchill Livingston, London.

Kardas, E.P. (2003) Integration: All-or-none and summation. *Lecture at Southern Arkansas University, Magnolia; Department of Behavior and Social Sciences*. Delivered as Biology 260 Lecture on Sept. 25, 2002, pub.2003@http://peace.saumag.edu/faculty/Kardas/Courses.

Kawakami, Y. et al.(2002) In vivo muscle-fibre behaviour during counter-movement exercise in humans reveals significant role of tendon elasticity. *Journal of Physiology*. 540:635-646.

Keitaro, K. et al.(2001) Influence of static stretching on viscoelastic properties of human tendon structures in vivo. *Journal of Applied Physiology*. 90:520-527.

Keitaro, K. et al. (2001) Influences of repetitive muscle contractions with different modes on tendon elasticity in vivo. *Journal of Applied Physiology*.91:277-282.

Keitaro, K., H. Kanehisa, et al. (2001) Effects of isometric training on the elasticity of human tendon structures in vivo. *Journal of Applied Physiology*.91:26-32.

Kenyon, T. and Essene, V. (1996) *The Hathor Material*. S.E.E.Publishing Co.

Kessler, R.M. and D. Hertling (1983) *Management of Common Musculoskeletal Disorders: Physical Therapy Principles and Methods*, Harper & Row, Philadelphia.

Khan, K.M. et al.(2000) Overuse Tendinosis, not tendonitis: a new paradigm for a difficult clinical problem. *The Physician and Sportsmedicine*.28:38-48.

Khan, K.M. et al. (2000) Where is the pain coming from in tendinopathy? It may be biochemical, not only structural, in origin. *British Journal of Sports Medicine*. 34(2):81-84.

Kiely, D.K., et al.(1994) Physical activity and stroke risk: The Framingham Study..*American Journal of Epidemiology*. 140:608.

Kimmel, D.B. and R. R. Becker et al. (1990) A comparison of the iliac bone histomorphometric data in post-menopausal osteoporotic and normal subjects. *Bone Mineralization*. 11: 217-235.

Kirk, A. et al. (2003) Increasing physical activity in people with type 2 diabetes. *Diabetes Care*. 26(4):1186-1192.

Klages, Ellen(1991) *Harbin Hot Springs, Healing Waters Sacred Land*. Harbin Springs Publishing.

Kleerekoper, M. et al.(1994) Reference data for bone mass, calciotropic hormones, and biochemical markers of bone remodeling in older (55-75) postmenopausal white and black women. *Journal of Bone Mineralization*.9(8):1267-1276.

Korostoff, E.(1977) Stress generated potentials in bone: Relationship to piezoelectricity of Collagen. *Journal of Biomechanics*. 10: 41-44.

Kravitz, Len and Jerry J. Mayo(1997) *The Physiological Effects of Aquatic Exercise*. Aquatic Exercise Association.

Kraushaar, B, and R. Nirschl. (1999) Tendinosis of the elbow (tennis elbow): clinical features and findings of histological, immunohistochemical, and electron microscopy studies. *Journal of Bone and Joint Surgery*. 81(2):259-278.

Lamb, Horace(1993) *Hydrodynamics*. Dover.

LaMothe, J. and R. Zernicke (2003) Strain rate influences periosteal bone formation. *Abstract*. Published at www.cihrmatrix.ca, University of Calgary.

Lanyon, L.E. (1984) Functional strain as a determinant for bone remodeling. *Calcified Tissue International*. 36:S56-S61.

Lanyon, L.E. et al. (1984) Static vs. dynamic loads as an influence on bone remodeling. *Journal of Biomechanics*. 17:897-905.

Law, R. and H. Bukwirwa (1999)The Physiology of Oxygen Delivery. *Update in Anaesthesia*. Issue 10; Article 3; World Federation of Societies of Anaesthesiologists. www.nda.ox.ac.uk/wfsa/html.

Lazio, J. and P. Kannus (1997) *Human Tendons:Anatomy, Physiology, and Pathology*. Human Kinetics.

Ledbetter, W.B.(1992) Cell matrix response in tendon injury. *Clinics in Sports Medicine Vol. II*.3:533-577.

Lee, I.M., C.Z Hsieh, and R.S.Paffenbarger Jr.(1995) Exercise and longevity in men. The Harvard Alumni Study. *Journal of the American Medical Assoiciation*.273(15):1179-1184.

Levine, Peter (1997) *Waking the Tiger*. North Atlantic Books.

Liedloff, Jean (1985) *The Continuum Concept, In Search of Happiness Lost*. Addison-Wesley, New York.

Leklem, J. (1994) Vitamin B6. In *Modern Nutrition in Health and Disease* 8th ed. ,Shils, M.E. et al. (Eds). Lea and Fibiger.

Liburdy, J.(1992) *Evaluation of the Aquatoner Performance*.Clemson , SC. (in Nalu Appendix).

Lieb, Robert (2003) Adaptive physiological processes of the human body during a one hour aquatic treatment, particularly in relation to the blood, heart, circulation and the lymphatic systems. Translated thesis in *Aquatic Writings*. La Mesa, Ca. Published at http://aquaticwritings.tripod.com.

Liebenson, C. (1996) *Rehabilitation of the Spine: A Practitioner's Manual*.Williams & Wilkins.

Little, Kitty (1973) *Bone Behavior*. Academic Press.

Liu, S.H. et al.(1995) Collagen in Tendon, Ligament, and Bone Healing. *Clinical Orthopedics and Related Research*. 318:265-278.

Locker, Thomas (1997) *Water Dance*. Art/Science. Harcourt Brace & Co.

Lodish, Harvey,et.al.(1999) *Molecular Cell Biology*.W.H.Freeman & Co.

Lowe, W.W.(1995) *Functional Assessment in Massage Therapy*. Massage Education & Research Institute.

Maffulli, N.,K.M.Kahn et al. (1998) Overuse tendon conditions: time to change a confusing terminology. *Arthroscopy*.14(8):840-843.

Mahan, L. K. and S. Escott-Stump (2000) *Krause's Food, Nutrition, & Diet Therapy*. 10th ed. W.B.Saunders Co.

Makara, G. et al. (1980) The endocrine hypothalamus and the hormonal response to stress. *Selye's Guide to Stress Research*. Hans Selye,(Ed.) Rinehold.

MapQuest.com (2004),R.R.Donnelley & Sons, Lancaster, PA.

Manson, J.E. et al (1991) Physical activity and incidence of non-insulin dependent diabetes mellitus. *Lancet*. 338(8770):774-778.

Marcus , R. (1996) Mechanisms of exercise effects on bone. *Principles of Bone Biology*. Bilezikian, John P.(Ed.) Academic Press.

Marieb, Elaine Nicpon (2000) *Human Anatomy and Physiology*. 5th edition. Benjamin/Cummings.

Martin, Bruce and David Burr(1989) *Structure, Function, and Adaptation of Compact Bone*. Raven Press.

Martin, Bruce, D. Burr and N. Sharkey (1998) *Skeletal Tissue Mechanics.* Springer Verlag.

Martini, Frederic et al. (2001) *.Fundamentals of Anatomy and Physiology.* 5th edition. Prentice Hall.

Mayol, Jacques (1999) *Homo Delphinus.* Idelson-Gnocchi Publishing.

McKinney, R. and R.E.Andersen(2000) Exercise benefits patients with osteoarthritis. *The Physician and Sportsmedicine.* 28:10.

McLeod, K.J. and C.T. Rubin (1990) Frequency-specific modulation of bone adaptation by induced electric fields. *Journal of Theoretical Biology.* 145: 385-396.

McNeill, A.R.(2002)Tendon elasticity and muscle function. *Comprehensive Biochemistry and Molecular Integrative Physiology.*Dec;133(4):1001-1011.

Meydani, M. et al, (1993) Protective effect of vitamin E on exercise-induced oxidative damage in young and older adults. *American Journal of Physiology.* 264(33)R992.

Melton, L.J.,III(1995) Perspectives: How many women have osteoporosis now? *Journal of Bone Mineralization.* 10, 175-176.

Meredith, C.M. et al. (1989) Dietary protein requirements and body protein metabolism in endurance-trained men. *Journal of Applied Physiology.* 66:2850.

Mertz, W. (1993) Chromium in human nutrition: a review. *Journal of Nutrition.* 123:626.

Meyer, Richard E.(1982) *Introduction to Mathmatical Fluid Dynamics.* Dover.

Michaud, T.J. et al. (1995) Comparative exercise responses of deep water and treadmill running. *Journal of Strength and Conditioning Research.* 9:104.

Michell, Keith(1987) *Practically Macrobiotic.* Healing Arts Press.

Mikesell, Norman (1985) *Structured Water: Its Healing Effects On The Diseased State.* http://naturealternatives.com/lc/mikesell.html.

Milne-Thompson, L.M.(1996) *Theoretical Hydrodynamics.* Dover.

Mindell, Arnold (1993) *The Shaman's Body.* Harper & Row. San Francisco.

Misner, Charles W. et al.(1973) *Gravitation.* W.H.Freeman & Co.

Moore, J.S.(1992) Function, structure, and responses of components of the muscle-tendon unit. *Occupational Medicine.* 7(4):713-740.

Morgan, Elaine (1994) *The Scars of Evolution,* Oxford University Press.

Mougios, V. and A. Deligiannis (1993) Effect of water temperature on performance, lactate production and heart rate when swimming at maximal and submaximal intensity. *The Journal of Sports Medicine and Physical Fitness.* 33:27-33.

Morales, A.J. et al. (1994)Effects of replacement dose of dehydroepiandrosteine in men and women of advancing age. *Journal of Clinical Endocrinology and Metabolism.* 78 (6): 1360-1367.

Murray, R. (1987) The effects of consuming carbohydrate-electrolyte beverages on gastric emptying and fluid absorption during and following exercise. *Sports Medicine.* 4:322.

Murray, R. et al. (1989) The effects of glucose, fructose, and sucrose ingestion during exercise. *Medicine and Science in Sports and Exercise.* 21:275.

Murtagh, J. (1991) Bicipital tendonitis. *Australian Family Physician.* 20(6):817.

Narby, J. and F. Hurley, Eds. (2001) *Shamans Through Time.* Putnam.

Narlikar, J.Vishnu (1996) *The Lighter Side of Gravity.* Cambridge University Press.

NASA (1967) *Gemini Summary Conferenc. NASA SP-138.*

National Academy of Sciences(1989) *Recommended Dietary Allowances,* 10th ed. National Academy Press.

National Research Council (1982) Executive summary: Diet, Nutrition, and cancer. *Nutrition Today.* 17(4):20.

National Research Council (1989)*Diet and Health: Implications for reducing chronic disease risk.* National Academy Press.

Nei, Masatosh, and Sudhir Kumar (2000) *Molecular Evolution and Phylogenetics.*Oxford University Press.

Nessbaum, S.R. and J.T. Potts (1994) Advances in Immunoassays for parathyroid hormone: Clinical applications in skeletal disorders of bone and mineral metabolism. *The Parathyroids.* (Bilezikian, J.P. et al., Eds). pp.157-170. Raven Press.

Noakes, T. (2002) IMMA-AIMS advisory statement on guidelines for fluid replacement during marathon running. *New Studies in Athletics:IAAF.*17(1):7-11.

Nolte, John (2002) *The Human Brain: An Introduction to It's Functional Anatomy.* Mosby Year Book.

Odent, Michel (1995) *We Are All Water Babies,* Celestial Arts, Berkeley.

Ogden, David (2002) *The Unpredictable Command Technique.*DSL, Ltd.

Ozaki, J. et al.(1989) Recalcitrant chronic adhesive capsulitis of the shoulder: role of contracture of the coracohumeral ligament and rotator interval in pathogenesis and treatment. *Journal of Bone and Joint Surgery.* 71(10):1511-1515.

Pal, B. et al.(1986) Limitation of joint mobility and shoulder capsulitis in insulin and non-insulin dependent diabetes mellitus. *British Journal of Rheumatology.* 25(2):147-151.

Pardy, R.L. et al. (1984) The ventilatory pump in exercise. *Clinical Chest Medicine.* 5(March):35-49.

Parfitt, A.M. (1977) The cellular basis of bone turnover and bone loss. *Clinical Orthopedics.* 127: 236-247.

Parfitt, A.M. (1983) The physiological and clinical significance of bone histomorphometric data. *Bone Histomorphometry Techniques and Interpretation,* (R.R. Recker, Ed,).145-223. CRC Press.

Peckenpaugh, Nancy J. and C. M. Poleman(1995) *Nutrition Essentials and Diet Therapy.* W.B.Saunders & Co.

Pennington, S. Ed.(2001) *Proteomics: From Protein Sequence to Function.* Springer Verlag.

Pirnay, F. et al.(1987) Bone mineral content and physical activity. *International Journal of Sports Medicine.* 8: 331-335.

Placzek, J.D. et al.(1998) Long term effectiveness of translational manipulation for adhesive capsulitis. *Clinical Orthopedics.* Nov. 356:181-191.

Pocock, N.A. et al.(1987) Genetic determination of bone mass in adults. *Journal of Clinical Investigation.* 80: 706-710.

Pollack, M.L. et al.(1998) The recommended quantity and quality of exercise for developing and maintaining cardiorespiratory and muscular fitness and flexibility in healthy adults. *Medicine and Science in Exercise and Sports.* 30(6):975-991.

Pollack, M.L. et al. (2000) Resistance exercise in individuals with and without cardiovascular disease. Council on Clinical Cardiology, *American Heart Association.* 101(7):828-833.

Poor, G, and E.J. Atkinson et al. (1995) Age related hip fractures in men: clinical spectrum and short-term outcomes. *Osteoporosis International. 5(6):419-426.*

Prandtl, Ludwig et al.(1957) *Fundamentals of Hydro — and Aeromechanics.* Dover.

Rambaut, P.C. (1979) Prolonged weightlessness and calcium loss in man. *Acta Astronaut.*6:1113-22.

Rayment, I. et al. (1993) Three-dimensional structure of myosin subfragment-1: a molecular motor. *Science.* 261:50-58.

Reeves, N.D. et al. (2003) Effect of strength training on human patella tendon mechanical properties of older individuals. *Journal of Physiology.* 548.3, pp.971-981.

Reginster, J.Y. et al.(1999) Promising new agents in osteoporosis. *Drugs R D.* 1(3):195-201.

Riley, G.P.et al.(1994) Tendon degeneration and chronic shoulder pain. *Annals of Rheumatic Disorders.* 53(6):359-366.

Rivenburgh, D.W.(1992) Physical modalities in the treatment of tendon injuries. *Clinical Sportsmedicine.* 11A(3):645-659.

Rizk, T.E. et al.(1991) Corticosteroid injections in adhesive capsulitis: investigation of their value and site. *Archives of Physical Medicine and Rehabilitation.* 72(1):20-22.

Robinson, T.L., et al. (1995) Gymnasts exhibit higher bone mass than runners despite similar prevalence of amenorhea. *Journal of Bone Mineralization.* Res.10:26-35.

Rogers, J.M. and Dieppe, P.A. (1989) Symmetrical erosive arthritis in Ohio woodland indians. *Journal of Rheumatology.* 16(7):1012-3.

Romanov, Nicholas (2002) *Pose Method of Running.*Pose Tech. Press.

Rosen, Vicki and R. S. Thies (1995) *The Cellular and Molecular Basis of Bone Formation and Repair.* Landes Co.

Rothfeld, Glenn S. and Suzanne LeVert (1996) *Natural Medicine For Back Pain.* Rodale Press.

Rothschild, B.M. and Woods, R.J. (1990) Symmetrical erosive disease in Archaic Indians: the origin of rheumatoid arthritis in nthe New World. *Seminars in Arthritis & Rheumatism.* 19(5):278-284.

Rothschild, B.M.and Woods, R.J. (1992) Character of precolumbian North American spondyloarthropathy. *Journal of Rheumatology.* 19(8):1229-1235.

Rothjschild, B.M. and Woods, R.J. (1993) Geographic distribution of calcium pyrophosphate deposition disease in pre-Columbian North America: independent validation of CPPD criteria. *Clinical & Experimental Rheumatology.* 11(3):315-8.

Ruegemer, J. et al.(1990) Differences between prebreakfast and late afternoon glycemic responses to exercise in IDDM patients. *Diabetes Care.* 13(2):104-110.

Ruoti, Richard G., Morris, David M. and J. Andrew (editors 1996) *Aquatic Rehabilitation* Lippincott, Williams & Wilkins.

Sadler, Michelle (1999) *Encyclopedia of Human Nutrition.* 3 volumes. Academic Press.

Safran, M.R. et al. (1998) Biceps tendon injuries. *Manual of Sports Medicine.* 347-349. Lippincott Williams & Wilkins.

Salem, Lionel (1987) *Marvels of the Molecule.* VCH Publishers.

Samarskii, A.A. and A.N. Tikhonov (1990) *Equations of Mathematical Physics.* Dover.

Sander, R. and S. Brone (2000) Exercising the Frozen Shoulder. *The Physician and Sportsmedicine.* 28:9.

Sanders, M. et al.(1997) A comparison of results of functional water training on field and laboratory measures in older women. *Medicine and Science in Sports and Exercise.* 29:S110.

Sawyer, David (1999) *Birthing the Self.* Self-Published. Source: B. Courtney.

Schmitz, K. (2000) Exercise and cancer. *University of Minnesota Cancer Center.*

Schnirring, L. (2001) New formula estimates maximal heart rate. *The Physician and Sportsmedicine.*29:7.

Schroter, P. and A. Brunschwiler (1996) *Wassertanzen,* Aurum Verlag, Braunschweig.

Secher, N.H. et al. (1977) Central and regional circulatory effects of adding arm exercise to leg exercise. *Acta Physiol Scand.* 100(July):288-297.

Seely, Richard R., Trent Stephens and Philip Tate (2002) *Anatomy and Physiology.* McGraw Hill.

Seibel, M.J.(1999) *Dynamics of Bone and Cartilage Metabolism.* Academic Press.

Selye, H.(1956) *The Stress of Life.* McGraw Hill.

Sethi, N. et al. (1999) Disorders of the long head of the biceps tendon. *Journal of Shoulder and Elbow Surgery.* 8(6):644-654.

Shadwick, R.E. (1990) Elastic energy storage in tendons: mechanical differences related to function and age. *Journal of Applied Physiology.* 68: 1033-1040.

Shephard, R.J. (1966) The oxygen cost of breathing during vigorous exercise. *Journal of Experimental Physiology.* 51:336-350.

Sherman, W.M. (1987) Carbohydrate, muscle glycogen and improved performance. *The Physician and Sports Medicine.* 15(2):157.

Short, C.L. (1974) The antiquity of rheumatoid arthritis. *Arthritis & Rheumatism.* 17(3):193-205, May-June.

Sieg, Kay W. and S. P. Adams (1996) *Illustrated Essentials of Musculoskeletal Anatomy.* 3rd edition. Megabooks.

Silver, F.H. et al.(2001) Molecular basis for elastic energy storage in mineralized tendon. *Biomacromolecules.* Fall;2(3):750-756.

Silverberg, S.J. et al.(1996) *Osteoporosis* (R. Marcus, Ed.). pp716-723. *Academic Press.*

Simkin, Ariel, and Judith Ayalon.(1990) *Bone Loading.* Multimedia Books Ltd.

Smith, J.W. and R. Walmsley (1959) Factors affecting the elasticity of bone. *Journal of Anatomy.* 93,503-522.

Smolin, Lee(2001) *Three Roads to Quantum Gravity.* Basic Books.

Starr, Victor (1968) *Physics of Negative Viscosity Phenomena.* McGraw Hill.

Steele, D.G. and C. Bramblett (1988) *The Anatomy and Biology of the Human Skeleton.* Texas A&M Press.

Stein, B.R.(1989) Bone density and adaptation in semiaquatic mammals. *Journal of Mammology.* 70:467-476.

Stone, Ronald G.(1996) *Effects of Exercise on Bone Mineral Density.* School of Occupational Therapy and Physical Therapy, University of Puget Sound, Tacoma.

Stout, S. and D.J. Simmons(1979) Use of histology in ancient bone research. *Yearbook of Physical Anthropology.* 22:228-249.

Sturesson, B. et al.(2000) A radiostereometric analysis of the movements of the sacroiliac joints in the reciprocal straddle position. *Spine.* 25(2):214-217.

Tanaka, H., et al. (2001) Age-predicted maximal heart rate revisited. *Journal of the American College of Cardiology.* 37(1):153-156.

Taaffe, D.R. et al., (1995) Differential effects of swimming versus weight-bearing activity on bone mineral status of eumenorrheic athletes. *Journal of Bone Mineralization.* 10(4):586-593.

Tajima, F. et al.(1988) Renal and endocrine responses in the elderly during head out immersion. *American Journal of Physiology.*254:R977.

Tate, et al.(1998) In vivo tracer transport through the lacunocanicular system. *Bone.* 22:107-117.

Templeton, M.S. et al. (1996) Effects of aquatic therapy on joint flexibility and function ability in subjects with rheumatic disease. *Journal of Orthopaedic and Sports Physical Therapy.* 23:376-381.

Thompson, D.D.(1980) Age changes in bone mineralization, cortical thickness, and Haversian canal area. *Calcified Tissue International.* 31:5-11.

Tilton, F.E. et al.,(1980) Long-term follow-up of Skylab bone demineralization. *Aviation and Space Environmental Medicine.*51(11):1209-1213.

Tortora, Gerard J. et.al.(2000) *Principles of Anatomy and Physiology.* John Wiley & Sons.

Traber, P.G. (1995) Carbohydrate assimilation. In *Textbook of Gastroenterology,* T.Yamada. (Ed.).J.B.Lippincott.

TRI (2004) Touch Research Institute, University of Miami School of Medicine www.miami.edu/touch-research/home.html

Turnland, J.R. (1994) Copper. In *Modern Nutrition in Health and Disease*, 8th ed. vol.1.Shils, M.E. et al. Eds. Lea and Fiberger.

Van Baar, M.E. et al. (1999) Effectiveness of exercise therapy in patients with osteoarthritis of the hip or knee: a systematic review of randomized clinical trials. *Arthritis and Rheumatism*.42(7):1361-1369.

Van de Graaff, Kent M. and Stuart Ira Fox(1995) *Human Anatomy & Physiology*. Wm. C. Brown.

Van der Wiel, H.E. et al. (1995) Additional weight bearing during exercise is more important than duration of exercise for anabolic stimulus of bone. *Bone*. 16, 73-80.

Van Mechelen, W.(1992) Running injuries: a review of the epidemiological literature. *Sports Medicine*. 14(5):320-335.

von Franz (1980) On Active Imagination. *Inward Journey: art as therapy*. La Salle and London. pp 125-133.

Wall, W.P.(1983) *The correlation between high limb-bone density and aquatic habits in recent mammals*. Journal of Paleontology. *57(2):197-207*.

Warner, J.J. et al.(1996) Arthroscopic release for chronic refractory adhesive capsulitis of the shoulder. *Journal of Bone and Joint Surgery*. 78(12):1808-1816.

Weinbaum, S.,S.C. Cowan, and Y. Zeng (1994) A model for the excitation of osteocytes by mechanical loading-induced bone fluid shear stresses. *Journal of Biomechanics*. 27:339-360.

Weyerer, S. (1992) Physical inactivity and depression in the community. *International Journal of Sports Medicine*. 13:492-496.

Westling, L.(1992) Temporomandibular joint dysfunction and systemic joint laxity. *Swedish Dental Journal*. 81S:1-79.

Weyer, C. et al. (1999) The natural history of insulin secretory dysfunction and insulin resistance in the pathogenesis of type 2 diabetes mellitus. *Journal of Clinical Investigation*. 104(6):787-794.

Whalen, R.T.,D.R. Carter and C. Steele(1988) Influence of physical activity on the regulation of bone density. *Journal of Biomechanics*. 21: 825-837.

Williams, Sue Rodwell (1997) *Nutrition and Diet Therapy*. Mosby Year Book.

Wilmore, J.H. and D.L.Costill (1999) *Physiology of Sports and Exercise*.2nd ed. Human Kinetics.

Woo, S.L. et al. (1982) Mechanical properties of tendons and ligaments, II: The relationships of immobilization and exercise on tissue remodeling: *Biorheology*. 19(3):397-408.

Woods, R.J. and Rothschild, B.M. (1988) Population analysis of symmetrical erosive arthritis in Ohio Woodland Indians (1200 years ago). *Journal of Rheumatology*. 15(8):1258-1263.

Wyngaarden, James B. and Lloyd H. Smith, Jr. (1985) *Cecil Textbook of Medicine*. W.B.Saunders.

Yamada, H. (1970) *Strength of Biological Materials* (F.G.Evans, Ed.) Williams & Wilkins

Yokochi, Rohen(1993) *Color Atlas of Anatomy*. Igaku-Shoin Ltd.

Young, Warren C. et al.(2001) *Roark's Formulas for Stress and Strain*. 6th edition. McGraw Hill.

Weston, C. et al.(1987) Haemodynamic changes in man during immersion in water at different temperatures. *Clinical Science*. 73:613

Yung, C.et al.(2002) Sacroiliac joint pain syndrome in active patients. *The Physician and Sportsmedicine*. 30:11.

Zukav, Gary (1989) *The Seat of the Soul. p. 97*. Simon & Schuster.

Zeilik,Michael (1979) *Astronomy: The Evolving Universe*.2nd.ed. Harper & Row

Visual Credits

Milt Huffman-Lee *f56, 57, 59, 62-75, 130-149, 199, 201-203*
Bill Keough *f93A, 95, 96, 166, 174, 175B, 177-180*
Patti Loverock *f97*
Sky Dive Key West *f117*
Macromedia *f18*
Masaru Emoto *f19*
Emily Conrad *f24*
Dina Coyle   *Cover design, f60, 126-129, 154*
Corbis Corporation   *Background images for front & back covers*
Gabriella Detrich *f93B*
David Camplin *f93C*
Moody Castillo *f172A*
Sharon Walmuth *f75*
Igor Burdenko *f168*
Andreas Vesalii *f52*
Bill Eleazer *f103-116*
Ball (2000) *f151B*
Daugherty (1954) *f161*
Starr (1968) *f164, 165*
Zeilik (1979) *f160B*
University of Virginia
Molecular Biomechanics Lab *f58A-58E*
US Geological Survey, Paper 679-B *f157*

Michael Kesselring *f3, 98, 100, 169*
Barbara Courtney *f2, 6, 27, 30, 34A-34D*
Alexander Georgeakopoulos *f7, 9, 11B-14, 35-40, 43-50B*
Harold Dull *f8, 41*
Arjana Brunschwiler *f10, 11A, 42*
Richter-Colella Studios *f 15, 20-23, 25-28, 29, 31-33*
Mario Jahara *f16, 44*
School of Medicine
    Washington University at St. Louis, *f55A*
Hydrotone International *f182, 183*
Hydrofit *f184*
AquaTrend *f186*
Bioenergetics *f187*
Excel Sport Science *f188*
Eureka Mfg. Co. *f189*
RehabMed, Inc. *f191*
Pool Therapy, Inc. *f192*
Rio Swim Spa *f195*
SwimEx, Inc. *f196*
Biographical photos are from the contributing authors.
All other illustrations, drawings, photos, 3D charts & graphs are by Douglas Bedgood

Index

A

acetabulum   *168, 235*

acidosis   *245, 252*

ACTH   *355*

actin   *126-133, 263*

activating forces   *48*

activation frequency   *229*

activation rate   *229*

active healing   *47-49*

actomyosin   *129-133*

adduction   *151, 327*

adenosine triphosphate   *122, 129*

adhesions   *162, 362, 363*

adhesive capsulitis   *81, 182, 327*

adipose   *235, 261, 318, 361*

adrenal medulla   *355*

adrenalin   *355, 356, 366*

adrenocorticotropic hormone   *355*

aerobic   *26, 65, 133-150, 193-200, 215, 253, 263, 270-274, 305, 324, 334*

aerobic potential   *135*

aging   *97, 212, 213, 220, 230, 247, 355*

Aikido   *36, 102, 109, 112*

Ali Shuffle   *340*

alpha state   *366, 367*

amino acid   *131, 133, 162, 178, 251, 254, 263-266, 271, 277, 354-356*

amoeba   *132, 133, 137, 138*

amphiarthroses   *168*

amylose   *258*

anaerobic   *133-139, 142, 144, 147, 149-150, 193, 196, 199-201, 252, 253, 255, 259, 263, 270, 274, 305, 359*

anaerobic threshold   *135*

annulus fibrosis   *237*

anti-inflammatory   *179, 274*

antioxidants   *270*

Aquajogger   *345*

aquatic bodyworker   *119*

aquatic endurance   *132, 185, 196, 198, 248, 251, 274,*

Aquatic Exercise Association   *26, 215, 328*

aquatic movement   *50, 53, 75, 96, 97, 326, 366*

aquatic practitioner   *88, 89, 93, 108, 113*

aquatic resistance   *135, 162, 168, 181, 195, 201, 202, 215, 216, 243, 301, 327, 354*

Aquatic Resonant Healing   *23, 69, 353*

Aquatoner   *17, 202, 203, 285, 286, 307, 312, 312-314, 316, 322-325, 343*

Aquatrend   *42, 56, 57, 73, 343, 345*

Arjana Brunschwiler   *21, 35, 36, 40, 101, 102, 110*

articulation   *105, 106, 115, 168, 184, 326*

arthritis   *17, 119, 179, 181, 245, 247, 293, 321, 323, 326, 331, 353*

Atlantis Rising   *24, 353*

ATP   *123, 128-139, 147-150, 194, 197, 266, 270*

atrophy   *154, 212, 215, 228, 248, 324*

attunement   *74*

authentic expression   *53*

autonomic nervous system   *321, 355, 358*

Awareness Portals   *51*

axon   *129, 132, 150*

Q

R

W